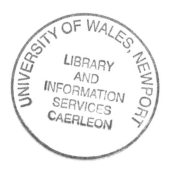

Amplification for the Hearing-Impaired

Amplification for the Hearing-Impaired
Second Edition

Edited by **Michael C. Pollack, Ph.D.**

with an Introduction by Raymond Carhart, Ph.D.

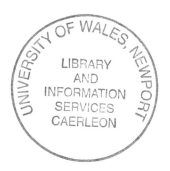

Grune & Stratton
A subsidiary of Harcourt Brace Jovanovich, Publishers
New York London Toronto Sydney San Francisco

Grune & Stratton, Inc.
111 Fifth Avenue
New York, New York 10003

Distributed in the United Kingdom by
Academic Press, Inc. (London) Ltd.
24/28 Oval Road, London NW 1

Library of Congress Catalog Number 79-24024
International Standard Book Number 0-8089-1212-7

Printed in the United States of America

Those of us who learned from him, were intellectually stimulated by him, and saw many advances in Audiology arise as a result of his research and teaching are indebted to Dr. Raymond Carhart. To his memory this book is dedicated.

Michael C. Pollack

Contents

4. Practical and Philosophical Considerations   143
Joseph P. Millin

5. Hearing Aid Selection for Adults   177
Henry D. Schmitz

6. Hearing Aid Selection for Preverbal Hearing-Impaired Children   213
Mark Ross and Carole Tomassetti

8. Speech Signals and Hearing Aids   309

Daniel L. Bode

11. Business Aspects of Hearing Aid Dispensing   393

Melvin J. Sorkowitz

12. Professional Relationships   423

Kenneth E. Smith

Appendix   435

Index   447

Contributors

Kenneth W. Berger, Ph.D.
Director of Audiology
School of Speech
Kent State University
Kent, Ohio

Daniel Bode, Ph.D.
Department of Audiology
Gallaudet College
Kendall Green
Washington, D.C.

Joseph P. Millin, Ph.D.
Professor of Audiology
School of Speech
Kent State University
Kent, Ohio

Ron Morgan
Westone Laboratories, Inc.
Colorado Springs, Colorado

Michael C. Pollack, Ph.D.
Director, Audiological Services
Pacific Hearing Services
Upland, California

Mark Ross, Ph.D.
Professor of Audiology
Department of Speech
University of Connecticut
Storrs, Connecticut

Derek A. Sanders, Ph.D.
Associate Professor
Department of Communicative Disorders and
    Sciences
State University of New York
Buffalo, New York

Henry Schmitz, Ph.D.
Hearing and Speech Associates of
    Orange County
Orange, California

Kenneth E. Smith, Ph.D.
Hearing Associates, Inc.
Prairie Village, Kansas

Melvin J. Sorkowitz
Vicon Instrument Company
Colorado Springs, Colorado

Carole Tomassetti
Director of Audiology
Willie Ross School for the Deaf
Longmeadow, Massachusetts

Preface

In the four years since the publication of the first edition of this book, several changes have taken place in our field. Many more audiologists are now involved in the dispensing of hearing aids; so many, in fact, that the Academy of Dispensing Audiologists was formed to meet and represent their needs and interests.

New experimental methods are now being utilized to provide us with better approximations of real ear responses of hearing aids.

KEMAR data have greatly altered many traditional views of earmold acoustics and hearing aid responses.

Improved earmold and hearing aid technologies have led to new developments in both areas, allowing us to do a better job for our patients.

The FDA and FTC have been actively involved in promulgating regulations of the hearing aid industry.

All of these changes led me to realize the need for an updated edition of this book. It is quite different from the first edition and also quite similar. A new chapter has been added on the business aspects of audiology, and many of the new contributions have brought forth new perspectives. Our orientation in this edition is more toward the dispensing audiologist.

Raymond Carhart

Introduction

Dr. Carhart completed the introduction to our first edition shortly before his death. As far as I know, it was his last completed work. It is reprinted here essentially intact as a memorial to him. The only changes I have made are deletions of references to material in the first edition that are not included in this edition.

MCP

Let us start with some obvious but necessary remarks. First, a hearing loss becomes a handicap only when it keeps the listener from perceiving sounds of importance to him. Second, modern techniques of amplification offer the best single means of combating most such handicaps. Third, since people move from one environment to another, the wearable hearing aid brings particularly versatile help. For this reason, a great deal of attention has been given this past third of a century to the development of good wearable hearing aids and to refining the art of finding hearing aids that are well suited to individual users. Now there is need for a clear summary of what we have learned. This book gives such a summary. It draws together the experiences of three decades in a way which makes those experiences useful to the student of hearing, to the clinical audiologist and to the interested layman. In this sense the book is a guide to the selection and use of hearing aids.

While the book contains much positive information, there is still a great deal to learn about how best to use amplification, including wearable hearing aids, with auditorily-impaired children and adults. This fact also permeates the focus of the chapters which follow. These chapters review current knowledge while recognizing need for further progress. The book starts with a history of hearing aid development. It next examines how hearing aids are constructed, how they work, how their performance is measured, and how they are coupled to the ear. There then follow discussions on practical and philosophical considerations in choosing a hearing aid, on selection procedures for adults, on selection procedures for preverbal children, on special hearing aid applications, on factors affecting aided reception of speech and on the search for the so-called master hearing aid. The book terminates by considering the problems of counseling and by orienting the hearing aid user to the methods that have been developed for dispensing hearing aids to users, as well as to the relationships between audiologists and other groups who also serve the hard of hearing population.

Described in another way, this book focuses heavily on clinical procedures and concerns. In this sense it is a "how to do it" volume. One of its advantages is that a number of authors have contributed chapters. This fact increases the scope of the experience on which the book is based. In general, these writers agree. However, they also express differences of opinion, as is necessary and expected in a field which is still evolving. The reader must recognize at the outset that some of the basic questions about hearing aids are still unresolved and therefore remain the subject of controversy. This fact means that the book is dealing with a maturing, expanding field which promises us a richer future than its present.

A good illustration of a question that is as yet unresolved centers around the issue of selective amplification. This issue emerged in its simplest form with the advent of the wearable vacuum tube hearing aid. A little known anecdote from the late 1930s highlights the controversy neatly. Walter Huth, a conscientious hearing aid engineer, decided to produce a wearable instrument with as high fidelity as he could achieve. With pride, he showed his hearing aid to C.C. Bunch, who was the most experienced audiometrist of that time. Bunch's reaction was negative. He said, "Your hearing aid is designed for normal listeners rather than hard of hearing persons." "Look at this batch of audiograms from persons with hearing loss." "See how their hearing deficits slope in different directions." "You should build a whole family of hearing aids each of which is the reverse of one of the characteristic slopes in hearing loss." Huth took Bunch's advice. Because of this encounter Huth reversed his philosophy, and the companies with which he was associated marketed instruments designed to compensate for several distinctive hearing loss contours.

Bunch's idea of compensating for each patient's audiometric contour soon lost popularity for two reasons. Large programs for rehabilitation of hearing-impaired service personnel were organized during World War II. The workers in these programs were unable to demonstrate that superior performance with hearing aids was linked uniquely to selective amplification. Concurrently, an experimental study at Harvard (Davis et al., 1946) showed that patients with different contours of loss tended to do better with a system having a frequency response slope that ranged between being flat and a 6 dB per octave rise. Highly comparable results were obtained at about the same time in Great Britain (Medical Research Council, 1947). Thus it would seem that the issue had been settled: that other aspects of hearing aid performance were the more critical ones once a standard frequency response that would be suitable for most patients was achieved.

But time has not let that verdict stand. Berger's discussion of the master hearing aid in Chapter 9 makes this clear. Variable frequency response is a feature that has consistently been built into such instruments. Berger would include several frequency responses in an ideal master hearing aid to help give it the flexibility in amplification characteristics currently found among wearable hearing aids. Clinical audiologists today are consciously modifying frequency responses of hearing aids to meet special needs, and for many clinicians the ultimate goal is prescription fittings. In Chapter 3, Pollack and Morgan discuss the use of venting ear molds and of open molds as methods for reducing emphasis. Other mentions of the role of selective amplification are found in Chapters 4, 5, and 6. To generalize, we have moved from an era where selective amplification was unpopular to a philosophy where many audiologists remain alert to the patterns of hearing loss exhibited by their patients and keep in mind a variety of ways for modifying the frequency pattern of the amplification the patient is receiving. Thus, the art of selective frequency modification has become a commonly used tool of the clinical audiologist. However, the fact is that the procedures involved are still in the realm of a poorly understood "art." Clinical audiology has not yet formulated any systematic general theory as to the role and proper applications of selective amplification. We operate by rule of thumb rather than by scientifically confirmed principle. The task ahead is to develop a new level of sophistication. There already are a number of indications that research with insight will move us rapidly in this direction.

For example, consider a recent finding that awaits practical application. Clinicians have not currently become adept at utilizing the results which Thomas and Pfannebecker (1974) obtained: namely, that discrimination in quiet is clearly improved for many persons with sensorineural loss by substantially filtering out low frequencies. Since these investigators found large variations in performance from one subject to another and since these variations are not clearly related to audiometric configuration, no clinically applicable generalization is as yet possible. Moreover, there is need to discover whether the advantages of high pass filtering also apply to noisy environments. These are questions that future investigation must answer. Once these matters are clarified, it may be possible to specify much more wisely which hearing aid a patient should have.

Or again consider experimentation that is being carried out at Central Institute for the Deaf (Pascoe, 1974). Here a variety of systematically differentiated response characteristics is being tried with selected hearing-impaired subjects. The limited information available to date suggests that there may soon emerge principles stating much more definitively what modifications in aided frequency response will most enhance speech understanding, although we must recognize that these principles may not call for a different selective amplification for each patient.

There also are hints that proper control of other dimensions of performance will add importantly to more successful hearing aid use in ordinary life situations. As mentioned in Chapter 6, Villchur (1973) reported using a two channel amplitude compressor to improve the intelligibility for speech sounds achieved by six subjects with sensorineural loss. He adjusted the compression in each channel to compensate for abnormalities in the loudness scale of each subject. Another possibility, which is radical by contemporary opinions, regarding the detrimental role of harmonic distortion is that a combination of frequency shaping and peak clipping may benefit some hearing-impaired persons. The rationale for this statement comes from the work of Thomas and Sparks (1971). They found that subjects with sensorineural loss experienced improved intelligibility for monosyllables in background noise if the incoming signals underwent high pass filtering and infinite amplitude clipping. The clinical applicability of this and other combinations of filtering and amplitude limiting await careful exploration, but the point brought forth by these examples is clear. There is a real probability that we are emerging into a new era of understanding as to which characteristics of hearing aids are clinically desirable. The performance features of future instruments and the method by which they are selected for a patient may be very different five or ten years hence than they are now. Consider as a final thought in this regard the fact that contemporary expertise in microcircuitry allows highly sophisticated signal filtering and manipulation to be achieved, so that frequency and amplitude responses could be adjusted independently at third-octave intervals or less. The technology for processing signals in much more sophisticated ways is here. The only unanswered requirement is that audiology must learn enough about the needs of individual patients to specify what it wishes this sophisticated technology to achieve in the way of hearing aid design. For example, studies on speech perception by the hearing-impaired, such as urged by Bode (Chapter 8), are essential to this achievement.

The foregoing comments must be interpreted properly. They emphasize that we can expect substantial progress in the future. Of course, such developments will not in the meantime lessen the capabilities we already have, and it is with these capabilities that the present book is concerned. Thus, in the context just expressed the present book becomes a needed and highly practical progress report. It deals with a contemporary situation which may be expected to last for considerable time and to change through evolution rather than through abrupt reorganization. Moreover, the contemporary situation is beset by issues and interactions that are not exclusively investigative or clinical. Practical forces and conflicts modify contemporary circumstances and therefore must also be considered.

One issue that stands out involves the conflicts among audiologists as to how hearing aids should be selected for patients. Let us look backward briefly. During World War II clinical audiology assumed the responsibility for guiding hard of hearing persons in selection of hearing aids. It added the responsibility to carry out these services in environments free from commercial pressure and business interest. Such services were first offered extensively in military programs for aural rehabilitation, but they soon spread to nonmilitary centers too. A major decision, which had to be made at this point in time, was the choice of the techniques on which to base selection of the preferred hearing aid for a given patient. Two major philosophies, which are relevant today, emerged. Each had its proponents and these proponents tended to form camps, which too often expended their energies in argument with one another rather than in resolution of basic research issues. Many subviews emerged, as the reader will encounter in such chapters as 4, 5, and 10. The end result, as discussions throughout the book either state or hint, is that an uneasy truce exists. For example, in Chapter 5 various procedures for hearing aid selection are outlined, but then the reader is left to choose the clinical course he will follow. The reader can not help but emerge with the feeling that clinical audiology does not have a positive stand, but that any method for which an audiologist can present a thoughtful argument is probably as good as any dissimilar method for which another audiologist can present a comparably thoughtful argument. The implication is that the two methods are of equal merit. Such indecisiveness can not be considered the mark of maturity in the profession. Clinical research of sufficient rigor and extent must be conducted to resolve the underlying issues. Clinical audiology must assume responsibility for dealing directly and positively, and as a total profession with the issue of the relative merits of alternative methods for hearing aid selection.

In this regard, we must remind ourselves that intensive research into problems of hearing aid efficiency can not be carried on merely as an adjunct to the routine management of clinical cases. Systematic attack on a research question requires a scope and control of observation which goes beyond the practical constraints that exist in most clinical situations. When a patient is being studied clinically there are restrictions on the number and variety of amplification characteristics with which he can be tested. Moreover, his needs must take precedence over the scientific curiosity of the clinician, so that the characteristics of hearing aids tested must be controlled primarily by contemporary knowledge as to how to meet the patient's needs. Full evaluation of the subtleties of interaction between the details of hearing impairment and the variabilities of hearing aid performance must be sacrificed to the exigencies of the patient's immediate requirements. Do not misunderstand. The competent clinical audiologist, as is apparent later in this book, has developed, to a high degree, the art of guiding his or her patients in selection of effective hearing aids. However, practicing the contemporary art of hearing aid selection involves taking shortcuts and making intuitive decisions that preclude obtaining the full array of information needed to generate the science of hearing aid selection. Clinical audiology must develop new investigative methods capable of generating such a science and must employ these methods vigorously.

Despite the arguments and disagreements just mentioned, the art of hearing aid selection rests on several stalwart principles. There is a series of clinical goals to be reached provided these goals are obtainable within the constraints of contemporary technology and the patient's hearing disorder. Most clinicans recognize four achievements as the minimum to be sought (see Chapter 5): namely, (1) restore to the user an adequate sensitivity for the levels of speech and environmental sounds he finds too faint to hear unaided; (2) restore, retain, or make acquirable the clarity (intelligibility and recognizability) of speech and other special sounds occurring in ordinary, relatively quiet environments; (3) achieve the same potential insofar as possible when these same sounds occur in noisier environments; and (4) keep the higher intensity sounds that reach the hearing aid from being amplified to intolerable levels. There are children and adults whose auditory impairments are so severe that they preclude these individuals from fully reaching these goals; but the goals themselves stand as appropriate clinical aspirations and the recognition of their importance permeates many parts of this book.

These minimum goals can be achieved for many hard of hearing persons if they wear single hearing aids. But the goals do not represent full restoration of auditory efficiency. There are other dimensions of hearing that are desirable to recapture. The question is how to do so. Many clinicians feel that binaural hearing aids offer the answer. However, as one can deduce from the resume on binaural hearing aids in Chapter 7, the situation is not that simple. There is realtively little definitive information regarding the benefits of binaural aids. Here we have another instance where the art of guiding hard of hearing patients must currently proceed on the basis of clinical intuition and limited experimental evidence. Again, the task that lies ahead for clinical audiology is to isolate clearly each of the several dimensions of binaural efficiency that are disturbed by hearing losses and then to determine the effect which the wearing of two hearing aids has on each of these dimensions. In other words, there are principles underlying each dimension which must be defined more precisely, so that each facet of binaural function can be employed to the individual hearing aid user's best advantage.

Let us pursue this topic further, because the complexities of aided binaural hearing exemplify intricacies which exist in other realms as well. We will concern ourselves for the moment with ear-level hearing aids. In such a case the role of the "head shadow" emerges as one preeminent determinant of efficiency. We know that a person wearing only one hearing aid will encounter many everyday situations in which his head is between the microphone of his hearing aid and the source of the sound to which he wishes to attend. The head blocks the sound and reduces its intensity at the microphone. Sometimes the effect is great enough to make it harder to hear even in a quiet background. However, the situation is made worse when there is also background sound and when this sound is not similarly "shadowed" by the head because it comes from the side nearer the microphone. Since at such a moment the background sound is not also reduced in level, the ratio of wanted sound to background sound is momentarily made less favorable. Extra masking occurs because the single hearing aid is on the wrong side of the head. The situation may be reversed an instant later, but meanwhile, a temporary hardship has occurred. A second hearing aid eliminates such unpredictable disadvantages. Now, one of the two hearing aids will always be advantageously placed. This aid will be free from sound shadow and will temporarily give the superior reception. In the presence of competing sounds, the advantage thus gained in signal-to-competition ratio can be as much as 13 dB (Tillman *et al.*, 1963; Carhart, 1970).

Not everyone recognizes that it must still be demonstrated as to how and to what degree the other presumed advantages of binaural hearing are achievable with contemporary hearing aids. Unfortunate interactions between a patient's hearing loss, the nature of the acoustic environment, and the characteristics of hearing aids may erase for some patients the presumed benefits of binaural aids. Nábělek and Picket (1974), for example, found that normal hearers got a 3 dB binaural gain when listening through two hearing aids to test words said against a background babble. Five hard of hearing subjects averaged only half as much binaural gain because some did not receive any binaural help while others received the normal benefit. Moreover, we must remember that there are limits to the amount of binaural gain even normal hearers may expect. This gain depends on the masking level differences achieved at those frequencies that are most important to the speech sample of the moment. (See Chapter 8, Carhart *et al.*, 1967; Levitt and Rabiner, 1967). The threshold for intelligibility of connected speech is improved for normal listeners in the presence of competition only about 7 dB by optimal binaural conditions. Precise discrimination of consonants benefits 2 or 3 dB less, even though the threshold for mere detection of a single sentence said repeatedly may be increased by about 13 dB (Kock, 1950). These benefits are not large but their importance for normal unaided hearers is not to be discounted. Unfortunately, these benefits represent boundaries which only a fraction of the hard of hearing population can fully reach with binaural instruments.

Furthermore, there are a number of other questions which must be clarified about each person who seems, on the basis of conventional audiometry, to be a good candidate for two hearing aids. For example; "Can this person fuse the signals received at the two ears via hearing aids into a single wound image and, if so, can he or she retain this fused image over a satisfactory range of sound intensities?" The work of Wright and Carhart (1960) would indicate that such a fusion of images is sometimes a transient and ephemeral phenomenon for hard of hearing subjects listening via two aids.

Another question is, "Can a binaural hearing aid user experience true localization of sound sources as do normal hearers, and, if not, what impressions of directionality can he or she attain?" Data reported by Bergman and his associates (1965) illustrate the problem. They had hearing-impaired subjects balance two hearing aids so that a loudspeaker in front of the listener was perceived "somewhere along the midplane either directly in front of him, in his head, or directly behind him. . . ." (p. 36). A person who perceived the image "in his head" was obviously not localizing it fully, neither was a person who experienced an external projection of the image that seemed very close to his head rather than at the proper distance from it. One must conclude that some of Bergman's subjects experienced crudely lateralized images as opposed to fully localized ones. Our point here is not to criticize the Bergman study but rather to stress that clinicians must not assume that binaural hearing aid users are achieving greater benefits than they actually are. In this regard, still other questions are "Can the binaural hearing aid user obtain as much escape from masking in multi-source environments as do normal two-eared listeners?" "Can such a user achieve normal efficiency in fluctuating sound backgrounds, and, if not, what is the scope of his or her deficit?" "Can such a person resist the degradation of an acoustic environment produced by reverberation as effectively as can a normal hearer, and, if not, how serious is the added problem?" And so on.

We have pursued the topic of binaural hearing aids far enough to realize our limitations of understanding. Considering the fact that this book deals with contemporary practices and knowledge, however, it is somewhat unjust to point out these limitations. The way to eliminate the limitations is to glean new information through research. But this demand for research is in a sense unfair to practicing clinicians. They are bedeviled each day by the specter of imperativeness in a way that even the clinical researcher is not. The researcher can gather fact after fact at his leisure until he has a sufficient edifice of evidence to answer his question with surety. How different the clinican's task. He, too, is an investigator but the question before him is, "What can I do *now* about the needs of the person who is seeking my help at this moment?" The clinican proceeds to gather as much data about his client as he can in a clinically reasonable time. He does not have the luxury to wait several months or years for other facts to appear. The decisions of the clinican are more daring than the decisions of the researcher because human needs that require attention today impel clinical decisions to be made more rapidly and on the basis of less evidence than do research decisions. The dedicated and conscientious clinician should bear this fact in mind proudly. His is the greater courage.

Remembering that the clinical responsibility of today must be met today, this book offers an inclusive guide to the highly diverse array of issues that converge on contemporary audiology. It offers the student excellent coverage of present day opinion, information, and practice. It is thus a very suitable medium for launching the advanced student into the mazes and vicissitudes of the current hearing aid field. But as the student proceeds into this maze, there are cautions for him to keep in mind.

For example, there is a subtle imbalance in this book. It is more oriented to the problems of adults than to those of children. Only Chapter 6 deals directly with children's needs. This imbalance of emphasis merely recapitulates past history. Adults have always comprised the major segment of the hearing aid market. Therefore, design objectives of engineers have primarily pointed toward the needs of adults. It has become an implicit assumption, accepted by almost everyone, that the potential psychoacoustic capabilities of a child with a hearing loss can be deduced from what is known about adults with comparable loss. This presumption needs confirmation. Do clinicians typically ask whether a child who has congenital deafness of the Mondini variety with consequent gross malformation of the inner ears might also have important disturbance of psychoacoustic functions within his remaining range of audibility? Or again, is a wider frequency response needed to learn to understand speech than that which is required to continue to understand it once it has been learned? In other words, the point at issue insofar as children are concerned is that clinical audiology has not attacked many aspects of their needs incisively. There are of course notable exceptions, one of which is to be found in the excellent presentation on hearing aids for preverbal children in Chapter 6 of this book. But the plea at this point is that, while we have learned to use hearing aids on children with results that are often acceptable, we can do our best for children only if we change our basic focus and stop defining what we think hearing aids should do for them largely in terms of the needs and responses of hearing-impaired adults.

Another subject requiring careful thought is the relation of the actual hearing aid performance achieved in living situations to that of the physical measurements obtained in anechoic chambers and acoustic test boxes. This topic is discussed at the end of Chapter 2, but it warrants additional comment here.

To explain, it has long been traditional to determine the sound output of a hearing aid earphone in a standardized 2cc coupler. Many clinicians react to the resultant record as though it were an accurate description of the relative responsiveness of the hearing aid when worn by a listener. However, for several reasons the response in the 2cc coupler gives an imperfect estimate of the frequency response when the instrument is in actual use (see Chapter 2). First, the hearing aid output as measured in a closed 2cc coupler is not the same as the output in a closed human ear canal (Nichols et al., 1945; Martin, 1971). Another factor which modifies frequency response appears when measurements are obtained while the aid is not worn on the head or body, as it would be in real life. In these latter circumstances, diffraction effects and so-called "baffle" effects (see Chapter 2) occur which change the sound intensity at the hearing aid microphone (Nicholas et al., 1947; Olsen and Carhart, 1975). Such effects modify hearing aid output and the meaning of measurements, which are made when such effects are not included, such as occurs in a standard "test box."

Another variable which is often ignored in the clinical world is ear canal resonance, with the consequence that compensation for loss of this resonance is frequently not taken into account when defining the effective frequency response of a hearing aid. To explain, the normally open ear canal functions as a tube which increases the effective sound pressure at the eardrum relative to the pressure at the entrance to the ear canal. This enhancement extends over a substantial band of higher frequencies in the speech range and can reach about 20 dB in the neighborhood of 3000 Hz (Wiener and Ross, 1946). Since plugging the canal with a hearing aid earpiece disturbs this resonance, accurate plotting of the effective frequency response requires compensating for the resulting disruption of ear canal resonance. Enough data relating to the variables involved have been gathered so that an estimate of total correction needed to compute the true sound pressure levels at the eardrum can be made from frequency response curves obtained via 2cc coupler. Any clinician, however, who fails to make this correction, but still presumes he is reproducing the equivalent of open ear reception on the basis of responses measured in a 2 cc coupler, is misguided (Knowles and Burkhard, 1975). Moreover, the degree of his inaccuracy will depend upon many variables which he may find difficult to assess, a point which is touched in a somewhat different way in Chapter 4.

Stated conversely, the clinical audiologist must continuously remember that traditionally obtained frequency response curves do not accurately describe the performance of the hearing aid while in use. Failure to keep this principle in mind may be one of the reasons that the risk of reaching solid generalizations about the relationship between frequency response and clinical effectiveness has been so slow.

A somewhat similar caution is necessary when considering the interpretation of other electroacoustic measurements. The following example will illustrate this point. During World War II excellent data on the technical performances of contemporary hearing aids became available from the Harvard Electroacoustic Laboratory (Nichols *et al.*, 1945). These hearing aids were much larger than the instruments of today but their electroacoustic excellence was sufficiently comparable for our example still to be pertinent. During 1945 a study was conducted at Harvard's Psychoacoustic Laboratory. This study used hearing aids on which data from the Electroacoustic Laboratory were available. The study demonstrated how much gain persons with normal hearing, when temporarily masked to simulate a prespecified degree of sensorineural hearing loss, could achieve with each of a number of the aforementioned hearing aids (Hudgins *et al.*, 1945). It so happened that the rehabilitation program at Deshon General Hospital was concurrently using these same hearing aids with quite a number of its patients. The Deshon staff was able to assemble groups of patients who had been tested with exactly the same fittings as had been used in the Harvard study. The startling fact which emerged was that the clinical patients achieved notably less gain with these aids, hearing loss for hearing loss, than did the masked normal hearers. There clearly were detrimental interactions which made the benefits of using a hearing aid less when suffering a true hearing loss than when simulating a comparable sensorineural impairment through masking. The point is that if clinicians are not aware that such detrimental effects can occur, they will fail to use with fullest insight the laboratory data available to them.

A serious deficiency of contemporary clinical audiology is the inadequacy of its methods for speech audiometry. This topic per se is not given much attention in this book, although the role of speech audiometry as a help in hearing aid selection is mentioned often. The fact is that speech audiometry as practiced clinically for hearing aid selection is relatively archaic and unrevealing. It needs improvement in several ways if its results are to be of greatest help to hearing aid users. For one thing, we are still awaiting a definitive validational study of the relationship between formal scores obtained via speech audiometry and work-a-day hearing aid efficiency. Some attempts, beginning with those of Davis (1948), have been made to correlate performance in life situations with formal test results, but the relations between test scores and efficiencies in the work-a-day world still await adequate description. Furthermore, although there has been a substantial proliferation of speech tests since 1950, this proliferation has often tended to preserve existing weaknesses in test design rather than to eradicate them.

Consider one example of clinical inefficiency in measuring speech discrimination. The W-22 test, which is widely used, contains many test words that are easily discriminated by most patients (Carhart, 1965). Time is therefore wasted on these items, and patients' scores tend to cluster at the high end of the scale. Elpern (1961) suggested that the waste in time could be reduced if the test were shortened to half its original length. In many clinics this procedure is now followed. However, Elpern's approach was to cut the total number of items in half rather than to discard the easiest 50 percent of them. The final effect is to reduce the precision (reliability) of the test without expanding significantly the range over which scores distribute themselves. When applied to evaluating a person's performance with hearing aids, the half list procedure importantly lessens the credence which can be given to each score obtained and hence reduces the confidence with which a clinician can advise a potential hearing aid user.

Another criticism of speech audiometry is that as currently practiced in many places it does not adequately simulate everday listening situations. This criticism is probably particularly telling when it comes to the evaluation of hearing aids. Test administered in quiet or in a steady state noise can fail to reveal detrimental interactions which can occur between hearing loss, hearing aid, and acoustic environment (see Chapter 8). There is now substantial evidence that such unfavorable interactions can occur (Tillman et al., 1970). Moreover, a review of considerable data from several laboratories suggests that the adverse interaction is most pronounced if the background is composed of human speech.

It would thus seem that conscientious clinical practice would require selecting a hearing aid in part on the basis of performance in such a speech background. Certainly, the impressions we have gained from observations of aided performance in white noise, in speech spectrum noise, or in quiet are not fully applicable.

One of the relatively unpublicized paradoxes in the field of aural rehabilitation is that the transition from military audiology to civilian audiology brought about a sharp but still somewhat incompletely recognized change in the philosophy of patient management.

Early American hearing aid programs emerged as crash ventures. The armed forces established comprehensive rehabilitation centers for deafened service personnel. A point that is often forgotten is that each patient was in the rehabilitation program much longer than is practical today, except for those in a few military and Veterans Administration hospitals. Thus, the selection of a hearing aid in the early days could be made part of an intensive sequence in rehabilitation that could last two or more months. At Deshon General Hospital (Carhart, 1946), for example, the rehabilitation procedures accomplished two goals that we usually fail to achieve today. First, the patient became sophisticated in what to expect from hearing aids as a class, because he was required to wear a number of different instruments in daily life before his final instrument was issued. He learned what problems hearing aids could pose for him, with the outcome that he would no longer blame his final instruments as being individually defective in these regards. Second, he discarded through everyday use those instruments obviously unsuited to his needs. Eventually three or four aids emerged as particularly good for him. His final hearing aid was then chosen from among these instruments. Formal tests were used at this point, but the important thing to remember is that these formal tests were merely the last stage in a long procedure of winnowing out undesirable aids and of habituating the patient to wearable amplification.

The captive thousands of patients for whom weeks and months of training in military hospitals could be ordered disappeared after World War II, even among the main core of veterans with service connected hearing impairment. These veterans and patients from the civilian sector were seldom willing to accept the prolonged and intensive regimes developed in military rehabilitation centers. In many locations the typical patient now had to be processed in hours rather than weeks. Clinicians, facing this pressure for accelerated procedures, drifted toward the view that hearing aid selection was a relatively independent function. Even though audiologists continued to claim that the hearing aid must be integrated into a total rehabilitation program, this integration very often took place poorly. No one can do extensive rehabilitation on a patient who will not agree to participate as often or as long as the program requires. Therefore, shortcuts and compromises were necessary. A new goal emerged: namely, to assess the patient's needs for amplification rapidly, and, if he was found to need amplification, to discover a good hearing aid for him, also quickly. Associated with this new goal came the necessity to shorten and thus greatly weaken the rehabilitational procedures for adjusting patients to hearing aids.

The future will certainly modify the views and practices of clinical audiology in sociologic and economic areas, as well as in the realms of technology and patient management. Moreover, it is well to remember that such changes may possibly come very fast because critical issues are currently under controversy. Chapter 12 is in part concerned with matters of this type. For one thing, the attitudes of clinical audiologists regarding themselves and the field they represent are of prime importance. One sometimes gets the sense that clinical audiologists are willing to settle for the classification of second class professionals. It may be reassuring in this time of conflict to consider the American Speech and Hearing Association as a haven and rallying point. It may be essential to preserve this rallying point in order to win legal privileges and to protect professional territory. But careful evaluation of the scientific and educational issues involved makes clear that the person who has achieved certification in Audiology from ASHA has emerged as a professional whose recognized competency is defined by the Master's degree and a moderate amount of supervised clinical experience. There are historical reasons for this situation. However, the point is that as long as either ASHA or clinical audiology are satisfied to accept only this definition as describing competence in clinical audiology, the field can not expect to be recognized as equal to professions that hold the doctorate as one of their inviolate requirements. This situation is particularly unfortunate when one recalls the caliber of the tasks and responsibilities inherent in top notch clinical audiology.

One effect of the tendency of audiologists to define their field largely in clinical terms is that by so doing they have functioned primarily as consumers of the research performed by others. There is a handicap in being a consumer of scientific information rather than a producer of it. The consumer does not greatly determine the direction of progress. He works with what is at hand, that is, with what others have made available to him. As some of our earlier comments implied, such a limitation seems to have existed in the technology of wearable hearing aids. The fact that audiologists have not seriously researched hearing aid needs has probably restricted the variety of hearing aid characteristics that have been commercially available. It has been the manufacturing industry whose major spurs to action have consisted of intra-industry competition and feedback from dealer experience that has supplied the variety of hearing aids available in the United States. Clinical opinions have had sporadic impact, but these opinions themselves have not always been consistent. Thus, although one can point to a few examples of effective interaction between manufacturing and clinical groups, as in the case of the early development of CROS and its companion systems (see Chapter 7), clinical audiologists have been forced to "make do" with whatever hearing aid stock was contemporarily available. Even now, as is subtly apparent at points in this book, clinicians do not have the feeling of being even partially in control of this aspect of the situation.

Just a word now about the boundary between hearing aid dealers and clinical audiologists. Many persons of integrity, compassion, experience, and competence are found in each group. These individuals have strong motivations to help hard of hearing people. Consequently, we should expect coordination and cooperation between the two groups. Unfortunately, positive interactions develop on a person-to-person basis rather than permeating group attitudes. At this writing, tensions between the commercial and the clinical camps are fairly high. The problem appears on the surface to be largely jurisdictional. However, there is an underlying philosophical cleavage which gives the two groups conflicting frames of reference.

What, then, is the philosophical disparity?

There are two premises from which the clinical audiologist ordinarily starts. First, he sees his main task as coping with the full array of communicational problems brought about by impaired hearing. Without going into detail, this task requires the following steps: (1) assessing communicational capacity thoroughly; (2) determining what communicational, educational and/or rehabilitational needs must be met; (3) planning programs to do so; (4) participating in the appropriate phases of these programs; and (5) arranging for whatever other forms of help are needed. The tasks of assessing the role of a hearing aid for an individual and of helping this person find a suitable instrument are only part of the work to be accomplished in the first two of the aforementioned five steps. The recognition that the clinical audiologist has five major responsibilities clearly leads to the premise that the total endeavor is of sufficient complexity and diversity, and therefore requires a large amount of formal training and clinical experience in order for it to be carried out competently. There is too much to be learned to presume that it can be mastered by informal study and undirected contact with hearing-impaired persons.

Individuals in the hearing aid business often have a different outlook. Their rehabilitative goal is more restricted, aimed primarily at finding effective wearable amplifiers for persons with hearing impairments, helping these persons in the initial adjustments to their instruments, and supplying the follow-up services that will keep the instruments functioning well. Although there are a few individuals in the business who have embarked on broader approaches, the fact remains that the hearing aid business has not seen its task as that of requiring extensive formal academic preparation. In general, its philosophy has been that field training with supplementation from correspondence work, company workshops, and other short courses can assure competence. Where licensure of hearing aid dealers is involved, the ground rules may be laid down fairly precisely by state law, but the basic approach still seems to be that the hearing aid dealer is a business man who must have some special knowledge so that the public will be protected as he goes about his business.

Finally, we must mention a less well known, but extremely important, recent development that will probably greatly affect everyone involved with hearing aids. This development potentially can have a massive influence on both the availability of hearing aids and on their performance characteristics. For instance, it is possible that forthcoming legislation will place hearing aids under the jurisdiction of the Federal Food and Drug Administration. If so, a series of regulations governing the specifications and tolerances that manufacturers must meet will probably go into effect. It does not now appear that specific performance characteristics will be required, except for a few boundaries of electroacoustic response which will be designated. Thus, the manufacturer can probably continue to select his own design objectives. Once he has done so, however, all his instruments of that particular model will probably have to fall within relatively narrow tolerances. In this sense he will have to manufacture to tight specifications.

It is hard to foresee the impact that will occur if the aforementioned regulations are promulgated. Past experience with the quality control that has existed in the hearing aid industry suggests that the new regulations may be very hard to meet on a mass production basis. Each new instrument may need to be given rather extensive tests and substantially greater care may need to be taken in matching components. Such factors will drive up the cost of hearing aids. Furthermore, manufacturers may choose to produce fewer types of instruments. They may be slow to incorporate innovative components as these appear. Manufacturers will probably also be constrained from developing highly unconventional hearing aids.

The development just described is only one example of the way in which the hearing aid business may be curtailed by increasing government regulation in the years ahead. Remember that the Federal Trade Commission has been concerned with practices in the hearing aid field for a number of years. Now hearing aid manufacturers are on the verge of being supervised and held to externally imposed standards by a second regulatory agency. The point at issue is not whether the public should be protected. Of course, it should be protected. The point at issue is that regulation may make it very hard for businesses to continue producing improved hearing aids at accpetable prices. Such difficulties could eventually effect detrimentally the array and versatility of the hearing aids that are clinically available. The end result could be to reduce the help which can be given the hard of hearing public via wearable amplification.

Such a turn of events must challenge clinical audiology to pick up the gauntlet that has been lying at its feet for years. During these years clinical audiology should have been developing more definitive methods for using amplification to the best advantage of hearing-impaired children and adults. The record to date is not a proud one. Now other forces are emerging which have the power of final decision as to what hearing aids shall or shall not be. These forces may not have either the clinical experience or the audiological orientation to exercise the best judgment in regards to the needs of the hearing-impaired population. Clinical audiology can remain a viable force in the hearing aid field only if it accepts the responsibility for initiating the research needed to clarify the many unanswered issues which are threaded through this book. The interests and endeavors of many investigators must be enlisted. Substantial funding, some of which has already been committed, must be available. After clinical needs and requirements have been clarified through such research, the other persons involved will undoubtedly be easily persuaded to support these needs and requirements—whether such persons be manufacturers, the promulgators of regulations, or other individuals who are both interested and influential.

This introduction comes to a close by emphasizing again the paradoxes before us. Hearing aids are now of great benefit to a great many people. Proper clinical insight and management can enhance that benefit. The book which follows is a knowledgeable guide to current practices and procedures for doing so. But the book also bares the contemporary controversies and unresolved clinical uncertainties which will affect the future. It will be interesting to see whether this book becomes an epitaph to a profession's inability to marshall its intellectual capabilities or the prelude to a manifesto of that profession's capabilities to meet its challenges fully.

BIBLIOGRAPHY

Bergman M, Rusalem H, Malles I, Schiller V, Cohan H, McKay E: Auditory rehabilitation for hearing-impaired blind persons. ASHA Monographs 12 1-46, 1965

Carhart R: A practical approach to the selection of hearing aids. Trans Amer Acad Opthalmol Otolaryngol Jan-Feb: 123–131, 1946

Carhart R: Problems in the measurement of speech discrimination. Arch Otolaryngol 82:253–260, 1965

Carhart R: Problems of the hearing impaired in noisy social gatherings. Oto-Rhino-Laryngology. Excerpta Medica International Congress Series No. 206, 564–568, 1970

Carhart R, Tillman T W, Johnson R: Release of masking for speech through interaural time delay. J Acoust Soc Am 42:124–138, 1967

Davis H: The articulation area and the social adequacy for hearing. Laryngoscope 58:761–778, 1948

Davis H, Hudgins C V, Marquis R J, Nichols R H Jr, Peterson G E, Ross D A, Stevens, S S: The selection of hearing aids. Laryngoscope, 56:85–115, 135–163, 1946

Elpern B S: The relative stability of half-list and full list discrimination tests. Laryngoscope 71: 30–36, 1961

Hudgins C V, Peterson G E, Hawkins, J E, Ross D A: Performance tests of hearing aids. Section II of Evaluation of Hearing Aids, Office of Scientific Research and Development, Division 17, Section 17.3, OSRD Report 4666, 1945

Knowles H S, Burkhard M D: Hearing aids on KEMAR Hearing Instruments 26: 19–21, 41, 1975

Kock W E: Binaural localization and masking. J Acoust Soc Am 22:801–804, 1950

Levitt H, Rabiner L R: Predicting binaural gain in intelligibility and release from masking for speech. J Acous Soc Am 42:820–829, 1967

Martin M C: Are frequency characteristics important? Scand Audiol Supp. 1, 93–98, 1971

Medical Research Council: Hearing Aids and Audiometers. Report of the Committee on Electroacoustics. London, His Majesty's Stationery Office, Special Report Series, No. 261, 1971

Nabelek A K, Pickett J M: Reception of consonants in a classroom as affected by monaural and binaural listening, noise, reverbation, and hearing aids. J Acoust Soc Am 56:628–639, 1974

Nichols R H, Jr., Marquis R J, Wiklund W G, Filler A S, Feer D B, Venaklasen P S: Electro-acoustic characteristics of hearing aids. Section I of Evaluation of Hearing Aids, Office of Scientific Research and Development, Division 17, Section 17.3, OSRD Report 4666, 1945

Nichols R H, Jr, Marquis R J, Wiklund W G, Filler A S, Hodgins C V, Peterson G E: The influence of body-baffle effects on the performance of hearing aids. J Acoust Soc Am 19:943–951, 1947

Olsen W O, Carhart R: Head diffraction effects on ear-level hearing aids. Int Audiol 244–258, 1975

Pascoe D P: Frequency responses of hearing aids and their relation to word discrimination by hard-of-hearing subjects. J Acoust Soc Am 56:S46A, 1974

Thomas I B, Pfannebecker G B: Effects of spectral weighting of speech in hearing-impaired subjects. J Audio Engin Soc 22,:690–693, 1974

Thomas I, Sparks D W: Discrimination of filtered/clipped speech by hearing-impaired subjects. J Acoust Soc Am 49:1881–1887, 1971

Tillman T W, Carhart R, Olsen W O: Hearing aid efficiency in a competing speech situation. J Speech Hear Res 13:789–811, 1970

Tillman T W, Kasten R N, Horner J S: Effect of head shadow on reception of speech. ASHA, 5, 778–779, 1963

Villchur E: Signal processing to improve speech intelligibility in perceptive deafness. J Acoust Soc Am 53:1646–1657, 1973

Wiener F M, Ross D A: The pressure distribution in the auditory canal in a progressive sound field. J Acoust Soc Amer 18: 401–408, 1946

Wright, H N, Carhart R: The efficiency of binaural listening among the hearing-impaired. Arch Otolaryngol 72: 789–797, 1960

Amplification for
the Hearing-Impaired

Kenneth W. Berger

1
History and Development of Hearing Aids

In terms of the length of time there has been any interest in disorders of hearing, electric hearing aids are relatively new, having been available commercially only since the early 1900s. Prior to the introduction of electric amplification, the hearing-impaired individual had to rely on mechanical devices, some of which were quite bizarre by today's standards. In this chapter, Ken Berger traces the development of mechanical and electrical amplification devices, putting a good deal of emphasis on the evolution of the electric hearing aid. Of particular interest is the chronology of hearing aid "firsts" that is included.

The primary importance of this chapter, in my views, is that by becoming familiar with the past, one can develop a better appreciation for the present level of hearing aid technology and can more reliably judge the strengths and weaknesses of today's hearing aids.

MCP

The history of electric hearing aids is not yet a century old. Yet, historic data about and references to early electric hearing aids are scarce. Even more rare are historic facts about pre-electric hearing devices, their manufacture, and their acoustic characteristics.

A number of authors make the statement that mankind's first hearing "aid" was the hand cupped behind the ear. Although the statement is made only on the basis of guessing, without supporting evidence, it might well be true. Then we might suppose that at some still prehistoric time someone with either normal hearing or with a hearing loss found that an animal horn or a broken seashell served to better focus sound into the external auditory canal. The earliest historic references to hearing aids suggest that the animal horn and seashell were the first hearing devices.

In attempting to determine the early history and development of hearing aids one is faced with a number of hurdles. First, patent records do not date back to the early development of hearing aids and some of the earliest patents on nonelectric hearing aids clearly suggest that these were refinements from older basic models. Second, the history of the education of the deaf might be expected to offer some insights into the development of hearing aids, but until the advent of electronic instruments there were few, if any, that greatly benefited the deaf. Therefore, education of the deaf was largely concerned with speechreading or manual communication, and teaching the deaf child to talk. Third, the few very early printed references to hearing instruments are generally within philosophical or medical discussions rather than in published articles or books about the instruments themselves. Thus, the history of pre-electric hearing aids is, at best, sketchy and incomplete. More recent developments in hearing aids are largely unheralded.

SOUND COLLECTORS

As suggested above, the first historic references to aids for hearing were sound collectors. Animal horns appeared to be the most common devices used. These were hollowed and the tip end placed toward the ear, so as to better collect sound and direct it into the external ear. A lesser number of references to the history of hearing aids mention seashells as serving the same purpose.

Curiously, the first published scientific communications on hearing instruments were concerned with *speaking trumpets* and *hearing trumpets* for use by persons with normal hearing. Only later did it become obvious to persons working with the hearing-impaired individual that the same principles could be applied as an aid to hearing impairments. Thus, large ear trumpets were used by ship captains to receive oral messages transmitted from shore or from another ship, and speaking trumpets were merely the same ear trumpets used in reverse. That is, the speaker used the small end to speak into, similar to the way a cheerleader at a football game uses a megaphone. These early speaking and listening trumpets were made of metal or glass. Ear trumpets for people with hearing impairments were most commonly made of thin metal or tortoise shell, although a few economy models were mere cardboard cones or tubes. Rather soon in their development, ear trumpets were made collapsible and could be carried more easily; one may also note early efforts to disguise the trumpets.

It may be surmised that gradually a number of instrument makers developed the art of manufacturing speaking and listening trumpets. A few of these artisans, perhaps encouraged or assisted by physicians, surely specialized in such instruments for the deaf. Most of the early manufacturers of "deaf aids" seem to be individuals or firms that manufactured surgical instruments. The earliest firm known to have manufactured hearing aids on a commercial basis was established in London about 1800 by F. C. Rein and Son. Rein manufactured hundreds of different nonelectric hearing instruments, most of them in limited quantities (Berger 1974).

The well-known *acoustic throne* was made by Rein in 1819 for King Goa (John) of Portugal. This instrument is shown in a number of books on hearing aids, and is now on display at the Amplivox factory north of London. The throne consists of hollowed armrests, carved into lion's heads at the front. The armrest cavities lead to a resonant box located in the seat of the throne, and the sound is then heard via a hearing tube connected to the resonator. In addition to the more common type of ear trumpet, the Rein firm also manufactured acoustic urns, ear trumpets with large silver resonators, acoustic devices hidden in the hat or by the beard, and speaking tubes for churches.

Before the twentieth century a number of firms in Europe and the United States began to manufacture an assortment of hearing aids and to innovate them. Still, pre-electric hearing aids had extremely limited effects in helping those with hearing impairments. Small, quite flat metal or tortoise shell trumpets were popular and were usually referred to as ear cornets. Other writers use the terms trumpets and cornets as synonyms. Ear trumpets and cornets provided amplification in a narrow frequency range, which assisted the hard-of-hearing user to some extent.

Figure 1-1 shows the acoustic gain of several ear trumpets which were popular in the pre-electric hearing aid era. These curves are based upon free-field unaided versus aided test comparisons (Sabine 1921). The responses shown are

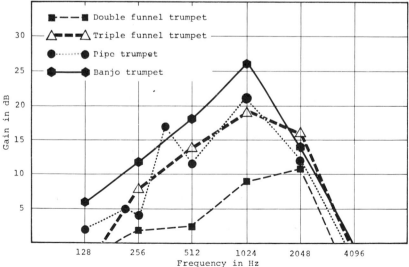

Fig 1-1.   Acoustic gain of ear trumpets.

for a funnel-shaped trumpet that collapsed from two sections and a longer funnel trumpet which collapsed from three sections. The banjo trumpet was a conical instrument with a rather small cross-section which had a scoop or dish-like collector attached to it. The pipe trumpet resembled a large tobacco pipe. It consisted of a conical section which bent and expanded to a large collector area. The frequency responses shown in Figure 1-1 are considerably smoother than those actually produced by ear trumpets, since relatively few frequency points were used in the testing.

BONE CONDUCTORS

Bone conduction hearing devices are mentioned occasionally and appeared rather early in hearing aid development. Most of these were little more than strips of wood or rods of iron. One end of the strip or rod was often held between or touching the teeth of the speaker, and the other end was held in the same manner by the person with a conductive hearing loss.

Numerous individuals over a long period of time "discovered" the usefulness of these rods, sticks, and similar objects as bone conduction hearing devices. Figure 1-2 shows an interesting modification of the rod device which was made by Giovanni Paladine (1842—1917) in 1876. He called this a *Fonifero*. At one end of the rod is a curved portion, almost a complete semicircle, which was rested against the throat of the speaker. The listener's end of the Fonifero was placed against the teeth, the forehead, or the mastoid area. This end of the rod was similar to a small cup. In cases of conductive hearing loss this and similar devices were quite effective but cumbersome. In Paladino's instrument the speaker and listener had to maintain a specific distance from each other. The original illustration of the Fonifero was not clear, which may explain why the drawing of the device in the otolaryngology handbook of Politzer (1878) shows the listener's end shaped like a hook rather than a cup. Several subsequent articles and books evidently used Politzer's illustration as a model and also incorrectly showed the listener's end of the device (Berger 1976c).

In 1879 Richard Rhodes, of Chicago, invented and patented a hearing fan, which he called Rhodes Audiphone. This device consisted of a thin piece of pliable material shaped like a fan. The upper edge of the fan was held against the user's upper teeth or clasped between the teeth. A system of cords permitted the user to increase or decrease the tension on the fan itself, thereby allowing for some adjustment in sound pick-up. For approximately the following 5 years, many individuals obtained similar patents for hearing fans of various sizes, shapes, or materials. They also incorporated ideas for folding the fan when it was not in use. These hearing fans did collect sound, and they evidently served their purpose for those with a mild to moderate conductive hearing loss, provided that the user had a good set of teeth! (Berger, 1974).

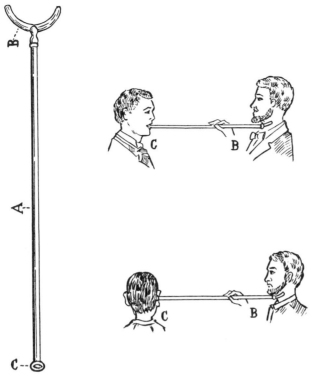

Fig 1-2. The Fonifero.

Since women frequently carried fans before the turn of the last century, hearing aids built into or resembling partially collapsed fans were in vogue. The bone conduction fan was discussed above. Another popular version of it had a small ear trumpet built into a half-open fan. Figure 1-3 shows a fan with an ear trumpet built into it. Still another model was made of metal and was merely held behind the ear to direct sound into the ear.

EAR INSERTS

A large number of types, styles, and sizes of ear inserts have been designed in an effort to aid hearing. Some of these ear inserts were much like the metal ear specula used by otologists. Others were more expanded at the external end, so as to collect sound a little better. Most of the ear inserts provided little or no amplification, and it is apparent that their sole value was for individuals who had a collapsed external auditory canal.

Adam Politzer (1835−1920), who gained world renown as head of the Vienna ear clinic, designed an interesting ear insert device. This is shown in

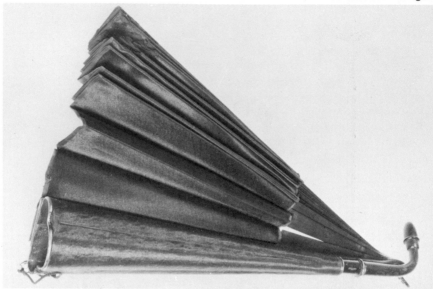

Fig. 1-3   Hearing fan (courtesy of the Smithsonian Institution).

Figure 1-4. Politzer's device was made of vulcanite and was shaped like a tiny alpine horn. The circular opening was directed to the rear. Several sizes were available, the largest being 2.5 cm long with a 12-mm diameter mouth opening and a 5-mm diameter insert end. In the late 1870s Politzer modified this device by removing the material from the inner angle. This resulted in an L-shaped instrument with a trough. In his book on diseases of the ear, nose and throat, written in 1891, the noted New York otolaryngologist St. John Roosa stated that he had not found any marked benefit from this Politzer device.

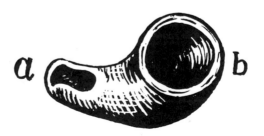

Fig. 1-4.   Politzer ear insert.

THE CARBON TRANSMITTER

The invention of the telephone in 1876 by Alexander Graham Bell spurred the interest of many toward the development of a device that would not merely collect sound but also amplify it. If speech could be transported across considerable distance, could not the same speech be amplified for the deaf individual?

In many discussions about the history of hearing aids Alexander Graham Bell is credited with inventing the electric hearing aid for his mother (or his sweetheart, both of whom had a hearing loss) but he gave up the effort to use the ideas to invent the telephone. The facts cast doubt on all such statements, since the electric hearing aid did not appear until almost a quarter of a century after the telephone was invented (Berger 1976a).

Rather than working on an electric amplifier for the deaf, Bell was actually attempting to refine and modify the "singing flame" or manometric flame of König, hoping that this would give the deaf a visual indication of their own speech efforts. Bell, it may be recalled, was a speech teacher. A statement by Bell at the twenty-fifth anniversary celebration of the Horace Mann School for the Deaf, in Boston in 1894, clearly indicates his efforts during the early 1870s regarding an instrument to assist the deaf:

> My original skepticism concerning the possibility of speech reading had one good result; it led me to devise an apparatus that might help the children . . . a machine that should render visible to the eyes of the deaf the vibrations of the air that affect our ears as sound. . . . It was a failure, but the apparatus in the process of time became the telephone of today.

In his classic textbook on otolaryngology, published in 1945, Chevalier Jackson credits Dr. Ferdinand Alt with producing the first electric hearing device in 1900. Alt was an assistant at the Politzer Clinic in Vienna. The instrument is said to have consisted of a carbon microphone, a magnetic earphone, and a battery. Jackson was evidently quoting Max Goldstein, who in his book *Problems of the Deaf*, published in 1933, pictures this instrument. Alt noted that his instrument was of little use if the speaker was more than 2 ft away. It might also be argued that the illustration in Goldstein's book shows an instrument of more recent vintage than 1900, as witness the size, wiring, and connectors (Berger 1970b). My own belief is that the 1900 date is an incorrect reading by Goldstein or a misprint for 1906.

Even accepting the year 1900 for Alt's instrument, I have recently uncovered good evidence that the first electric hearing aid was publicly shown in 1898, or at the latest in 1899, and may have been made in an experimental version as early as 1895. This was a table model instrument with a carbon microphone and up to three pairs of earphones. The apparatus was called an Akoulallion (coined from the Greek verbs "to hear" and "to speak") and was manufactured in limited quantities by the Akouphone Co., of Alabama. The inventive genius behind the instrument was Miller Reese Hutchison, perhaps better known to most people by his invention of the klaxon horn.

About 1900 the Akoulallion was modified in somewhat smaller dimensions as the Akouphone, and is pictured in the article by Berger (1970b). Several articles in the literature on the education of the deaf at that time noted that neither instrument had sufficient power to help those with severe hearing loss. Thus, like the nonelectric hearing instruments, the first electric hearing aids, as made by Alt and by Hutchison, helped only those with a mild to moderate hearing loss.

The Miller Reese Hutchison patents for several hearing aid devices were manufactured and marketed by a series of firms which, with a number of reorganizations, ultimately became the Dictograph Products Co. and used the Acousticon tradename. The third generation hearing aid made by Hutchison was called the Acousticon. A factor which contributed to popularizing Hutchison's inventions was the use of one of his instruments by Queen Alexandra of England at her coronation in 1902 (Berger 1974).

Within a decade, a number of hearing aid manufacturers began making carbon-type hearing aids: C. W. Harper, of Boston, made an "Oriphone" beginning late in 1902; Mears Radio-Hearing Device Corp. was inaugurated in 1904 by Willard Mears, who had previously been associated with Miller R. Hutchison; Globe Ear-Phone Co. began a long and successful business in 1908; the Williams Articulator Co., of Chicago, was established in 1909; Deutsche Akustik-Gesellschaft, of Germany, was established in 1910; Siemens & Halske, of Germany, began hearing aid manufacture on a limited basis in 1910; and the Gem Ear Phone Co., of New York City, was established in 1912. Still other manufacturers of hearing aids were established and were successful for a brief span of years.

Of the various hearing aid firms mentioned above, it may be noted that only Acousticon and Siemens are still making hearing aids. In tracing hearing aid history, one can readily note older firms disappearing and new ones forming as each major change in technology transpired: nonelectric to carbon, carbon to vacuum tube, and vacuum tube to transistor.

The carbon hearing aid consisted of a carbon granule or carbon shot microphone—more properly called a carbon transmitter—an earphone, and a battery. Beginning about 1930, a bone vibrator was used in place of the earphone with some models. Also, the earphone was later reduced dramatically in size and an eartip was used to direct the sound to the ear canal, at which point in time it became appropriate to use the term *hearing aid receiver*. Soon thereafter the eartip was replaced with stock vulcanite earmolds, and then with custom-made vulcanite ones, and finally with plastic earmolds (Berger 1976b).

Carbon hearing aids with single microphones and without boosters produced limited gain. A strong resonant peak is seen in the frequency responses. Figure 1-5 shows responses from a Globe carbon aid that was popular around 1916

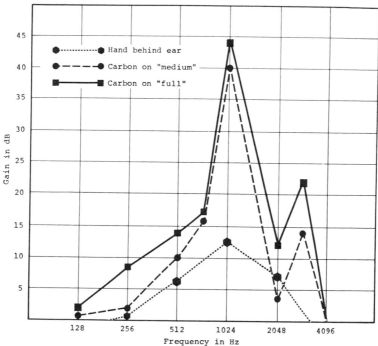

Fig. 1-5. Acoustic gain of carbon aid compared to hand held behind the ear.

(Sabine 1921). Like the frequency responses of ear trumpets shown earlier, those for a carbon aid are a comparison of free-field aided and unaided responses. For comparison purposes Figure 1-5 also includes gain data for the same subject, with the hand behind the ear. The carbon aid response is shown for the instrument with the volume control (a sliding resistance) set at both medium and full gain. Like the responses shown for ear trumpets, those for the carbon aid were sampled at a limited number of test frequencies, which obscured the many peaks and valleys of the actual response.

Carbon hearing aids were available in table models or as wearable instruments. The former often had multiple microphones and often included large collecting cones and resonant cavities. The size and shape of the microphones varied, and the instruments designed for persons with a greater hearing loss usually employed two or more microphones united electrically and often physically. A sliding resistance volume control was an early addition to the basic instrument, and later a booster (or amplifier) was available. Essentially, the booster was an enclosed double diaphragm that permitted some additional gain for the instrument, but usually at the expense of greater distortion.

Carbon microphones were somewhat temperamental, and efficiency was easily reduced in humid and dusty environments. The microphone, and particularly the booster, would often operate imperfectly if the wearer made any gross body movements. However, the instruments were relatively inexpensive, and with proper care they lasted a long time. Carbon hearing aids were popular from the first decade of the present century through the late 1930s. In fact, one still finds, on rare occasions, an elderly individual wearing a carbon hearing aid, preferring it to the more recent developments in amplification.

VACUUM TUBE INSTRUMENTS

The major problem with carbon hearing aids was that the amount of acoustic gain possible with them was limited and the frequency response was narrow. What was needed was a device that could greatly raise the power of the speech signal. The vacuum tube amplifier accomplished this goal very well.

In much of the world the vacuum tube is called a valve, and in its simplest form it does act as a valve, much like a resistor operating in one direction only. With the invention of the triode vacuum tube in 1906, Lee DeForest added a grid to the cathode and plate of the older diode. The small wire mesh, or grid, permitted control of the electrons from the cathode to the plate. This control, so important in the design of amplifiers, permitted the development of the first electronic hearing aids.

The first vacuum tube hearing aid was developed by Earl C. Hanson and patented in 1921. The instrument, larger than a box camera, was battery-powered and employed a single triode. It is unfortunate that discussions of the history of hearing aids almost uniformly give credit to persons other than Hanson for the first vacuum tube hearing aid. Soon large vacuum tube hearing aids were marketed by L. Gaumont of France, Marconi of England, the Western Electric Co., and Radioear Corp. (Berger 1972). All of these instruments tended to be cumbersome, and were quite expensive. In addition, the triode was notorious for its lack of stability. Because of the size, cost, and difficulties with the amplifier, these earliest vacuum tube hearing aids were not much competition for the carbon instruments available at the time.

In 1931 the pentode vacuum tube, which consisted of a plate, a cathode, and three grids, was perfected. The pentode was stable in performance, had a relatively long life, and readily permitted amplifier stages to be coupled so as to obtain virtually as much increase in power as was desirable. Thus, the first practical and popular vacuum tube hearing aids began to appear in the mid-1930s. These earliest vacuum tube hearing aids, which were wearable, were later referred to as two-piece instruments since typically there was a microphone-amplifier portion and, separately, a battery pack. Most of the two-piece vacuum tube hearing aids were larger and heavier than the existing carbon hearing aids, but they permitted substantially more gain in the signal than did the carbon instruments.

It should be clearly recognized that the first hearing aids which were powerful enough to assist those with a severe to profound hearing loss did not appear on the market until around 1936. Since hearing aids powerful enough to assist the deaf (as opposed to the hard of hearing) did not appear until relatively recent years, it is understandable that oral programs for the deaf did not generally become oral-aural until the 1940s or later.

That the vacuum tube hearing aid did not quickly replace the carbon model can be seen from numerous statements in the professional literature. Weille and Billings, in their 1937 electroacoustic study of hearing aids, employed only carbon instruments "because the average patient wears only a carbon microphone aid." It was estimated that in 1937 approximately 95 percent of the hearing aids in use were carbon instruments (Hayden 1938). Writing in 1940, Hayden still questioned whether vacuum tube aids "will supplant the carbon type hearing aid or vice versa, or whether each will eventually occupy its own definite field."

Soon after the introduction of two-piece vacuum tube hearing aids, hearing aid manufacturers were able to miniaturize their instruments so as to allow for one-piece wearable hearing aids. Miniature vacuum tube technology was pioneered in England and wearable electronic hearing aids, manufactured by Amplivox, Multitone, and other British firms, first made their appearance there. Arthur M. Wengel of Madison, Wisconsin is credited with manufacturing the first wearable vacuum tube hearing aid in the United States. (Also see his involvement with master hearing aids in Chapter 9.) Early one-piece, or monopack, hearing aids were made in the United States by Beltone, Vacolite, Paravox, and Mears.

Crystal Microphone and Receiver

The purpose of a microphone is to transduce the acoustic signal into an electric signal as faithfully as possible. The carbon microphone was more correctly a transmitter in that it transduced the acoustic signal but could not generate a signal. The crystal microphone, so useful with the vacuum tube hearing aid, actually generates a voltage when pressure is applied to the crystal; this action is known as the piezoelectric effect.

The typical crystal microphone consists of two small slices of crystal cemented together. A small rod connects the diaphragm to the crystals. When changes in sound pressure move the diaphragm, this movement is transmitted to the crystals through the connecting rod and causes the crystals to generate an electric signal that fairly faithfully follows the original acoustic signal. This electric signal is led to the amplifier proper for amplification.

The crystal microphone responds to a larger frequency range than did the carbon microphone and is not as easily damaged by dust or dirt. Nor do position changes of the wearer affect its response. However, the crystal microphone, like the carbon microphone, performs poorly in extreme temperature and humidity conditions.

Once the amplifier in the hearing aid has performed its work, the electric signal needs to be transduced back to acoustic energy. This transduction is accomplished by the earphone or receiver. It has been common practice in the hearing aid industry to use the term receiver to refer to a small earphone (about 1.0 in. or smaller in diameter) to which an earmold is attached.

A receiver is essentially a microphone in reverse. In the case of the crystal receiver, the amplified electronic signal is fed to the crystal. When electric impulses are passed through the crystal, it will vibrate mechanically, setting up airborne sounds that are sent on to the ear.

Magnetic microphones and receivers were also used with vacuum tube hearing aids, particularly later in the vacuum tube hearing aid era. The magnetic microphone is not as fragile as the crystal one. In addition, bone conduction vibrators for hearing aids have been of the magnetic variety in the carbon, vacuum tube, and transistor eras.

Batteries

Carbon hearing aids used one or several batteries, in series. Vacuum tube hearing aids required an "A" battery to warm up the filament of the tube and a "B" battery (plate battery) to achieve amplification. As noted above, the first wearable vacuum tube hearing aids required a separate battery pack. The battery pack was either carried in the pocket or fastened to the underclothing. Persons wearing two-piece vacuum tube instruments can truthfully be said to have been wired for sound.

The cost of batteries for vacuum tube hearing aid users was rather high. To lengthen the life of a battery it was recommended that their use be rotated to allow time for recuperation. Storage of batteries required a cool dry place for best savings. It was possible to recharge the battery, but this did not seem to have been a common practice with vacuum tube hearing aid users.

TRANSISTOR INSTRUMENTS

Hearing aid technology has had some dramatic changes in a relatively brief span of years. The carbon hearing aid was little more than 25 years old when the much-improved and acoustically more flexible vacuum tube hearing aids appeared on the market in wearable versions. The vacuum tube hearing aid was only about 25 years old when the transistor appeared on the scene.

The transistor was invented at the Bell Telephone Laboratories in December 1947 by J. Bardeen, W. H. Brattain, and W. B. Shockley. The inventors were later awarded the Nobel prize for their work. The first transistors were the point-contact type and were not useful in hearing aids. A refinement, the *geranium junction transistor,* soon appeared and its first commercial use was in hearing aids. Beginning in 1952 a few hearing aid manufacturers began using junction transistors in place of the output vacuum tube in hearing aids, which required a minimum of circuit change. These were the so-called hybrid transistor hearing aids. Even this slight change, however, resulted in substantial battery savings to the hearing aid user.

Soon all-transistor hearing aids appeared on the market, and within a year or two the vacuum tube wearable hearing aid disappeared entirely. It will be recalled from previous discussion that the vacuum tube gradually replaced the carbon hearing aid, over a period of some years. In the case of the *transistor,* however, it completely replaced the vacuum tube in hearing aids within 2 or 3 years. In comparison with the vacuum tube, the transistor is smaller, more sturdy, requires virtually no warm-up period, and operates well on a single battery of small size. The smaller transistor size and lower battery voltage requirements permitted dramatic miniaturization in the size of the hearing aid.

The body style (or conventional, or pocket aid) could now be made substantially smaller than the older vacuum tube hearing aid. The transistor also permitted other styles of hearing aids to be introduced, such as the behind-the-ear and the hearing aid built within eyeglass temples. Patents for these styles antedate the transistor by many years, but reducing the size of the hearing aid could not be achieved so that the design could not be made practical until the transistor was perfected.

A number of claims for "firsts" in the hearing aid industry has been made by various manufacturers. Dating these firsts depends to some extent upon fixing the date a certain instrument or feature was patented, when it was introduced to the manufacturer's dealers, when it was first advertised, and when it was first placed on sale. Early all-transistor hearing aids were placed on the market by Microtone, Maico, Unex, and Radioear. These appeared in January and February of 1953. The first transistor hearing aids were somewhat more expensive than the latest vacuum tube models, and initial difficulties were encountered in the quality of the transistors themselves. In a short period transistor quality control was achieved, and the dramatic savings in batteries in the transistor instruments quickly spelled the end of the vacuum tube era.

By late 1954 the first eyeglass hearing aids, with the amplifier and microphone enclosed in the temples, made their appearance. Akumed of Germany and Otarion of the United States were the first to market such instruments. Because hearing aid technology at that time did not permit ideal miniaturization, the eyeglass hearing aids contained a microphone and part of the amplifier in one temple. Wiring ran forward and around the lens frame to the other side, and the remainder of the amplifier, leading to a receiver, was in the opposite temple. Barrettes that were marketed during the vacuum tube and transistor eras had much the same arrangement, with the wire leading across the headband.

Within several years, it was possible to house the microphone, amplifier, and internal receiver in a single temple, which permitted binaural ear-level hearing aid fitting. Although the early eyeglass hearing aid wiring arrangements had no special name, it should be noted that, in the 1960s, for special fittings this arrangement was essentially reverted to under the name CROS. For further discussion of CROS and other across-head routing arrangements, see Chapter 7.

Another hearing aid style permitted by the transistor and smaller battery requirements was the *behind-the-ear model*. This has also been called the post-auricle and over-the-ear style. The behind-the-ear style readily permitted binaural fitting, and the acoustic power of these instruments is now sufficient to reach almost all hearing losses. Many hearing aid manufacturers make eyeglass and behind-the-ear style instruments with the same acoustic responses, so the prospective purchaser may choose either ear-level style desired.

The latest hearing aid style is the in-ear hearing aid. These instruments began appearing in the latter part of the 1950s in rather large dimensions, and might be better described as at-ear rather than in-ear. In-ear hearing aids are presently available built either within a custom earmold or merely as a small device with a canal portion.

In-ear hearing aids have been made practical by the latest development in amplifiers, *the integrated circuit*. The integrated circuit is a refinement and development of the silicon planar transistor. The integrated circuit consists of transistors, resistors, and "wiring," all on a tiny wafer of silicon or similar material. The integrated circuit has permitted further miniaturization of hearing aids, and is inherently low in power needs as well as being relatively robust. The first hearing aid with an integrated circuit, however, was not an in-ear model but rather appeared in a behind-the-ear style made by Zenith and introduced in 1964. It may be expected that further miniaturization and improvement in the hearing aid amplifier will follow, since the brief history of electronic hearing aids has largely been directed toward miniaturization.

Presently the most space-occupying part of the hearing aid is not the amplifier but the power supply, microphone, and receiver. Reduction in the size of these components may permit the hearing aid to be placed well within the ear canal, out of sight. An appropriate name for such an instrument would be ear canal aid. A number of experimental designs have been tried in reference to transducers and power supplies, but none has appeared to be practical as of this writing. Research in this direction and in the area of implanted hearing aids continues.

Microphones

The crystal microphone was popular with vacuum tube hearing aids. With the advent of the transistor instruments, a microphone of lower impedance was needed. The magnetic microphone, which made its appearance with some vacuum tube instruments, became the one of choice with transistor hearing aids. The magnetic microphone has a rather ideal frequency response over the range of frequencies most important for speech. Very high and very low frequencies, however, need to be sacrificed, particularly when the magnetic microphone is made in extremely small dimensions.

With research and development, a version of the crystal microphone, the ceramic microphone, was perfected. The high impedance problem of the ceramic microphone was solved by employing the field effect transistor (*FET*). The ceramic microphone offered some of the advantages of the older crystal microphone, but unlike the crystal microphone it is virtually free of humidity and temperature problems. The ceramic microphone permitted extended low-frequency amplification of hearing aids.

Condenser microphones have long been the standard of excellence in the broadcast and recording industry. Unfortunately, condenser microphones have a large voltage need and do not permit miniaturization. The perfection of the FET for ceramic microphones and the discovery of electret-like characteristics of some thin-film plastic materials permitted the development of the electret condenser microphone. An electret is a permanently electrically polarized material, but I shall follow the convention of referring to the electret microphone rather than the longer and more technically correct name *electret condenser microphone*.

The electret microphone has an extremely broad and quite flat frequency response. Like the ceramic microphone, it is rugged and sensitive. The electret microphone is virtually free of problems associated with mechanical feedback or with clothing rub. The electret microphone has replaced the magnetic and the ceramic microphone in most hearing aids.

The latest development in microphones for hearing aids is the directional microphone. In 1969 Willco, at that time a German affiliate of Maico Electronics, Inc., introduced the first hearing aid with a directional microphone. This microphone has both front and rear openings. Sound impinging from the rear is attenuated a significant number of decibels, sufficient for the wearer to focus on sound coming from the front. Directional electret microphones are employed by a number of hearing aid manufacturers around the world.

Power Supply

Technically, a battery consists of two or more cells. The words *battery* and *cell,* however, are used interchangeably in reference to hearing aids. With carbon and vacuum tube hearing aids, the zinc oxide battery was employed. These needed to be fairly large in order to be practical. The zinc cell had a sloping discharge characteristic. That is, with use it gradually produces a smaller and smaller voltage. Users had to turn up the volume control of the hearing aid as voltage was reduced. Earlier it was mentioned that for ideal use these batteries needed time for rest and recuperation, and hot weather reduced their life.

During World War II, the mercury cell was developed by Dr. Samuel Ruben. At the close of that war, mercury cells found a ready market with hearing aid manufacturers and users. Mercury cells as compared to zinc cells are smaller and more robust. More important, for hearing aid use the discharge characteristic is such that the voltage drops significantly only at the very end of the cell's useful life. Furthermore, the mercury cell operates under wider temperature ranges and needs no time for rest and recuperation (that is, *depolarization*). The voltage of mercury cells is also rather ideal for transistor needs. With the introduction of transistor hearing aids, the mercury cell was the one most commonly used. The popular no. 401 mercury cell was introduced in 1952.

With the advent of silicon transistors, a battery with more restricted operating voltages was required. To solve this problem, the silver oxide cell was developed. Soon thereafter *silicon planar transistors* were developed which operate on either mercury or silver cells. The more popular cell sizes are now made in both mercury and silver oxide versions. At present, the choice of mercury or silver oxide cell depends primarily upon hearing aid gain requirements.

In addition to the popular mercury and silver cells, rechargeable cells are available. The rechargeable cell, sometimes referred to as an accumulator, is considerably more expensive than other types. However, they may be recharged many times, so that over a long use period the cost per hour of hearing aid wear is somewhat lower than for the mercury or silver cell. Rechargeable cells are more popular in Europe and Asia than in North America. The infamous advertising phrase "no batteries to buy" usually refers to a rechargeable cell. However, the phrase is untruthful because ultimately the cell must be replaced.

Just as continuing research in transducers and amplifiers for hearing aids goes on, so do experiments with different types of batteries. At present, lithium cells seem to offer promise for future use in hearing aids. It is probable that in the future batteries for hearing aids will be made in various shapes so as to fit in the hearing aid case wherever there might be room.

COMMENTS

In this brief review of the history of hearing aids, it can be noted that the overriding goal of the manufacturer appears to be more power and a smaller hearing aid. In the 50-year history of the electronic hearing aid, great progress has been made in both of those directions. At the same time, it is disheartening to note that the acoustic fidelity of the product and flexibility in manipulating the output and frequency response have not received as much attention or publicity.

The hearing aid manufacturer seems to have heeded the desires of the hearing aid wearer for a more readily concealed aid and the request of his local dealers for more power in a smaller package. The audiologist has undoubtedly been remiss in not making known his desires for a more flexible hearing aid amplifier and one with greater fidelity. Much of the remainder of this book discusses problems of hearing aid fitting and attempts to overcome those problems so that the ultimate goal—prescription hearing aid fitting—may be achieved. Until hearing aids can be accurately applied to specific hearing loss needs, hearing aid fitting is likely to remain more of a slipshod art than a science.

BIBLIOGRAPHY

Berger KW: The vactuphone—pioneer vacuum tube hearing aid. Natl Hear Aid J 23:27−29, 1970a

Berger KW: The first electric hearing aids. Hear Dealer 21:23−38, 1970b

Berger KW: Western electric hearing aids. Hear Dealer 23:18−20, 1972

Berger KW: The Hearing Aid: Its Operation and Development, ed 2. Livonia, Michigan, National Hearing Aid Society, 1974

Berger KW: From telephone to electric hearing aid. Volta Rev 78:83−89, 1976a

Berger KW: The earliest known custom earmolds. Hearing Aid J 29:5, 10, 35, 1976b

Berger KW: Early bone conduction hearing aid devices. Arch Otolaryngol 102:315−318, 1976c

Goldstein M: Problems of the Deaf. St. Louis, The Laryngoscope Press, 1933

Hayden AA: Hearing aids from otologists' audiograms. J Am Med Assoc 111:592−596, 1938

Hayden AA: Hearing aids—tube or carbon? J Am Med Assoc 115:191−193, 1940

Jackson C, Jackson CL: Diseases of the Nose, Throat, and Ear, ed 2. Philadelphia, WB Saunders, 1959

Paladino G: Dell'arrivo della voce e della parola et laberinto a traverso le ossa del cranio. G Int Sci Med 2:850−854, 1880

Politzer A: Lehrbuch der Ohrenheilkunde. Stuttgart, Verlag von Ferdinand Enke, 1878

Sabine PE: The efficiency of some artificial aids to hearing. Laryngoscope 31:819−830, 1921

Weille FL, Billings BH: A study of the efficiency of carbon microphone hearing aids. N Engl J Med 216:790−794, 1937

APPENDIX

Chronology of Hearing Aid Development

1551	Cardano described a bone conduction device consisting of a metal shaft or spear.
1640	Artificial eardrum made by Banzer of Germany.
1657	Hoefer, Germany, mentioned ear trumpets in use in Spain.
1670	Sir Samuel Moreland, England, invented a large speaking trumpet.
1673	Kircher wrote a book in which several hearing instruments are illustrated.
1677	Conyers of England worked on modifying Moreland's speaking trumpet.

1757	Jorrisen of Germany rediscovered the bone conduction rod as a hearing aid.
1790s	Townsend trumpet; a metal cone, developed in London.
1800	The firm F. C. Rein, trumpet makers in London, was established.
1805	F. C. Rein manufactured a speaking tube.
1808	Mälzel of Germany began making ear trumpets, including several for the composer Beethoven.
1812	Itard of France used a wooden rod as a bone conduction device.
1820	Duncker of Germany invented a speaking tube.
1826	Arrowsmith of England rediscovered the bone conduction rod for hearing.
1836	First known British patent for a hearing aid.
1853	Toynbee of England developed an artificial eardrum device.
1855	First patent for a hearing aid issued in the United States.
1869	Hawksley & Son of London is established; still in business.
1876	Telephone invented by Bell.
1879	The Audiphone, a bone conduction hearing fan, was invented by Rhodes of Chicago. Many similar devices were developed between 1880 and 1890.
1887	Ear trumpet with diaphragm earpiece patented by Maloney in the United States.
1890	Kirchner & Wilhelm of Stuttgart is established. Makers of hearing instruments; still in business.
1892	First patent for an electric hearing aid issued in the United States to A. E. Miltimore of Catskill, New York.
1898	(or 1899). First hearing aid made by M. R. Hutchison of Mobile, Alabama, which led to the Acousticon tradename.
1898	Marage compared hearing aid responses using the manometric flame.
1899	First Hutchison patent for a hearing aid.
1900	Electric hearing aid said to have been developed by F. Alt, Vienna.
1902	C. W. Harper of Boston began manufacturing electric hearing aids.
1906	Triode vacuum tube invented by DeForest.
1912	First volume control for an electric hearing aid.
1912	Zwaardemaker of The Netherlands measured hearing aid amplification, using calibrated instrumentation.
1920	First vacuum tube hearing aid patented by E. C. Hanson. Manufactured at the beginning of 1921 by Globe.
1923	Marconi of England and Western-Electric of the United States introduced vacuum tube hearing aids.
1923	First electric bone conduction vibrator. A. G. Pohlmann and F. W. Kranz.
1923	First in-ear electric hearing aid patent, Germany.

1924	Vacuum tube hearing aid manufactured by Radioear.
1926	First patent for a custom earmold.
1931	First electric hearing aid eyeglass patent.
1935	The Selex-A-Phone, introduced by Radioear, the first "master hearing aid."
1936	First AGC in a hearing aid; Multitone of London.
1936	First hearing aid with a telephone coil, United States.
1936	First wearable vacuum tube hearing aids appeared in England.
1937	First wearable vacuum tube hearing aid made in the United States.
1938	First audiometer built to hearing threshold, Maico.
1942–44	First one-piece vacuum tube hearing aids, by Paravox, Mears, and Beltone.
1945	The word audiology was "coined" by Canfield and by Carhart.
1946	The so-called Harvard Report was published.
1947	First electronic "master hearing aid;" introduced by Beltone.
1947	Transistor invented in December at Bell Telephone Laboratories.
1948	First hearing aid with a printed circuit; Solo-Pak.
1948	International Hearing Aid Association organized, which in 1952 became the Society of Hearing Aid Audiologists, and in 1965 the National Hearing Aid Society.
1952	First hearing aid that employed a transistor; vacuum tube and transistor hybrid circuit.
1953	First all-transistor hearing aid: Microtone, in January.
1954	First commercially manufactured electronic hearing aid eyeglasses manufactured, Otarion.
1955	First at-ear hearing aid, Dahlberg.
1958	First known report of an implanted hearing aid, France.
1959	First hearing aid dealer state licensing law passed, Oregon.
1960	ANSI (then ASA) standard for the measurement of electroacoustic characteristics of hearing aids was published.
1961	HAIC standard method for describing hearing aid performance was published.
1962	CROS described by Wullstein and Wigand; reported and actually named in 1965 by Harford and Barry.
1964	First hearing aid with an integrated circuit, Zenith.
1969	First directional microphone in a hearing aid, Willco.

Michael C. Pollack

2
Electroacoustic Characteristics

In order to work effectively with hearing aids, it is necessary to understand how they work and how their performance is measured. In this chapter, I present information in a practical manner about the electroacoustic characteristics of hearing aids. I have included comments indicative of my biases throughout the chapter. Among the newer ideas presented are measurements using KEMAR and battery drain data. The main thrust of these ideas is not to allow yourself to become rigidly caught up in the aspects of hardware, but to carefully consider your patient and his or her use of that hardware.

MCP

Perhaps the most significant advancement in hearing aid technology has been the development of the transistor. Its small size and versatility, coupled with the development of miniature transducers of high-quality performance capabilities such as the electret microphone, have permitted the miniaturization of hearing aids. This miniaturization allows the aid to be worn at or in the ear and yet provide the listener with a signal quality equal or superior to that of body-worn vacuum tube instruments.

Today, the countless styles, components, power capabilities, and applications of amplification for the hearing-impaired present a confusing and complex array of options to the many professionals concerned with the hearing aid. What are the limitations of the various styles of aids? What are the many basic and optional components of amplification systems? How do they work? How does one measure the performance of a hearing aid? What do these measurements mean? What can go wrong?

STYLES OF PERSONAL AMPLIFICATION SYSTEMS

Prior to the introduction of the transistor, hearing aids were, because of their size, worn only on the body. Since the early 1950s, three other basic configurations have been introduced in addition to the body aid with locations at (A) ear-level; (B) eyeglass (both air- and bone-conduction versions); (C) all-in-the-ear. Typical instruments for each of these styles are presented in Figure 2-1.

Body Aids

Until the mid 1960s the body style (also referred to as conventional, on-the-body, or at-the-body style) was the most common type of aid available. Today, it is generally recommended only for the most severe and profound hearing losses. Body-worn instruments, most often rectangular in shape, are either worn in a short pocket or special harness, or clipped to the clothing. A wire cord runs from the aid to the air- or bone-conduction receiver at the ear.

Ear-Level Aids

Also known as over-the-ear, behind-the-ear, at-the-ear, and post-auricular instruments, ear-level hearing aids rest behind the pinna, with a plastic "elbow" fitting over the anterior edge of the ear, connecting with a plastic tube that leads to the concha. Most of the hearing aids sold today are of this type. Table 2-1 presents data from the Hearing Industries Association regarding sales of hearing aids by style from 1963 to 1978. You can see how the percentage of body aids

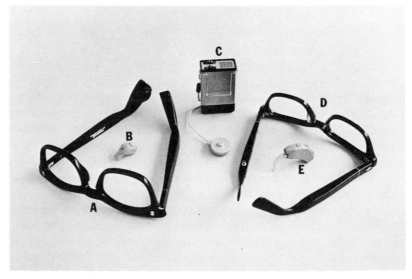

Fig. 2-1. Typical hearing aid styles. *A*, Bone-conduction eyeglass; *B*, In-the-ear; *C*, Body; *D*, Eyeglass; *E*, Ear-level. (Courtesy of Dahlberg.)

Table 2-1

Trends in Hearing Aid Sales

	Percent Sold			
Year	1963	1974	1977	1978
Body aids	20.0	7.1	3.0	4.1
Eyeglass aids	34.5	22.9	10.0	10.1
Ear-level aids	43.4	67.4	56.2	56.3
In-the-ear aids	2.1	2.6	30.8	29.5
CROS-type aids*		4.7	3.0	2.3

*Includes both ear-level and eyeglass versions. Figures extrapolated from total eyeglass and ear-level figures above.

has decreased dramatically as the power levels of behind-the-ear instrumentation have increased over the years. This is also reflected in the increase in ear-level aid percentages over the 15-year period.

Eyeglass Aids

Many ear-level aid responses are available in comparable eyeglass-temple models. This mode is very well suited to CROS-type aids (see Chapter 7). Besides the obvious advantage of this arrangement for some persons who must wear glasses, the somewhat greater distance from the microphone to the ear in an eyeglass aid, as compared to a behind-the-ear instrument, permits the use of more gain without the problems of feedback. This is explained in greater detail in the "Feedback" section of this chapter.

Recently, at least one hearing aid manufacturer has introduced a specially designed adapter to couple an ear-level aid to the user's eyeglasses. Figure 2-2 shows this adapter. It is very convenient as an approach for a person who wants an eyeglass aid, but for whom a better set of hearing aid characteristics is found in an ear-level instrument.

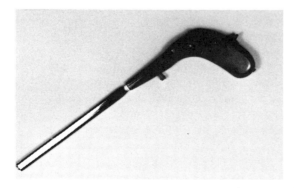

Fig. 2-2.   Siemens Hearing Instruments: Ear-level/Eyeglass adapter

When considering eyeglass hearing aids, you must remember that anytime the user removes his or her glasses, the hearing aid must also be removed. This can be very inconvenient for a person who does not wear the glasses during most waking hours.

In-the-Ear Aids

In recent years, there has been a great surge in sales of this type of hearing aid, as noted in Table 2-1. An intensive discussion of the advantages and disadvantages of in-the-ear instruments is presented as a separate section of Chapter 7.

Referring again to Table 2-1, these figures, and reports of trends in hearing aid recommendations by audiology clinics (Harford and Dodds 1974), indicate a decline in the use of body aids and an increase in the use of ear-level and in-the-ear aids over the years. This shift became apparent in the mid 1960s as more powerful ear-level aids became commercially available. Another probable factor in this trend is the increased sales of CROS-type instruments for individuals previously considered "unaidable." The figures in Table 2-1 are based on sales figures voluntarily provided by members of the Hearing Industries Association (HIA). Sales by non-HIA member manufacturers are not included in these data.

An important consideration relative to the various styles available is the amplification capability of each. Knowing the style of an instrument tells us very little about its acoustic performance, except that generally, the smaller the aid, the less powerful it is. This concept will be developed at some length later in this chapter.

OPERATIONAL OVERVIEW

Basic Components

Although technologic developments have resulted in many styles and applications, all electronic hearing aids operate basically on the same principle. In the broad sense, *a hearing aid is any device that more effectively brings sound to the ear*. A modern electronic hearing aid, however, is an amplifier whose function is to increase the intensity of sound energy and to deliver it to the ear with as little distortion as possible. Since the acoustic energy of sound cannot be amplified directly, it is necessary to convert it to an electrical signal. This signal is amplified and then changed back to acoustical energy.

To do this, any hearing aid contains four basic components (Fig. 2-3): microphone, amplifier, receiver, and power supply (battery). Additionally, there are three essential accessories and controls: volume control, earmold, and tubing or cord.

Block Diagram of a Simple Hearing Aid

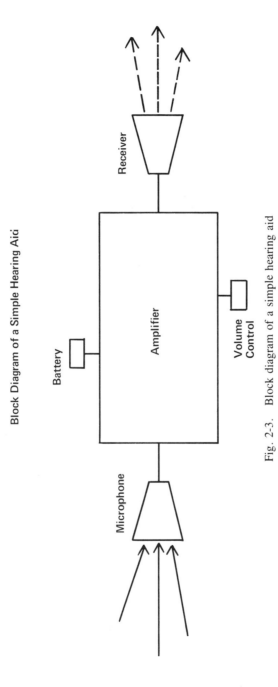

Fig. 2-3.   Block diagram of a simple hearing aid

25

MICROPHONE

A microphone is an energy transducer that converts the mechanical acoustic energy into an analogous, but weak, electric current. As described in Chapter 1, modern hearing aids use one of three types of microphones: magnetic, ceramic, or electret. A prerequisite for high-quality sound reproduction is the use of a good microphone, because the amplified signal can be no better than the signal received from the microphone. If that signal is of low quality, the output signal will also be of low quality. In other words, a hearing aid is no better than its microphone. An amplification system can be no better than its poorest component, and historically the microphone has been the weakest link in the hearing aid chain. However, with the advent of the wide spectrum microphones in use today (electret), the receiver has now taken on the rather dubious distinction of being the component limiting better hearing aid response.

AMPLIFIER

The weak electric signal generated at the microphone is coupled to the amplifier, which increases its amplitude (voltage). There are generally several stages to the amplification process. The more stages (transistors and associated circuitry) there are, the greater will be the amount of amplification. Two types of amplifier circuits are used in hearing aids.

A Class A or single-ended amplifier consists of three to five amplifier stages and is the most common type used in hearing aids. There is only one output amplifier stage, generally using one output transistor. It has a constant current drain independent of gain control settings and input level. Class A amplifiers are generally used in low and moderate output aids with an average output below 125dB SPL. Figure 2-4 is a schematic diagram of a single-ended amplifier.

The Class B or "push-pull" amplifier is used in high-output instruments with an average output greater than 125dB SPL. The amplified current is fed into a "phase splitter" that divides it into two signals of opposite phase. These signals are amplified separately by two different output stages and rejoined in the

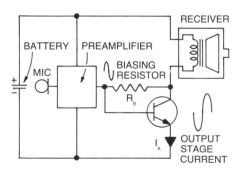

Fig. 2-4.   Class A (single-ended) output hearing aid circuit. (Reproduced with permission from Ely, 1978.)

push-pull receiver. Each output stage operates only during about one-half of the signal cycle. Battery current drain is dependent on volume control setting and input level. Because of this, drain is very low in quiet environments. The push-pull amplifier is also characterized by low distortion. Figure 2-5 is a schematic of this type of amplifier.

RECEIVER

In principle a microphone in reverse, the earphone or receiver converts the amplified electric signal into acoustic or sound energy and transmits it to the ear. Typically, hearing aid receivers are air-conduction transducers—presenting sound waves to the external auditory meatus. However, most body-style and some eyeglass aids can be used with bone-conduction receivers. These work in exactly the same way as the bone-conduction vibrator of an audiometer by presenting the signal directly to the mastoid process and theoretically bypassing the middle-ear conductive apparatus.

Conventionally, the receiver is located within the enclosure of the ear-level, eyeglass, and in-the-ear aids (internal receivers), but separate from the case of body aids (external receiver).

I mentioned above that the receiver is now often considered the "weakest link" in a hearing aid. This is due to the fact that today's electret microphones have a wider and flatter frequency response than either magnetic or ceramic microphones. One could then assume that the response of electret hearing aids would be greatly extended and flattened. This is not the case. While electret microphones have widened the low and high frequency ends of the spectrum to some extent, the overall response is very much limited by the response of the receiver. If the receiver has a narrow response, then the overall response of the instrument will reflect this.

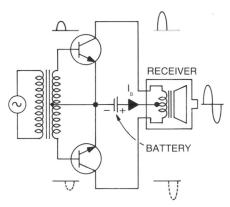

Fig. 2-5.   Class B (push-pull) output hearing aid circuit. (Reproduced with permission from Ely, 1978.)

Receivers in today's hearing aids are still magnetic, and, therefore, have a frequency response considerably narrower than that of the electret microphone. While electret-type receivers are available, they cannot, as of this writing, be used in hearing aids. They require a power supply considerably greater than that provided by conventional hearing aid batteries. Hopefully, within the near future, advances will be made that will allow the use of wider range receivers in hearing aids.

POWER SUPPLY

The battery provides the power for the amplification process. Compared to early vacuum tube batteries, the miniaturized cells, used with modern hearing aids, are relatively weak ($1.3 - 1.5$ V). One of the many advantages of transistors is that they require lower operational voltage for an acoustic output comparable to that of vacuum tube aids. A more detailed discussion of batteries is presented later in this chapter.

VOLUME CONTROL

It is often desirable for a hearing aid user to adjust the sound intensity he is receiving. For example, he may require less intensity in a very noisy environment. Most hearing aids have a dial or serrated wheel that serves as a volume control. It does not alter the input sound to the aid, but adjusts the amount of amplification of the input signal (gain). The volume control is a potentiometer or variable resistor (Fig. 2-6) consisting of a fixed resistance strip, usually a circular piece of paper or fiber, over which is placed a carbon compound. A sliding contact arm, connected to the external control, moves over this strip and varies resistance to the electric signal, with a corresponding change in the amount of amplification.

An infrequently considered, but nevertheless important, factor related to volume controls is their taper characteristic. This refers to the relationship between volume (gain) control rotation and amount of signal attenuation, i.e., how much of the maximum amplification is provided at various rotation points (25, 50, 75 percent, and so on).

A study by Kasten and Lotterman (1969) indicated that "the gain control taper does not provide a linear growth in gain." Their examination of 33 different hearing aids revealed a wide range of taper characteristics. Figure 2-7 presents five different tapers from their sample. A number of generalizations can be drawn from these data.

1. Relatively little gain is available once the volume control is beyond 50 percent of its total range. Most of an instrument's gain is delivered in the lower half of the control, while only a limited amount is available in the last half. For example, in Figure 2-7, aid A provides gain to within 5 dB of maximum by the time the control is rotated up to 50 percent, and only an additional 5 dB through the last half of its rotation. The implications of these

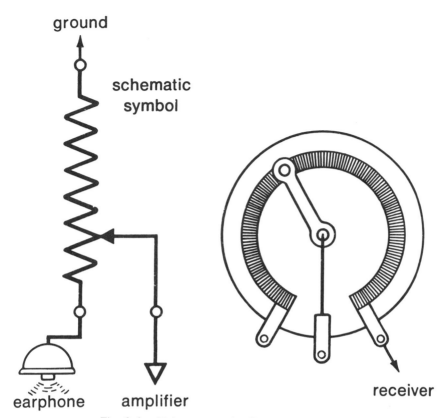

ground

**schematic
symbol**

earphone   **amplifier**

receiver

Fig. 2-6.   Volume control. (Courtesy of Zenith.)

data are that while a user may receive some additional amplification by rotating the gain control beyond a 50 percent setting, he may also encounter an unusually high increase in harmonic distortion that could decrease his aided performance (Lotterman and Kasten 1967b, Jerger et al. 1966, Kasten et al, 1967a).

2. The wide variety of taper characteristics and potentiometer ranges available in modern hearing aids may lead both the aid fitter and user to overestimate the amount of reserve gain available. For a group of higher power instruments (more than 45 dB average gain) the median value was 60 dB, but only 13 dB of gain remained above 50 percent rotation (Fig. 2-8). Some of the Kasten and Lotterman instruments achieved maximum amplification at or below the 50 percent point, leaving no reserve (Kasten and Lotterman 1969).

3. It is important for the clinician to know not only the taper characteristics of the aids he uses, but also the potentiometer ranges in order to have some

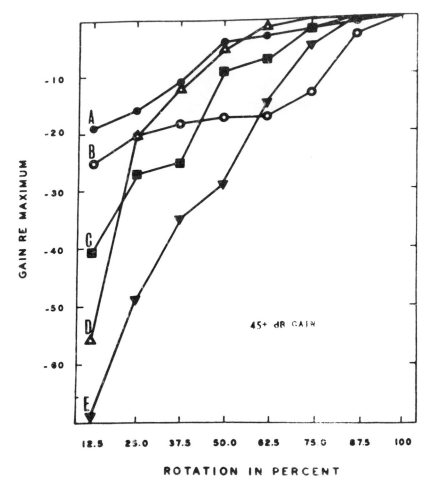

Fig. 2-7.   Sample volume control tapers. (Reproduced with permission from Kasten and
Lotterman, 1969.)

realistic expectations for hearing aids and their performance. It should be
noted that hearing aid manufacturers rarely provide this information on
model specification sheets.

EARMOLD

The importance of the standard earmold and its variations is presented in
Chapter 3 by Pollack and Morgan. Earmold importance in the hearing aid selection process is discussed in Chapter 5.

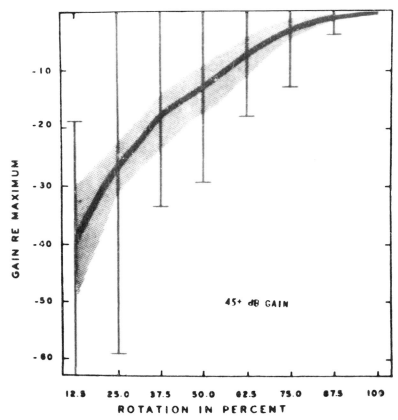

Fig. 2-8.   Variability of volume control tapers. (Reproduced with permission from Kasten and Lotterman, 1969.)

TUBING OR CORD

Ear-level and eyeglass hearing aids, with an internal receiver, require some means of delivering the amplified signals to the ear. Plastic tubing, connecting the elbow and earmold, is generally used for this purpose. The size, length, and condition of this tube can have appreciable effects upon the signal reaching the ear. These effects are described in the next chapter.

Body-style hearing aids, with the receiver external to the case, require a cord to deliver the amplified electric signal to the receiver. The condition of this insulated wire and its connections to the aid and receiver are important. The primary concerns are loose connections or a broken wire, which can cause an intermittent or total lack of signal.

Additional Components

While all aids contain the components described above, there are three additional electronic circuits available on most body-style and many ear-level and eyeglass models. All of them (tone control, telecoil, and output limiting control) affect the output signal in some manner.

TONE CONTROL

A tone control is generally thought of as a circuit designed to provide high or low frequency emphasis (such as treble and bass adjustments on a stereo). The circuit essentially does this, but by frequency suppression or filtering, rather than by emphasis or additional gain. The tone control is a filter network usually situated between stages of the amplifier. If high frequency emphasis (HFE) is desired, a high-pass filter network (low frequencies filtered) is used. Conversely, for low frequency emphasis (LFE), a low-pass filter network is employed.

This is an important concept to keep in mind because tone control labeling can be misleading. Controls are commonly marked H (HFE), N (normal response), and L (LFE), but the circuitry actually performs the opposite of what is suggested, i.e., low frequency filtering rather than additional high frequency gain. Figure 2-9 illustrates this.

Tone controls can be located on the outside or inside of the case, as a switch or screw adjustment. Some hearing aid manufacturers produce models with no adjustable tone control, but rather a series of different responses with varying degrees of low or high frequency filtering. When the aid is ordered, the response desired is specified and appropriate circuitry installed at the factory. An example of various responses available from one manufacturer is presented in Figure 2-23.

TELEPHONE PICKUP

Many hearing aids are or can be equipped with a special circuit to enhance use with a telephone. The circuit consists of a magnetic induction pick-up coil mounted inside the case. The telephone earphone is a magnetic receiver, which, through electromagnetic leakage, generates a magnetic field. If placed next to the telephone receiver, the induction coil picks up the magnetic field and converts it to an electric signal. It is then amplified and again transduced, this time into an acoustic signal. In other words, the telecoil takes the place of a hearing aid microphone as the input component of the aid.

Aids with this component have either a two- or three-position switch that allows use of the microphone alone (M), the telecoil alone (T), or both together (M/T). If the "T" position is chosen, the microphone is cut out of the circuit. The advantage of this is the ability to use the aid with a telephone without interference from sounds in the environment.

Newer telephones produced by Western Electric (Bell Telephone System),

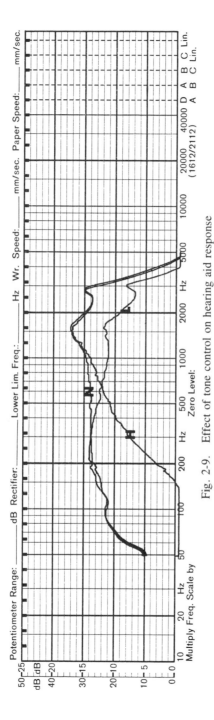

Fig. 2-9. Effect of tone control on hearing aid response

especially the push-button and trimline varieties, utilize a microphone-receiver system that allows too little electromagnetic leakage for use of hearing aid telecoils. After receiving a great many complaints from the public, the hearing aid industry, and audiologists, the Bell system developed a special adapter for use with telecoils. It is small enough to be carried in a pocket or purse, and attaches to the receiver of any telephone, making the induction coil–telephone pairing functional again (Bell System, 1974). It should also be noted that telephones used in the General Telephone System cannot be used with hearing aid telecoils, even if a special adapter is used. In those areas served by the General Telephone System, Western Electric receiver sets can be obtained for those individuals needing an electromagnetic telephone set.

OUTPUT CONTROL

Most body aids and many ear-level instruments have a screw or lever adjustment to reduce the maximum output intensity that can be generated. The rationales and techniques employed are discussed in the section on "Output Limiting" in this chapter.

FEEDBACK

At some time, most of us have experienced a squealing sound from a public-address system, tape recorder, hearing aid, or any other type of amplification system. This is one form of the phenomenon called feedback. Feedback can take many forms, both positive and negative, and has been a major engineering consideration in hearing aid design and production. Unfortunately, the professional literature in audiology and hearing aid technology contains little reference to and information about this major problem.

The usable power capability of aids commonly varies according to their size. Body aids are the largest and most powerful. In-the-ear aids are the smallest and provide the least gain and output. Ear-level and eye-glass instruments fit between these extremes. There is a very logical rationale for these relationships. Sound waves lose energy as they travel from the source. The further they travel, the greater the intensity loss. If there is any sort of signal leakage (acoustic, mechanical, or magnetic) from the receiver, the coupling systems, or both, the lower the intensity of the leaking sound when it reaches the microphone, the less are the chances that feedback will occur. Therefore, the farther apart the microphone and the receiver are, the greater amount of available output before feedback occurs and the less the energy reaching the microphone. With a body aid, the separation may be as much as 18 in, so higher amplification levels can be used. In-the-ear transducers may be separated by as little as 0.25 in, and are therefore the most likely to produce feedback at relatively low output levels. Thus, the power of these instruments is severely restricted.

Berger (1974), citing Wanink (1968), has described feedback as a phenomenon that ". . . may be said to be in operation in a system in which a specific output effect results from a specific input signal, where the output effect in turn, affects the input signal." For purposes of this discussion, four types of feedback will be considered: acoustical, mechanical, magnetic, and electronic.

Acoustical Feedback

What is acoustical feedback? To answer this question, we must look at the frequency response of a hearing aid. It is a graphic representation of the amount of amplification provided (gain) as a function of frequency. (This will be discussed at length later in this chapter.) Figure 2-10 shows a typical frequency response curve. Any system has one or more fairly prominent peaks in its response at which it is most sensitive. These peaks are the result of the individual or combined responses of microphone and receiver. If the amplification at that frequency is high enough and sound leakage occurs, the entire circuit may begin to oscillate, with resultant feedback. The fact that different hearing aids have peaks at different frequencies accounts for differences in the perceived pitch of the feedback from aid to aid.

This process is a cyclic one, occurring between the source of the leak and the microphone. Amplified sound escapes and is again picked up by the microphone and reamplified. In cases of low-to-moderate gain aids, the leaking sound has lost enough energy by the time it reaches the microphone to cause little problem. However, with higher powered instruments, a higher intensity signal reaches the microphone and the cyclic process of reamplification occurs—the sound is amplified again and again until its intensity at the appropriate peak frequency is great enough to set the circuit into oscillation. An interesting sidelight is that if the response of the system were perfectly flat, acoustical feedback would be unlikely because of the absence of resonant peaks. However, no such system exists in hearing aids; there are always peaks and the resultant feedback problem.

As is pointed out in the next chapter, the length and diameter of the tubing used with ear-level and eyeglass aids affect the resonant peaks of the system, either raising or lowering their amplitude and frequency of oscillation and perceived pitch of the feedback. It is hypothetically possible that length and diameter may determine, to some extent, the presence or absence of acoustical feedback. As of this writing, there is no research evidence either confirming or denying this hypothesis.

Acoustical feedback results from sound propagation through the air from the receiver-earmold coupling to the microphone. Two conditions are generally associated with this type of feedback: (A) direct leak of amplified sound from the medial side of the earmold to the outside and (B) poor acoustic isolation of the receiver, the microphone, or both. This permits the sound to radiate through the

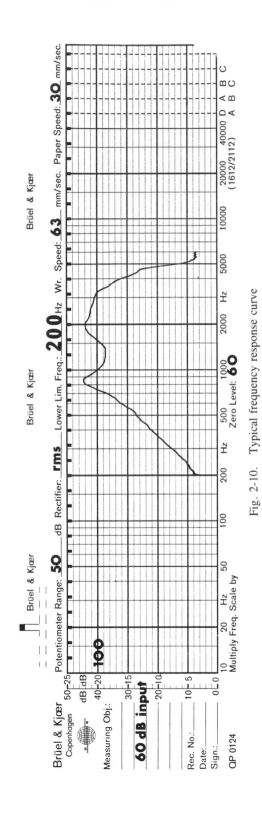

Fig. 2-10. Typical frequency response curve

36

hearing aid case of ear-level and eyeglass aids and be picked up by the microphone. The latter situation usually occurs only under high gain conditions. The direct leak can occur in a number of ways.

1. A poorly fitting earmold allowing sound to escape between the mold and the meatal wall. This is especially true with high powered ear-level and body instruments, due to the high intensity signals entering the ear canal. *Direct sound leakage is the most common cause of acoustical feedback.*
2. Improper connection between the receiver and earmold (body aids) or tubing and earmold (ear-level and eyeglass aids) allowing the sound to leak directly before it is delivered to the ear. This problem can generally be solved by inserting a fabric or plastic washer between the receiver and mold or cord-connector in the body aid, or recementing the tubing into the earmold in the ear-level aid. More recent receiver designs employ a double seal to prevent leakage through the connector plug holes.
3. A crack in the tubing between the internal receiver and earmold, again allowing a direct leak. The easiest solution is to replace the tubing.
4. A poor fit of the tubing to the elbow or receiver nozzle, allowing the direct leak. The best treatment is new tubing.
5. A poor fitting elbow at the receiver connection of ear-level aids. The cure is to replace the elbow.

A simple way to determine the cause of acoustical feedback is to check each of these factors, beginning with the earmold. First, place a finger over the canal opening of the mold and turn the volume control full "on." If no feedback occurs, but has occurred when the aid is worn, the cause is most likely a poorly fitting mold and a new one should be made. If feedback still occurs, check the tubing and its connections to the mold and receiver. In the case of body aids with external receivers, the next step is to insert a washer and repeat the first step. If feedback still is present after all connections have been checked, the problem is probably the result of poor receiver acoustic isolation. In this case, the hearing aid must be returned to the factory for repair.

The second condition is poor acoustic isolation of the receiver, or the microphone, or both, within the hearing aid case. Especially at high output levels, the walls of the receiver oscillate mechanically in a "pumping" action. This disturbs the air inside the case, generating a sound wave that travels through the air space to the microphone. Three approaches can be used to solve this problem: (A) maximize the space between microphone and receiver so that the sound pressure reaching the microphone is of lower amplitude; (B) use an interlocking wall between the microphone and receiver to block the sound transmission; and (C) place a rubber tube on the microphone port so that no sound from within the case can reach the microphone diaphragm. The tubing acts to attenuate the sound pressure reaching the microphone from within the case.

An intriguing finding, and one that may open avenues for additional re-

search, is that the acoustical feedback is essentially a high frequency phenomenon. There are two reasons for this.

1. Peaks in the response curve generally occur within the ranges of 1000—2000
    Hz for the primary peak and 3000—4000 Hz for the secondary peak. The
    former appears to be related to feedback resulting from acoustical radiation
    through the case, whereas the latter is related to direct leakage from the
    earmold, or tubing, or both.
2. Due to their shorter wavelengths, high frequencies can escape around a
    poorly fitting earmold with greater ease than can low frequencies. Combin-
    ing this with the above information, it can readily be seen why acoustic
    feedback is said to be a high frequency phenomenon.

This has recently presented considerable difficulty to hearing aid engineers.
Many manufacturers have been working on designs for extreme high frequency
emphasis instruments, but have had to keep gain relatively low because of
feedback problems. A possible solution to this might be to use the natural
resonant frequency of the external auditory meatus, 3800—4000 Hz. It appears
plausible to decrease some high frequency response in the aid to reduce feedback
and still provide high frequency emphasis by taking advantage of the resonance
characteristics of the meatus. This would have the effect of increasing the intensity of higher frequencies reaching the tympanic membrane at a rate of about 3
dB per octave, from 800 Hz upward. Additional research is needed on this
question.

Mechanical Feedback

Magnetic and ceramic microphones in all hearing aids, and the receiver in
ear-level, eyeglass, and in-the-ear instruments, are mounted inside the case on
rubber cushions to isolate them from each other and from the case. These cushions are employed to decrease vibration transmission and to protect the components from shock if the aid is dropped. If these isolators are improperly designed
or mounted, or have deteriorated, low frequency mechanical vibrations
(400—500 Hz) from the receiver can vibrate the case. These vibrations will be
picked up by the microphone and amplified. A "squeal" is heard that is lower in
pitch than that heard because of acoustical feedback. In fact, the distinguishing
auditory feature of mechanical feedback is its relatively low pitch. This is especially a problem with the ceramic microphone, which provides extended low
frequency response and is therefore more susceptible to mechanical feedback.
Electret microphones have a low-mass internal construction, which makes them
highly resistant to mechanical vibration. Increased miniaturization of hearing
aids has increased the problem of mechanical vibration feedback between the
microphone and receiver because of their proximity (Maxwell and Burkhard,
1969b). This is another reason for the relatively low gain of in-the-ear aids.

This problem can be solved in two ways. First, more compliant isolation supports for the transducers (better cushioning) are used to achieve high gain without vibrational feedback oscillation (Burkhard 1965, Nordstrom 1974). Second, microphones and receivers are oriented within the case with their directions of maximum vibration output and sensitivity at right angles to each other to take advantage of directional vibration damping properties (Maxwell and Burkhard, 1969a).

Magnetic Feedback

Magnetic feedback results from the coupling between the magnetic fields of the receiver and the telephone coil or magnetic microphone. The magnetic field from the receiver can "spill over" to the microphone or telecoil and be transduced to a feedback noise. This problem has been greatly reduced through the use of nonmagnetic microphones and improved receiver designs in more recently introduced aids.

Electronic Feedback

Electronic feedback is often used in amplifier circuits to help control the output of the hearing aid. A portion of the electric signal from the output stage of the amplifier is routed back to the input stage for self-regulatory functions, such as automatic volume control (AVC). Obviously, this is a beneficial form of feedback. Other controlled uses of feedback include giving some condenser microphones directional response characteristics and shaping amplifier response characteristics (Hillman, 1974).

There are two forms of electronic feedback that can have a detrimental effect on instrument performance. The first is *electrostatic feedback*. An electrostatic field is caused by a capacitive coupling from the output to the input stages of the amplifier, and becomes a problem when improper techniques are used to attenuate high frequency amplifier response. The resultant audible sound has a very high pitch, reported as a "hiss."

Electrical oscillation results from inadequate decoupling of battery and amplifier circuits. It is related to battery impedance in that as the usable battery voltage decreases, impedance increases and causes the amplifier circuit to oscillate. This is reflected in a low frequency "motorboating," which commonly sounds much like the buzz of a saw-tooth noise. The cure for electrical oscillation is to replace the battery and improve decoupling, making the circuit impervious to battery voltage changes.

Combination Effects

It is possible for more than one form of feedback to occur simultaneously. These combined effects are overlayed and more than one type of feedback is audible at the same time.

Conclusion

As pointed out above, many forms of acoustical feedback can be remedied by the audiologist or hearing aid dispenser by adjusting the earmold, the tubing, or both. If these modifications do not cure the problem, the instrument should be returned to the factory for appropriate repair. This is especially true for mechanical, magnetic, and electronic feedback problems, which ordinarily cannot be remediated outside a repair center.

ELECTROACOUSTIC MEASUREMENTS

History and Rationale

During the early period of electric and electronic instrumentation there was a lack of standardization of performance parameters including how to measure them and how to report them. Most often, each manufacturer used his own set of "standards" for sales promotion. As Berger (1974) states, "advertising slogans were the rule rather than statements based on scientific fact." Early attempts to achieve industry-wide standards met with little success. Romanow (1942) and Carlisle and Mundel (1944) produced some of the earliest extensive reports on hearing aid electroacoustic measurements. A committee of the American Hearing Aid Association compiled a *"Tentative Code for Measurement of Performance of Hearing Aids"* (Kranz, 1945), but it was neither sufficiently comprehensive nor widely accepted by the industry. For a thorough overview of attempts to standardize hearing aid measurements, the reader should consult Berger (1968 and 1974).

As hearing aid makes and models continued to proliferate, the need became apparent for a method to compare not only the performance of different models but of units of the same model as well. Without being able to describe performance characteristics in detail, a particular aid cannot be compared to others or to published characteristics of that model.

Standards

In 1959, the International Electrotechnical Commission (IEC) published their *"Recommended Methods for Measurements of the Electroacoustical Characteristics of Hearing Aids"* (IEC 1959). This European standard was slightly modified and adopted by the American National Standards Institute (ANSI, formerly the American Standards Association and United States of America Standards Institute) as American Standard S3.3 – 1960, *"Electroacoustical Characteristics of Hearing Aids"* (ANSI 1960). In 1961, the Hearing Aid Industry Conference (HAIC 1961) adopted the *"HAIC Standard Method of Expressing Hearing Aid Performance."* It was largely based on S3.3 – 1960. In the late 1960s, the HAIC standard underwent minor modification, and was adopted as ANSI Standard S3.8−1967, *"Methods of Expressing Hearing Aid Performance"* (ANSI, 1967). In essence, the IEC and early ANSI standards describe how to measure performance, while the HAIC and later ANSI standards specify not only how but *what* to measure.

In 1976, ANSI adopted new standards for hearing aids, S3.22−1976, *"Specification of Hearing Aid Characteristics"* (ANSI, 1976). This standard is presented as Appendix I at the end of this book. S3.22−1976 is essentially an update and expansion of S3.3−1960 and S3.8−1967. The main changes include the following.

1. A change in the frequencies measured to specify gain and output to 1000, 1600, and 2500 Hz, now called *High Frequency Average.*
2. For the first time, the standards include tolerances on the measured characteristics reported by manufacturers.
3. Also for the first time, an attempt to measure some characteristics at a volume control setting approximating a "use" setting known as *reference test gain.*

Testing Equipment

Lybarger (1961a, b) described the "typical situation for hearing aid use," as depicted in Figure 2-11. In this situation, the speaker and listener (hearing aid user) are some 3−15 ft apart. The average intensity of conversational speech is about 70 dB SPL at this distance. The speech signal not only reaches the hearing aid microphone through the direct air pathway but is also reflected from the walls, ceiling, and floor of the room in a rather random uncontrolled manner. Ambient noise in the environment also reaches the microphone and is amplified.

Obviously, this "typical" situation involves far too many uncontrolled variables for standardized measurements. Therefore, the standards specify the use of a free-field environment for testing (implying the use of an anechoic-type chamber) to eliminate reflected and standing waves and to reduce ambient noise levels. To further eliminate variables, the human speaker is replaced with a dynamic loudspeaker, having a "nearly uniform output over the 200−5000 Hz test band ordinarily used for hearing aids" (Lybarger, 1961b). Either a discrete or sweep frequency oscillator provides the test signal to the speaker. To insure a uniform signal to the hearing aid microphone, a monitoring condenser microphone is positioned in the test box enclosure. This microphone and its associated compressor amplifier automatically maintain a constant signal sound pressure within stated tolerances of ± 1.5 dB from 200−3000 Hz and ± 2.5 dB from 3000−5000 Hz.

Inside the test enclosure, the sweep or discrete frequency signal is amplified by the hearing aid, the output of which is delivered to a standard 2 cc coupler (artificial ear) that replaces the human ear for text purposes. From this point, the amplified signal is metered and, in automatic systems, printed out by a graphic

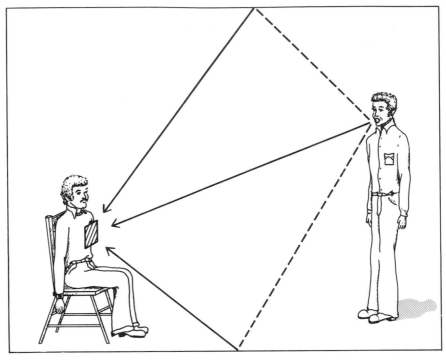

Fig. 2-11.   Typical situation for hearing aid use. (Adapted with permission from
        Lybarger, 1961.)

level recorder. Figure 2-12 is a block diagram of a complete hearing aid test
system. For detailed information regarding the specifications for a test system,
the reader is referred to the IEC (1959) or ANSI (1976) standards and to the Bruel
and Kjaer (B & K) "cookbook" (1973).

In recent years HC Electronics and Frye Electronics have introduced hearing
aid test systems considerably less expensive than a complete B & K system. With
the added complexity of hearing aids, it has become a necessity for every dispenser to have a test system to be sure all new aids perform as specified, to be
sure that repaired instruments work properly, to measure response changes made
by the dispenser, and to measure any deterioration in response over time of use.
The marketing of the less expensive systems has made test arrangements available to most dispensers.

Definitions and Standard Procedures

The performance characteristics most often measured are: Saturation Sound
Pressure Level (HFA−SSPL90); Reference Test Gain; Frequency Response;
Equivalent Input Noise Level; and Harmonic Distortion. Additional measures
include Battery Current and Automatic Gain Control (AGC).

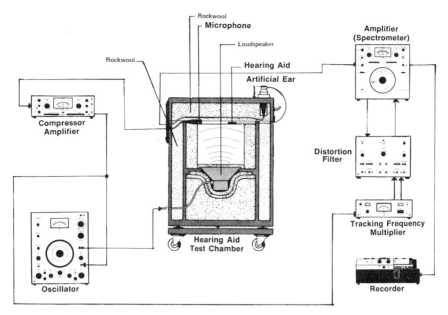

Fig. 2-12.   Hearing aid test system. (Courtesty of B & K Instruments.)

FULL-ON GAIN

As defined by ANSI (1976), full-on gain (FOG) is "the amount, in de-cibels, by which the sound pressure level developed by the hearing aid . . . exceeds the sound pressure level at the microphone opening of the hearing aid . . . ." This refers to the amount of amplification of the input signal. It is the decibel difference between input and output signals. For example, if the input signal is 60 dB and the output is 115 dB, the gain is 55 dB.

The FOG is measured with the volume control at its maximum (full-on) position and an input of 60 dB SPL (50 dB for AGC aids). The measurements can be made using either discrete-frequency signals or, preferably, a sweep-frequency signal. The output is plotted by hand or automatically, providing a curve describing gain as a function of frequency. From this curve the essential information can be extrapolated to specify the high frequency average FOG. To do this, the average gain at 1000, 1600, and 2500 Hz is determined.

This provides a limited impression of the amount of amplification through "speech frequencies." While better than the old average of 500, 1000, and 2000 Hz, the HF average can still be misleading, especially if the gain at one of the frequencies is appreciably higher or lower than the others. In this situation, one may receive a false impression of how much amplification the aid provides. For example, if the gain was 20 dB at 1000 Hz, 30 dB at 1600 Hz, and 65 dB at 2500 Hz, the HF average would be 45 dB. While this hypothetical instrument might be sufficient for an individual with a high frequency loss beginning at 1000 Hz, it would most likely not be adequate for someone with a relatively flat loss. This implies the importance of examining the FOG curve carefully.

In a later section of this chapter, some of the problems inherent in the ANSI standards are discussed, including proposals for considering the use of "speech" or "pink" noise rather than pure tones as the input signal and use of the Zwislocki coupler for a much closer approximation of real ear hearing aid response.

Another important bit of information, related to the gain curve and the average gain, is the gain-per-octave slope. In the example given above, the gain per octave between 1000 and 1600 Hz is 10 dB, but is 35 dB between 1600 and 2500 Hz. Referring to the discussion of that example, the value of these data is apparent. Unfortunately, few manufacturers routinely provide this information by itself or in a form that can be extrapolated, since they don't publishing true gain curves.

Of all hearing aid measurements, only the full-on gain curve shows the practical maximum gain of the instrument. It is easy to confuse this curve with the "reference test gain frequency response curve" (see below), but by carefully examining the measurement procedure one can see the differences. Some manufacturers obtain gain information from the frequency response rather than from the gain curve, resulting in a lack of standardized data reporting. Anyone reading hearing aid specifications should be aware of this. It is important to use standardized input levels to obtain data from which comparisons can be made.

REFERENCE TEST GAIN (RTG)

One of the major changes with the new ANSI standards is the inclusion of *reference test gain,* which simulates "use" position of the volume control. This is used for certain other measures including harmonic distortion, frequency response and range, and equivalent input noise level.

To adjust the gain control to RTG position, first determine the HF average SSPL-90 as described below. Then, using 60 dB input, adjust the control so that the average of the 1000, 1600, and 2500 Hz values is 17 dB less than the HF average SSPL-90. If the aid does not have enough gain to allow this adjustment, leave the control full-on. For AGC aids, set the control full-on. The rationale for this procedure is that the long-term average SPL for speech at 1 m is about 65 dB SPL, with peaks typically 12 dB above this value, or 77 dB SPL. Using a 60 dB SPL input and a 17 dB volume control setting back from the SSPL-90 value gives essentially the same value.

Another way to determine the RTG is to subtract 77 dB from the HF average SSPL-90. If the aid yields less gain than the value so specified, the RTG is determined with the gain control full-on.

SATURATION SOUND PRESSURE LEVEL (SSPL-90)

Also referred to as *acoustic output* or *maximum power output* (MPO), *saturation output is the greatest sound pressure level the aid is capable of producing, regardless of the amount of gain and the intensity of the input signal.*

Any amplification system can provide only a limited amount of output. A point is reached at which the amplifier cannot amplify further and the receiver cannot transduce a greater signal. If the input increases beyond the level at which saturation occurs, the output will not increase further, and may decrease, so that the signal will be considerably distorted. We have all experienced this when turning the volume control on a radio or TV to its maximum. Not only is the signal loud, but it is also obviously distorted.

The SSPL-90 is measured with the gain control at maximum and a 90 dB input. All other controls on the aid are adjusted to give the widest response. Using either a discrete- or sweep-frequency signal, plot a curve of output as a function of frequency between 200 and 5000 Hz. Using the three frequencies, 1000, 1600, and 2500 Hz, determine the HF average SSPL-90. Figure 2-13 shows a typical SSPL-90 curve.

It is vital to proper fitting to know the maximum output capability of a hearing aid for two reasons: (A) to be sure the instrument is producing a sound pressure level sufficiently above the user's threshold to be maximally useful; and (B) to insure that the aid does not produce a signal that exceeds the user's threshold of discomfort. In other words, the signal must not be too little or too much.

FREQUENCY RESPONSE CURVE

The most common curve on manufacturers' technical sheets is the basic frequency response, describing the relative amount of gain as a function of frequency. It is relative in that the frequency response is not based upon maximum gain.

For this measure, the gain control is set at reference test. With the control at this point and the input at a constant 60 dB, the signal frequency is varied and the curve recorded either automatically or manually. The reader is referred to Figure 2-10 for a typical frequency response curve.

To provide a consistent, undistorted graph of the frequency response, it must be plotted on a frequency-by-intensity chart in which the length covered by a 1-octave interval on the frequency abscissa is equal to a 13.5 dB length on the intensity ordinate. This scale is essentially the same as that in which one decade (i.e., 100–1000Hz) on the abscissa is equal to 50 dB ± 2 dB on the ordinate, as required in ANSI S3.8–1967.

The frequency response of any hearing aid depends on the respective responses of all its components: microphone, amplifier, and receiver. As was discussed earlier in this chapter, the amplifier and receiver can only process the signals they receive from the microphone. Therefore, the vital importance of the microphone in the system is evident. By the same token, the overall response of a hearing aid will reflect the characteristics of each component. If the amplifier works on only a restricted frequency range, the aid's response will reflect this, regardless of the characteristics of microphone and receiver. The same analogy holds true for the receiver. With this in mind, along with the difficulties inherent

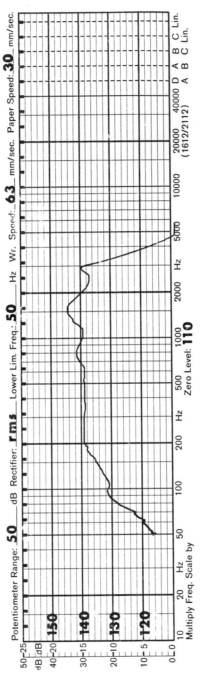

Fig. 2-13. Typical hearing aid output curve

in changing the responses of microphones and internal receivers, most intentional modifications of frequency response are achieved by altering the amplifier (tone control) or tubing-earmold coupling. The latter area is discussed by Ron Morgan and myself in the next chapter.

Distortion

An ideal amplification system is one that, among its other characteristics, reproduces an output signal identical to the input signal. However, no such system truly exists. Neither the microphone, amplifier, nor receiver is capable of producing an exact copy of the input signal. When the acoustic properties of the input signal are not reproduced exactly, the output is said to be distorted in comparison to the input. This distortion can take the form of resonant peaks or antiresonant valleys, decreased bandwith, or nonlinear frequency and/or amplitude reproduction. The ability of an amplification system to accurately reproduce the waveform of the input signal is referred to as fidelity—high fidelity for accurate or near accurate reproduction, and low fidelity for poor reproduction. In general, hearing aids are considered low fidelity systems.

For the purpose of this discussion, four types of distortion will be considered: nonlinear or amplitude distortion (including harmonic and intermodulation distortion), transient distortion, frequency distortion, and extraneous or noise distortion. The output of a hearing aid is said to be nonlinear when either the amplitude or frequency aspects of the waveform are not in the same relationship as they were in the input signal. The meaning of this will become apparent in the discussion to follow.

HARMONIC DISTORTION

Other forms of distortion that can affect hearing aid and user performance are often overlooked, making harmonic distortion the type most commonly considered in hearing aid technology. The reasons for this are that harmonic distortion is the easiest to measure and is the only type reported by manufacturers.

Harmonic distortion results when new frequencies are generated that are whole number multiples of the original or fundamental frequency, and that are not part of the input signal. For example, if a hearing aid distorts at 500 Hz, this indicates that in addition to the fundamental tone it amplifies and reproduces, the instrument also generates harmonic frequencies. Thus, in addition to the 500 Hz fundamental, the frequencies of 1000 Hz (second harmonic), 1500 Hz (third harmonic), and so forth, are also present in the output signal (Fig. 2-14).

Generally speaking, the greater the gain setting of an aid, the greater will be the harmonic distortion. Studies have shown high distortion at or near maximum gain in most aids, and lower distortion at reduced settings (Lotterman and Kasten 1967b, Kasten et al. 1967). These findings have serious implications in terms of hearing aid selection for the hard-of-hearing. In other words, it would be unde-

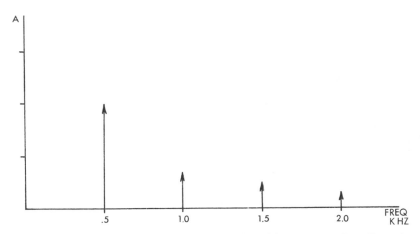

Fig. 2-14.   500 Hz fundamental plus second, third, and fourth harmonics. (Reproduced with permission from Ely, 1974.)

sirable to select for an individual an instrument that would have to be set at or near maximum gain in order to achieve a comfort level. In such case, the output signal would contain appreciable distortion, thereby probably lowering both the objective and subjective aspects of aided performance. Harmonic distortion appears to be an important determinant of the degree of success a hearing aid user may achieve with an instrument (Kasten and Lotterman, 1967).

If the amount of harmonic distortion is great, the effects can be serious in terms of speech intelligibility; that is, speech will be distorted and intelligibility will be reduced. Various investigations have shown that of all electroacoustic characteristics, harmonic distortion appears to be the one most closely related to aided speech discrimination ability. Results of these studies indicate that speech intelligibility decreases in an inversely proportional function to the level of distortion (Harris et al. 1961, Jerger et al. 1966, Olsen and Carhart, 1967, Olsen and Wilbur, 1968). However, these studies used rather severe levels of distortion. It is possible that as the harmonic distortion levels increased, other forms of distortion also increased, thereby reducing listener performance.

Two interesting observations arose from a study of a nonlinear distortion by Kasten and Lotterman (1967). First, there appeared to be an inverse relationship between level of distortion and frequency—as frequency increased, distortion decreased. This finding was supported by Lotterman and Kasten (1967a) and by Lotterman and Farrar (1965). Second, distortion level appeared to be inversely related to the power category of the aids, i.e., greatest distortion in mild gain instruments. Lotterman and Farrar (1965) and Lotterman and Kasten (1967a) also found that frequencies at which maximum distortion occurred were higher in ear-level than in body aids.

INTERMODULATION DISTORTION

Intermodulation distortion occurs when the output signal contains frequencies that are arithmetic sums and differences of two or more input frequencies. When two or more signal frequencies (as in speech) are applied simultaneously at the input, it is the result of amplifier nonlinearity. Speech intelligibility can suffer in the presence of intermodulation distortion due to unwanted frequencies distorting the primary message signal. When two frequencies are amplified by a nonlinear system, sum and difference tones can be generated. The same nonlinearity that generates harmonic distortion results in intermodulation distortion— harmonic distortion and intermodulation distortion result from the same source, amplifier nonlinearity. Figure 2-15 presents a typical simplified intermodulation distortion example in which are seen the fundamentals (500 and 700 Hz) and the sum (1200 Hz) and difference (200 Hz) frequencies. Figure 2-16 shows the same two fundamentals with the concomitant harmonic and intermodulation distortion frequencies.

TRANSIENT DISTORTION

Transient distortion occurs whenever the hearing aid is unable to duplicate the initial sharp attack (rise time) or the sudden decay (fall time) of a sound. In the latter situation, an alteration or lingering of the waveform often results in what is called "ringing." The way in which the output lags behind the input can be seen in Figure 2-17. This type of distortion appears to be closely related to the presence of sharp, resonant peaks in the response of the system. Speech intelligibility can be reduced by transient distortion, since the "ringing" of the output signal interacts with the transient nature of speech. This problem is compounded

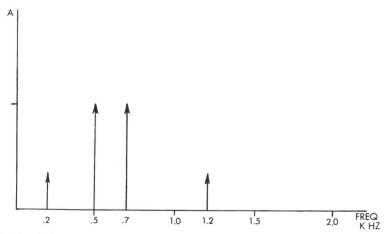

Fig. 2-15.   500 Hz and 700 Hz tones plus sum. (1.2K Hz) and difference (.2K Hz) intermodulation tones. (Reproduced with permission from Ely, 1974.)

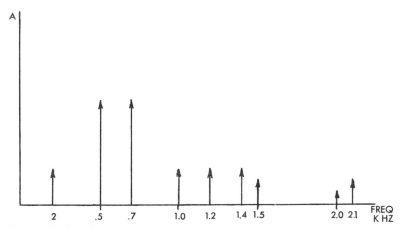

Fig. 2-16.   500 and 700 Hz tones plus harmonic and intermodulation distortion components. (Reproduced with permission from Ely, 1974.)

by the fact that speech is composed of many transients important to discrimination.

FREQUENCY DISTORTION

As considered earlier, the input and output signals are often not the same. If
the variations are related to the frequency spectrum of the signal, that is, if the
frequency response and bandwidth of the output are different from the input,
frequency distortion has occurred. This is related to the concept of fidelity.
Because the output signal from a hearing aid is so different from the input, in
terms of frequency response and bandwidth, hearing aids can reasonably be
called low-fidelity amplification systems.

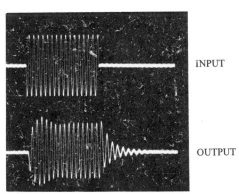

Fig. 2-17.   Transient distortion. (Reproduced with permission from Davis and Silverman, 1970.)

EXTRANEOUS DISTORTION

In body aids, if clothing rubs against the microphone opening or case, the friction can generate random noise, known as extraneous distortion. Also, at times the electronic circuitry of the aid can produce an inherent distracting noise. These kinds of extraneous distortion have the effect of decreasing the signal-to-noise ratio of the instrument, possibly "burying" the primary message signal in the noise.

Curran (1974) points out that we can not reasonably conclude that user performance will be satisfactory simply because published or individually measured harmonic distortion levels are low. As shown above, there has been no clear-cut, consistent relationship established between harmonic distortion and speech intelligibility. This may be due to the fact that harmonic distortion, by itself, may not significantly deteriorate intelligibility. Interaction effects, the appearance of multiple forms of distortion simultaneously, may be more detrimental than any one individual type of distortion. This is an area of much-needed research.

Distortion Measurements

At the time of this writing, the current American National Standard for the *Specification of Hearing Aid Characteristics* (ANSI, 1976) does not specify procedures for measuring any type of distortion other than harmonic. Even this procedure is not precise, calling for measurements at 500, 800, and 1600 Hz with a 70 dB SPL input level. However, the standards do not specify provisions or recommendations for methods of reporting distortion levels, i.e., at which gain setting distortion should be reported. For a complete review of these standards, refer to Appendix III of this book.

Harmonic distortion measurements are expressed in percentages and use the standard formula found in S3.3−1960 for total harmonic distortion (THD). The acceptable amount of distortion in a hearing aid is not standardized, although some investigators have shown that distortion values greater than 10% begin to have appreciably negative influences on speech discrimination (Lotterman and Kasten, 1967b, Jerger et al. 1966, Jirsa and Hodgson, 1970, Bode and Kasten, 1971). The Veterans Administration and others recommend rejection of any hearing aid with harmonic distortion over 10 percent (Jeffers et al. 1973).

One of the problems with harmonic distortion measurements is a lack of consistency regarding what is being measured. You can either plot the second harmonic of a number of frequencies, i.e., 500, 800, and 1600 Hz according to ANSI, or you can add all the harmonics (2nd, 3rd, 4th, and so on) at one frequency to calculate THD.

However, second harmonic distortion alone can be misleading, as is shown in Figure 2-18. In this example, we see frequency response, and second and third harmonic curves obtained at three input levels (60, 70, and 80 dB) with the same

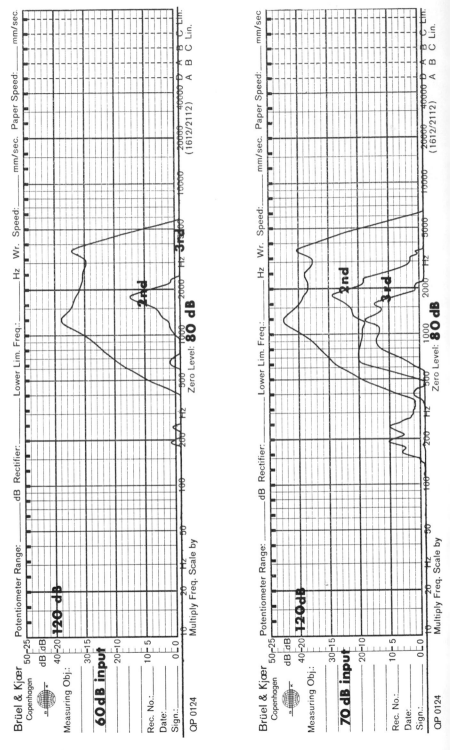

52

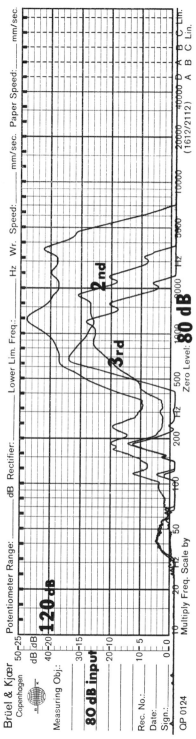

Fig. 2-18. Fundamental, second, and third harmonics of the same aid at three different input levels: *top*, 60 dB; *middle*, 70 dB; *bottom*, 80 dB. (Courtesy of HC Electronics.)

aid. As the input level increases, so do both harmonic curves, especially the third. In fact, third harmonic distortion begins to approxomate and exceed the second with the 80 dB input. If only second harmonic distortion was measured for the hearing aid used here, this situation could possibly pass unnoticed. THD measurements would pick it up.

Harmonic distortion is measured using a wave analyzer, distortion bridge, or filter set. The procedure involves filtering out the fundamental frequency from the output signal and measuring the intensity level of the remaining second or more harmonics. Using either the standard formula or conversion table, the intensity difference between the fundamental and harmonics is converted to a percentage value. Figure 2-12 includes an equipment model for harmonic distortion measurement.

This discussion on distortion measurement has been limited to harmonic distortion because, as I mentioned earlier, that is the only type for which there is even a semblance of an adequate and reasonable measurement protocol, much less an agreed upon one. Although frequency distortion is measured as frequency response, there is no means of quantifying it. Intermodulation distortion measurements require two input signals, has a more complex output, and lacks, at present, an acceptable procedure. This is another area ripe for investigation.

Output Limiting

It has previously been noted that all hearing aids have an inherent output limit, known as saturation output. One of the basic tenets in selecting a hearing aid is to choose an instrument that has sufficient, yet tolerable amplification. Especially for individuals with a reduced dynamic range, as in the case of a recruiting ear, it may be necessary to limit the output further, at least for high intensity inputs. Historically, three methods have been employed to achieve this additional limiting: peak clipping, automatic volume control, and curvilinear compression.

PEAK CLIPPING

This form of limitation is characteristic of all simple amplifiers and occurs when the output stage of the amplifier is driven beyond its power handling capability (past overload or saturation point). The peak clipping level can be fixed or variable. The saturation level described earlier utilizes peak clipping. If variable, the peak clipping level can be set below the saturation point to prevent intensities beyond tolerance limits from reaching a recruiting ear.

Figure 2-19 depicts the input-output (I-O) relationship of four different output limiting systems. By studying the curve labeled "conventional (linear)," it can be seen that the I-O ratio remains constant until the saturation or limiting level is reached. Further increases in input lead to overload and no further increase in output. Figure 2-20 displays the effect of this upon the signal

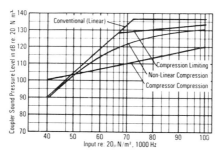

Fig. 2-19.   Input-output relationship of four limiting systems. (Reproduced with permission from Curran and Ely, 1973.)

waveform. As saturation is reached, the peak amplitude portions of the output signal are "clipped," flattening or squaring the waveform. This results in a physical distortion of the signal because its amplitude elements are now restricted relative to its low amplitude components.

Olsen (1971) reviewed the early literature and found suggestions that speech intelligibility is not disrupted appreciably by peak clipping and its resultant harmonic and intermodulation distortion. Staab (1972) indicated that even excessive peak clipping does not significantly decrease speech discrimination ability. Both reports indicate that there is a great reduction in sound quality when peak clipping is used as an output limiting device.

A brief consideration of acoustic phonetics can point out the logic of these reports. In English, vowel sounds are generally lower in frequency and higher in intensity than consonants. Consonants appear to be responsible for carrying the meaning of speech, while vowels carry the intensity. In peak clipping circuits, only the highest intensity components of the waveform are removed. Lower intensity elements are unchanged. Since the highest intensities in speech are the vowels, they are reduced, whereas the lower intensity meaning-carrying consonants are relatively untouched. Therefore, one would not expect speech intelligibility to suffer appreciably, but would expect sound quality to decrease.

AUTOMATIC VOLUME CONTROL

Also referred to as *automatic gain control (AGC), compression amplification,* and *linear dynamic compression (LDC), automatic volume control (AVC)* is a means of controlling amplifier gain. Such a system acts to decrease the gain as a function of the input level to prevent the output signal from reaching saturation when confronted with high inputs. AVC utilizes an electronic feedback principle for self-regulation in that a constant voltage from the output amplifier stage is circuited back to the input amplifier. The amplitude of this electric signal varies directly as a function of the input-output ratio. When it approaches saturation (high input-high output), a preset point is reached at which the AVC circuit is triggered and the gain is reduced automatically. When input decreases and nega-

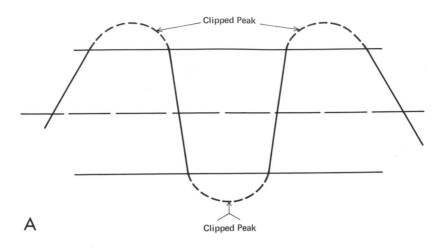

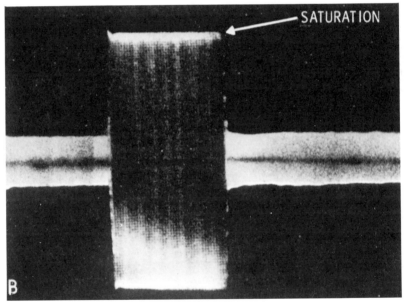

Fig. 2-20.   Effect of peak clipping on signal waveform. *A*, Diagrammatic view; *B*, Oscilloscopic view. (Courtesy of Audiotone.)

tive voltage decreases below the present point, the AVC circuit ceases to function and gain returns to its normal level.

Referring to the curve in Figure 2-19 labeled "compression limiting," it can be seen that an AVC input-output function is linear to the predetermined output level. Above this point, output is restricted because of a gain reduction. In this example, for inputs below about 65 dB SPL, the function is linear. Above 65 dB

SPL input, the AVC system operates to reduce the gain, reflected in only a slight additional rise in output.

Automatic volume control is not a new innovation. Davis *et al.* (1947) report that as early as 1944 recommendations were made to use compression amplification to limit high output levels as a preferred alternative to peak clipping. The primary advantage of AVC is that none of the signal is lost; the entire signal is compressed. The problem was one of size—making the circuit small enough for a wearable hearing aid. Hudgins et al. (1948) demonstrated the feasibility of using AVC in wearable aids. The first commercial wearable aid with it appeared in 1949 (Caraway and Carhart, 1967).

There are four critical variables in any AVC system: *Limiting level (LL), attack time (AT), release time (RT), and compression range (CR).*

Limiting level is the output intensity beyond which the system operates. It is represented by the 65 dB point, discussed above in relation to Figure 2-19.

The response of a compression system is not instantaneous; some period of time is required for it to operate. This is known as *attack time*. It is the time lapse from the moment signal amplitude (input) exceeds the limiting level to that instant when gain becomes stabilized at a reduced level. Because of the time lag, the output level will momentarily exceed the limiting level and may reach MPO (overshoot) and then immediately decrease as the circuit begins to reduce gain. Because the initial output is so high, the voltage to the AVC system is correspondingly high and, consequently, it may overcompensate to result in a momentary excessively low output (undershoot). After this point, the system stabilizes and continues to operate as long as the input level is high.

When the input level decreases, it takes a moment for the system to cut-off and restore the normal gain function. This time lag is referred to as *release time*. It is defined as the time from the moment input amplitude is decreased to that instant at which gain is again established at the precompressed level. During the lag, the gain remains reduced and, combined with the decreased input, the output momentarily drops. As soon as the appropriate correction is made, output function is restored.

Figure 2-21 is an oscilloscopic representation of the operation of an AVC system. Note the sections labeled "attack time" and "recovery time." Some of those working with hearing aids consider the time from initial high output to the start of AVC operation as the attack time and the remaining period until stabilization as recovery time. Others consider the entire period as attack time. I feel it is only a minor semantic point.

Compression range refers to the amount of gain reduction provided. Generally, this varies from 5 to 30 dB, depending on the system and the needs of the user. An important consideration is that if the input-output relationship becomes so high as to demand the circuit to compress beyond this range, the output signal will either become distorted or the limiting level will be exceeded.

Reference has been made to the time lags involved in AVC operation. Commonly, attack times vary between 5 and 100 msec, and release times be-

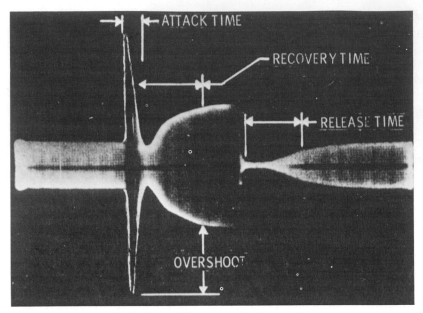

Fig. 2-21.   AVC system signal waveform

tween 40 and 150 msec, depending on the circuitry employed (Nunley 1973, Berger 1974). These time constants are critical in terms of speech intelligibility. Lynne and Carhart (1963) studied this variable and demonstrated that speech discrimination ability decreased as release time increased. A relatively intense speech component, such as a vowel, can cause the system to operate, with the resulting overshoot. If the circuit is operating, low intensity consonants can be reproduced too faintly during release, affecting intelligibility.

Most often, release time is longer than attack time in order to avoid what is called *AVC flutter*. This condition results when the system reacts to variations in the normal intensity of speech, perhaps even between syllables; constantly raising and lowering the gain causes a flutter effect. Flutter occurs most often if the release time is too short. An optimal release time is one between the point at which flutter may occur (usually less than 30 msec) and syllables are lost (over about 150 msec).

Thus far, only one form of compression, AVC, has been discussed. Two other types are gaining popularity in hearing aids: (A) *compressor compression* and (B) *curvilinear (nonlinear) compression*.

While AVC aids maintain a 1:1 input-output function until the limiting level is approached, the compressor compression circuit does not have a unity slope (not 1:1). For example, the curve in Figure 2-19 labeled *compressor compression* shows a 3:1 ratio. For every 15 dB increase in input, there is a corresponding output increase of only 5 dB. The slope of such a circuit can take many fixed I-O ratios, i.e., 2:1, 3:1, 10:7—almost any slope desired. Notice in the figure that the output never exceeds 120 dB SPL (considerably below saturation), even with an input of 100 dB. In this system, there is a constant degree of gain reduction; there is no 1:1 linear portion to the function. At 40 dB input, the gain is 60 dB; at 70 dB input, the gain is 40 dB: at 100 dB input, the gain is 20 dB.

Nonlinear or curvilinear compression is also known as adjustable AVC, logarithmic AVC, and compression limiting. With this circuitry, the I-O function is not fixed in a given ratio, but varies continually as a function of input level changes. In other words, the gain is continually decreasing as the input is increasing, as opposed to the linear AVC, which reduces gain by a fixed amount only as the limiting level is reached (Fig. 2-19). Curvilinear AVC provides constant and variable gain adjustment, minimum supression of low intensity inputs, and progressively greater compression with higher inputs. There is no specific limiting level; some limiting takes place at all input levels. Because of the constancy factor, this process involves no specific attack and release times.

All three of the compression modes have a number of things in common in terms of their advantages over peak clipping. Since none of the amplified signal is lost, as in peak clipping, compressed signals avoid the distortion factor. Output is limited to a level below saturation through a gain reduction to the entire signal. Also, these systems have the effect of expanding the dynamic range for the hearing aid user by providing a wider range of input levels to the ear; yet they do not exceed the tolerance limits of the ear.

Perhaps the most significant benefit in terms of speech intelligibility is that the original signal-to-noise ratio of the input signal is maintained. A compressor system decreases the signal and background noise equally. As noted earlier, in a peak clipping circuit only the highest intensity components (usually the primary speech signal vowels) are reduced. For example, consider an instrument with an MPO of 130 dB and a gain of 60 dB being used in an environment with 70 dB of ambient noise and a person speaking at a level of 90 dB (signal-to-noise ratio, +20 dB). If this hypothetical aid used peak clipping to achieve MPO, the +20 dB S/N ratio would be lost during amplification. The 70 dB noise would be fully amplified to 130 dB (60 dB gain). On the other hand, the speech would only be amplified 40 dB before it reached MPO and its peak intensities were clipped. The S/N ratio is now 0 dB; the noise is as loud as the speech. If the aid used a compression system, the +20 dB ratio would have been retained, since the gain of the entire input signal would have been reduced.

There is one last consideration regarding output limiting at the time of this writing. None of the standards for hearing aid measurements have complete recommendations for standardization of attack and release times or methods of performance measurements for these circuits. Additionally, the 1960 ANSI standard states "this standard does not apply when automatic gain control is in use." IEC (1959) states, "the automatic gain control (if any) shall be put out of action (during measurements)." The implication of these statements is that performance measurements made with an aid using a compression system may not be valid. For many instruments, outside the factory it is not possible to put the AVC "out of action."

During the past few years, some manufacturers have begun using a new compression system in some of their models, *input compression*. Most AGC aids compress the signal at the output stage. If the signal is monitored prior to the volume control, the amplifier has input-controlled AGC. In other words, if the monitoring takes place prior to the amplifier stage, it is input compression.

In this system, the gain of the amplifier is automatically reduced before the signal is amplified. Figure 2-22 schematically represents both types of compression circuits. One of the potential advantages of input compression is a deduction of distortion since the signal is compressed before it is amplified, rather than after, as in output AGC.

Problems with S3.22—1976

The new standards specify measurements over the range 200—5000 Hz. Many of today's new aids exceed this range on one or both extremes. One factor that will confound measurements on these instruments is that most commonly used hearing aid test boxes do not meet the needs for sound isolation and vibration dampening below 200 Hz. If low frequency noise levels (below 200 Hz) are high, the test system cannot adequately measure low frequency amplification of many newer aids. This can give a false impression that these frequencies are not amplified when they are, possibly resulting in misfittings of hearing aids in which low frequency masking effects could obliterate higher frequency information necessary for speech intelligibility. The implication here is that even if the standards are revised in this area, existing test chambers will not be adequate for the new measurements.

Another factor is that the 2cc coupler and microphone systems used in hearing aid measurements are not reliable at and above 5000 Hz, thus presenting obvious difficulties for high frequency measurements.

Another problem with S3.22—1976 is that it still specifies use of the standard 2cc coupler, which does not, and was never intended to, reflect real-ear response of a hearing aid. As is shown in another section, there is another system available to measure hearing aid responses that more accurately reflects how the instrument will perform in a human ear.

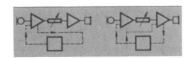

Fig. 2-22.   Schematic diagram of input compression. (Reproduced from Helle, 1978.)

Nonstandard Measures—Research Needs

The American hearing aid measurement standards ignore several electroacoustic factors related to speech transmission system integrity. Some of these are areas of presumed or demonstrated importance to hearing aid performance that have been completely ignored and/or are in need of further clarification through additional research and standardization. In general, they are self-explanatory.

1. Standardized characteristics of output limiting circuits—peak clipping, AVC, compressor compression, curvilinear compression—and methods of measuring their performance.
2. Measurement and expression methods for transient distortion, intermodulation distortion, and extraneous distortion.
3. Standardized means of measuring and expressing harmonic distortion.
4. Frequency response and sensitivity of the hearing aid using a telecoil.
5. Performance of bone-conduction aids.
6. Standardized expression of volume control taper characteristics.
7. Distortion as a function of battery voltage.
8. Effect of tone control position on speech intelligibility.
9. Measurement of hearing aid signal-to-noise ratios.
10. Accountability for head shadow and body baffle effects.
11. Clarification of the documented differences in hearing aid performance between the standard 2 cc coupler and the real ear (see the section of this chapter on Philosophies and Practicalities).

ALTERATION OF HEARING AID RESPONSE

There are various methods through which the frequency response of a hearing aid can be altered to meet the specific needs of the user. Modifications of earmolds and tubing, filter inserts, and variation of external receivers are described in the next chapter.

One method alluded to earlier in this chapter is modification of response through amplifier circuitry. Figure 2-23 presents the various amplification slopes available from one manufacturer. Any one of these slopes is available on most of that company's instruments. There are only a relatively few manufacturers with this service. Others prefer to alter responses using earmold/tubing modifications. However, such sloping can be extremely convenient when fitting for high frequency hearing losses.

Microphone Placement

Hearing aid microphones can be located in various positions in ear-level (top of ear and bottom behind the ear) and eyeglass instruments (temple piece forward and frame center of head). One factor not often considered is the effect

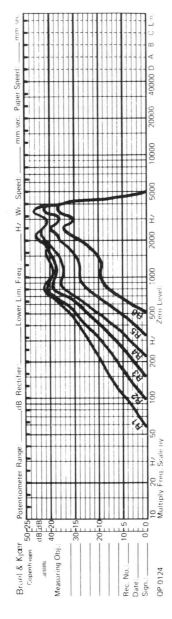

Fig. 2-23. Six different responses available in one hearing aid. (Courtesy of Audiotone.)

62

of microphone placement upon the frequency response of a hearing aid. Figure 2-24 demonstrates this with four microphone positions, showing the primary effect to be in the 1500–3000 Hz range. The most pertinent observation is the 8–10 dB advantage with the microphone placed at the top rather than at the bottom of the ear in the ear-level case. This can be an effective means of providing additional high frequency gain.

Body Baffle

Thus far, in this section I have briefly described ways to purposely alter the response of a hearing aid. There is, however, a condition that significantly changes the response characteristics undesirably. It is referred to as *body baffle*.

When an aid is worn on the body, its response is modified by the body and clothing. Both reflect and absorb sound. Erber (1973) described these effects, as follows, when a body aid is worn on the chest.

1. Sound pressure at the microphone is increased from 2 to 6 dB in the range 200–800 Hz.
2. Sound pressure at the microphone is decreased 5–15 dB in the range 1000–2500 Hz.
3. There is no significant change above 3000 Hz, except that output is decreased slightly in the high frequencies when the aid is covered by clothing.
4. Body baffle effects are 1–5 dB greater for adults than for children in the ranges 200–400 Hz and 1000–1500 Hz.

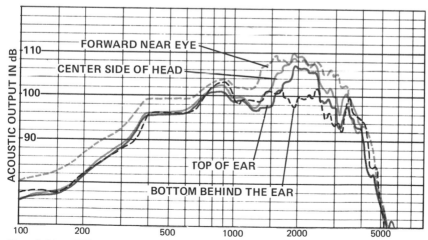

Fig. 2-24.   Effect of microphone placement on frequency response. (Courtesy of Zenith.)

These effects, while significant, can be compensated for if they are known. Unfortunately, body aid measurements in a test box are not the same as when the instrument is worn on the body. Since these effects are not included on specification sheets and are not commonly considered by those fitting aids, it is probable that many persons, especially children, since they are the population most often fit with body aids, are not receiving optimal benefit from their aids. It is important that additional research on body baffle be accomplished and that hearing aid manufacturers incorporate this phenomenon in their technical literature.

BATTERY LIFE

One of the most common questions asked of me by hearing aid users is "how long will the batteries last?." Reviewing manufacturer's technical sheets, every aid has a different battery life. The basic reason it is difficult to quantify battery life is that different aids have different power requirements and not all instruments use the same type of output circuit. The output circuit will, to a great degree, determine battery life and whether or not accurate predictions can be made.

Ely (1978) has presented a thorough overview of this question. In it he indicates that, in terms of battery drain and life, "the output stage . . . is the most important part of the hearing aid amplifier because it controls the majority of the energy consumed. . . ."

Earlier in this chapter I discussed the two primary types of amplifier circuits used in hearing aids today: single-ended (class-A) and push-pull (class-B). Figure 2-25 is a graphic representation of battery drain in a class-A amplifier under two conditions, with and without an input signal. Note that when the aid is turned on, but no signal is present, there is a constant *bias current* drain. When a signal is introduced, the current drawn varies about the bias value, but the average draw is still the bias value. Therefore, class-A amplifiers draw a fairly constant average current drain from the battery whether a signal is present or not. Thus, battery life is easily predicted using the following formula:

$$\text{Battery life (hours)} = \frac{\text{Battery capacity (milliampere} - \text{hours)}}{\text{battery current drain (milliamperes)}}$$

Current drain data are supposed to be presented on the specification sheet for each model. Table 2-2 summarizes battery capacity data for most commonly used hearing aid batteries.

The example below shows how to use the formula and capacity data from Table 2-2 for a class-A hearing aid with a specified maximum current drain of 1.2 milliampere-hours (MA-H) using a 675 P battery.

$$\text{Battery Life} = \frac{\text{capacity}}{\text{drain}}$$

$$= \frac{220}{1.2}$$

$$= 183.3 \text{ hours of use}$$

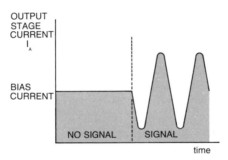

Fig. 2-25.   Class A output stage current. The shaded area shows the amount of battery current used. Reproduced with permission from Ely, 1978.

Table 2-2
Battery Capacity in Common Hearing Aid Batteries

	Rated Battery Capacities in Milliamp-Hours		
Size	*Mercury* *(1.3−1.35 V)*	*Zinc Air* *(1.25−1.35 V)*	*Silver Oxide* *(1.5−1.55 V)*
675	180−190	400	
675 P	215−220		
76			180−190
13	85	170	70−75
41	150−160	300	120
312	45		36−38
401	800		

This is an approximate figure subject to certain variables, such as variations among units of the same model, age of the battery, and whether or not the battery door is opened when not in use.

If we had used a silver oxide 76 battery in the above example, the result would be 158 hours. This reduced life is due to the higher voltage and resulting greater current drain of the 76, and the lower battery capacity of the silver oxide battery. In some aids, gain and output may be increased a few dB by using a 76 battery rather than a 675. *If performance is improved when using the higher power battery, it may be worth the lower battery life.* As Ely (1978) states, ''However, many newer stabilized hearing aid circuits show only small performance increases with the higher voltage battery, and this small difference may not be worth the resultant reduced battery life,'' and *probable higher cost per hour of use.*

The other type of circuit is class B or push-pull. Figure 2-26 shows the current drain characteristics for class-B, with and without an input signal. The *quiescent current* is the drain with no signal. It is generally a low drain, an advantage to this type of circuit. However, drain increases with output signal level until, at full output, peak current drain occurs. In other words, as the output of the aid increases, battery drain increases, as shown in Figure 2-26.

Although efficient from an energy usage point of view, such variance in battery drain makes accurate prediction of battery life almost impossible, because we cannot always predict the user's output needs and actual signal levels. If the manufacturer provides both quiescent and peak drain figures, you can, using the formula presented earlier, compute quiescent and peak drain battery life figures. It is safe to assume that the user's average battery life will be somewhere between these two figures.

Another factor to consider is the age of the batteries. As it ages over a period of some months, the battery's capacity will diminish. The user may notice a reduced battery life and fault the aid. I counsel my users not to purchase more than one package of batteries, per aid, at a time, and to buy them from us or some

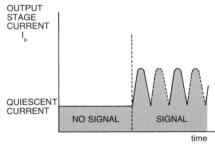

Fig. 2-26.   Class B output stage current. The shaded area shows the amount of battery current used. (Reproduced with permission from Ely, 1978.)

other reliable dispenser whose battery stock is fresh. *I discourage buying batteries at drug or discount stores because the age of the batteries is unknown.*

PRACTICALITIES AND PHILOSOPHIES

Interpretation of Response Information

Assuming that at least generalized specification sheets and, preferably, individual instrument response characteristics are available from the manufacturer, it takes practice to be able to interpret these data adequately. Most manufacturers use the testing equipment produced by the Bruel and Kjaer (B & K) Company of Copenhagen.

The chart paper has been described in terms of its intensity and frequency scales earlier in this chapter. The left side of Figure 2-27 is a reproduction of the legend area of the graph paper. The information contained therein is vital to accurate interpretation. *Measuring object* identifies the aid being tested and its conditions, i.e, tone control setting, tubing size and length, external receiver number, aid model and serial number, input level, and volume control setting. The latter two indicate immediately whether the curve is a gain or frequency response function. The differences between these have been described earlier in this chapter. The right side of Figure 2-27 is the frequency response curve obtained with the noted settings.

The spaces in the lower section are for information regarding control settings on the test equipment. "Zero level" indicates the intensity value assigned to the "O" baseline of the graph. This is extremely important, as normal B & K paper has an intensity (*potentiometer*) range of not more than 50 dB (0−50) on the ordinate. If a hearing aid produces more than 50 dB of gain at any frequency, and many do, the recording needle will run to the top of the graph and not give complete information. Referring to Figure 2-28, the top of the tracing line is flat, not revealing peaks and valleys in response. In this example, the zero level was 60 dB, so the potentiometer range was from 60−110 dB, but the aid put out a signal greater than 110 dB at some frequencies, resulting in a flattened curve. If the zero level is raised to 70 dB, the range is sufficient to give us the complete information. *Paper speed* (Paper Sp) is the speed with which the graph paper moves through the level recorder, in this case 30 mm/sec. Lower limiting frequency (L Lim Fr) indicates the starting point of the graphic recording, 200 Hz in this example. Potentiometer range (Pot) is either 25 or 50 dB. The latter is most commonly used for hearing aids. Therefore, the interval between horizontal lines on the paper is equal to 2 dB. *Writing speed* (Wr Sp) is the rate of the marking pen movement, 63 mm/sec in this example.

To determine the gain, output or frequency response, or range data from a graph, such as the one in Figure 2-27, one simply follows the procedures outlined

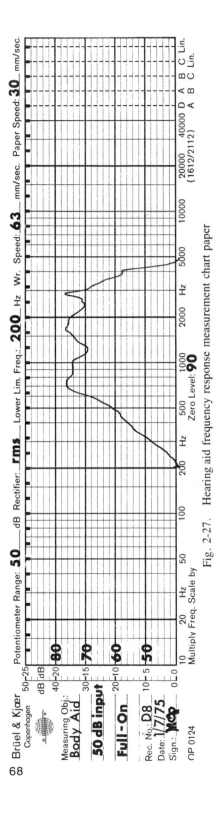

Fig. 2-27. Hearing aid frequency response measurement chart paper

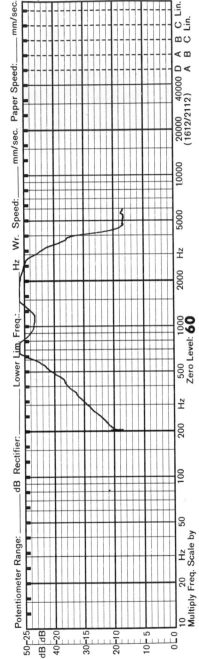

Fig. 2-28. Frequency response curve with inappropriate zero level

for that measure and reads the information off the graph. Note that the intensity scale figures can be read as either gain or output, depending on the reference point. For example, in Figure 2-27 the zero line is 90 dB, therefore the output at 1000 Hz is 90 + 34 dB (zero level plus graph reading) or 124 dB.

Practicalities

All manufacturers provide technical specification data sheets for each model of hearing aid they produce. These sheets contain all the required information, gain, output and frequency response, plus additional information in individual cases. These figures are average responses for the particular model. However, individual aids of that model may vary greatly in terms of gain, output, and frequency range, i.e., 10–15 dB variations in gain or output, more or less distortion, and volume control taper. Anyone who has measured hearing aid characteristics and compared those measurements to the manufacturer's technical sheets has seen discrepancies. Kasten et al (1967) demonstrated these differences experimentally.

Therefore, it is to the advantage of the audiologist or hearing aid dispenser to be provided with, or himself obtain, individual performance data on each aid. Most manufacturers do not provide these individual data. The American Speech and Hearing Association Conference on Hearing Aid Evaluation Procedures has stated:

> Since existing speech tests are often not satisfactorily able to differentiate the performances of various hearing aids, it seems of great importance to know the electroacoustic characteristics of the various aids . . . knowledge of certain acoustical characteristics of hearing aids is necessary for an evaluation. Therefore the three following considerations should be taken into account: (a) manufacturers' specifications may be incomplete or unavailable; (b) if not available, these specifications must be reported by the centers; and (c) if the center can not determine the characteristics of an aid through its own equipment and personnel, then some arrangement must be made to secure the necessary data (Castle 1967).

What happens to the response of an ear-level aid when the user's head is turned in various directions relative to a sound source? Figure 2-29 shows this relationship. In this example, an ear-level aid with forward-facing microphone was placed on the right ear of KEMAR and a sound source placed to the right of the head. It is obvious that maximum amplification is achieved when the head directly faces the sound source and minimal when it is faced away from the sound. The implication to be drawn from this graph is reinforcement of the concept that a listener should watch the face of a speaker. By doing this, the hearing aid user maximizes the response of his instrument.

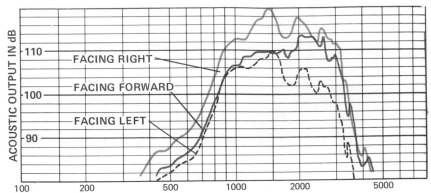

Fig. 2-29.   Effect of head turning on frequency response of an ear-level aid. (Courtesy of Zenith.)

Philosophies

As I wrote this chapter I became aware that the discussions that follow are, to me, the most important parts of any consideration of electroacoustic characteristics. If not for the fact that so much background information was necessary to make this section meaningful, I would have included it near the beginning of the chapter.

A close friend of mine is a transactional analyst. I recently spoke with him about some of my concerns regarding all of the technical aspects of electroacoustic measurements being related to hardware and not to the person who is going to wear the hearing aid. He described the lack of consideration for realistic hearing aid measurements as *bull-kaka*.

That term perfectly described my feelings. All measures of hearing aid function have no meaning unless they can be related to listener behavior. The standard measures do not tell us much, really. They are designed to describe hearing aids in the absence of the listener. If they are to have any meaning, we must be able to predict how they will affect the patient. Until a means of accurately predicting this is found, we have two isolated phenomena—hearing aid performance and listener performance. In chapter 4, Joe Millin presents some of his ideas on this and related matters. It is an important chapter and should be read carefully.

KEMAR

When the 2cc hard-walled coupler was developed some 30 years ago, *it was not designed to yield a response similar to that of the human ear*. The original intent was to provide a means of quality control (comparing the output of one unit of a hearing aid model with that of another unit of the same model) and a consistent electroacoustic measurement standard for the exchange of data between laboratories.

This was true for two reasons: (A) *the volume of a typical adult human ear between the medial end of an earmold and the tympanic membrane is about 1.2 cc, not 2 cc;* (B) *the hard-walled 2 cc coupler does not approximate the acoustic impedance of the human ear.* For these reasons, the acoustic energy transfer functions are significantly different for the 2 cc coupler and a real ear. The effects of these differences will be demonstrated below.

The 2 cc coupler was *never intended for use as a means of selecting a hearing aid* that is appropriate for a particular hearing loss. The typical B & K 2 cc coupler curves provided on manufacturers' specification sheets are not intended to reflect the response of the instrument in a user's ear. Yet, over the years, more and more such use has been made of these curves clinically, as well as in the literature. The various formulas for determining gain by frequency for a hearing loss (Berger, 1977) and nonspeech-based hearing aid selection approaches (Victoreen, 1973) are strongly based on 2 cc rather than real ear gain and output measurements.

Dalsgaard and Jensen (1976), in discussing the problems with 2 cc coupler measurements, have stated that they "are only of limited value in the clinical practice due to the large difference between the (2 cc) measuring conditions and the actual in situ (real ear) conditions of use for a hearing aid. . . . These differences are, however, generally overlooked in daily clinical work."

Differences Between 2 cc and Real Ear Measurements

Sachs and Burlchard (1972 a & b) have shown that, generally speaking, *comparisons of hearing aid responses measured in a 2 cc coupler and in a real ear demonstrate a pattern of consistent differences.*

1. Below 800 Hz sound pressure levels in the 2 cc coupler are about 4 dB lower than in the real ear.
2. Between 800 and 8,500 Hz, the average real ear/2 cc ratio increases with frequency at about 3.5 dB/octave. In other words, 2 cc coupler measurements are 5 dB less than real ear measurements at 1000 Hz, 12 dB less at 4000 Hz. The ratio increase is understandable at the higher frequencies because the effective volume of the tympanic membrane, which is a significant portion of the total effective closed volume, decreases. Therefore, the ear impedance does not decrease as rapidly with frequency as does the 2 cc impedance.

The upper two curves of Figure 2-30, show these differences. The top curve is the mean and range measurements of real ear hearing aid gain on 11 ears. The next lower curve is the same hearing aid response as measured in a 2 cc coupler.

Various clinical studies have also demonstrated these differences. As early as 1959, Van Eysbergen and Groen, based on 2 cc/real ear measurement dif-

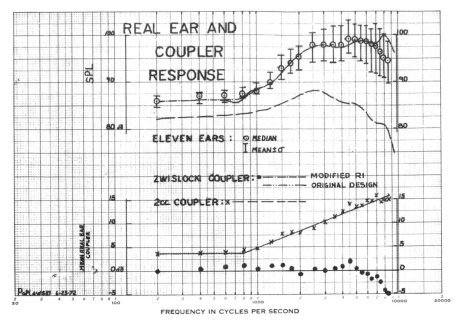

Fig. 2-30.   Real ear and coupler response. (Reproduced with permission from Sachs &
    Burkhard, 1972.)

ferences, recommended using the 2 cc coupler only for informational exchanges
between laboratories. Studebaker and Zachman (1970) and McDonald and
Studebaker (1970) showed that *the 2 cc coupler is not adequate for either
evaluation of hearing aids for clinical purposes or evaluation of earmold modification effects* (Chapter 3). The data of these two studies indicate that the measured differences leave many unresolved questions, particularly in higher frequency regions.

Studies by Tonnison (1975) and Pascoe (1975) provide data again indicating
that *2 cc coupler measurements do not adequately reflect real ear hearing aid
performance and could lead to erroneous conclusions about hearing aid performance.*

Zwislocki Coupler

The documented problems inherent in the use of the 2 cc coupler for clinical
hearing aid measurements and a general dissatisfaction with the 2 cc coupler as a
basis for predicting sound levels developed by hearing aids at the tympanic
membrane led Zwislocki (1971 A, B) to develop an alternative coupler. The
Zwislocki coupler reproduces the eardrum impedances of a typical adult human

ear. Its volume is close to estimates of the volume remaining when the meatus is occluded with an earmold, 1.2 cc.

The coupler has four side-branch resonators that synthesize the acoustic impedance variations in real ears. The "tympanic membrane" is a one-half-inch B & K condenser microphone (see Fig. 2-31). The four side-branches comprise inertance, resistance, and compliance of the ear canal to create what Zwislocki estimated to be an acoustic impedance approximating that of a normal human adult eardrum.

Referring back to the upper curve in Figure 2-30, the line is the response of a hearing aid measured in a Zwislocki coupler. You can see how closely it approximates the means of the measurements taken in real ears. According to Sachs and Burkhard (1972a), between 800 and 7,500 Hz, "the mean pressure in real ears and in the Zwislocki coupler differ by no more than 2 dB. . . ." Below

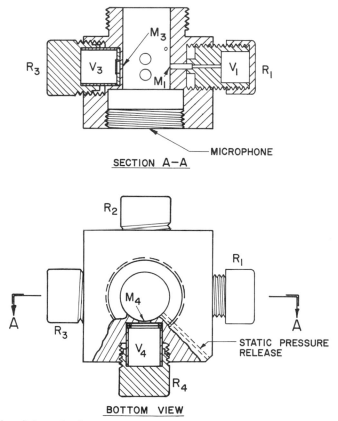

Fig. 2-31. Schematic diagram of the Zwislocki coupler. (Reproduced with permission from Burkhard, 1978.)

800 Hz, "pressure in the Zwislocki coupler is essentially identical to pressure in real ears (with no earmold leaks). . . ."

Kemar: A Manikin Using the Zwislocki Coupler for Hearing Aid Measurements

One of the major problems with the utilization of electroacoustic measurements in hearing aid fittings is the poor agreement between these measurements and behavioral measurements. The latter include the effects of the user—head diffraction and/or body baffle effects and ear canal resonances interacting with the physical characteristics of the hearing aid to influence the aid's performance on the person. Because of these strong interactions between the hearing aid and the wearer, it is important to include the diffraction and resonance effects in any hearing aid measurements that are to be considered in clinical hearing aid selection procedures. While this idea sounds good on the surface, many inherent problems exist that confound the situation. They will be discussed below.

As a result of these considerations, Knowles Electronics, Inc. developed an anthropometric manikin to facilitate in situ (on the head) measurements of hearing aid performance (Burkhard and Sachs, 1974). Named *KEMAR* (*K*nowles *E*lectronics *M*anikin for *A*coustic *R*esearch) the manikin utilizes the Zwislocki coupler to simulate the acoustic response of a human ear in a free field.

Figure 2-32 is a photo of the KEMAR manikin in an anechoic chamber. Figure 2-33 shows the Zwislocki coupler inside the head of KEMAR. KEMAR consists of a head and torso, and has the dimensions of an average human adult, including pinnae and ear canals. Using KEMAR it is possible to observe the effects of body and head diffraction on an acoustic signal traveling through a sound field to the ear.

According to Knowles and Burkhard (1975) and Burkhard (1977), a manikin has several other advantages for in situ hearing aid measurements:

1. It is a reproducible test subject that allows for uniformity between laboratories.
2. It can be stationary indefinitely for testing.
3. KEMAR can repeatedly be positioned in the same way.
4. Unlike human subjects, the manikin doesn't show response changes as a result of fatigue or other physiologic or psychologic changes.

Figure 2-34 depicts the response of the Zwislocki coupler in KEMAR. The input signal for this measurement was an acoustically flat sweep frequency tone at 60 dB SPL. The gain shown demonstrates the effects of diffraction and canal resonance. These data agree with Burkhard's (1977) real ear measures. We see different gain at the tympanic membrane (coupler microphone) as compared to sound pressure levels at the entrance to the canal, which results from standing wave resonances in the canal plus the resonances of the pinna and head shadow.

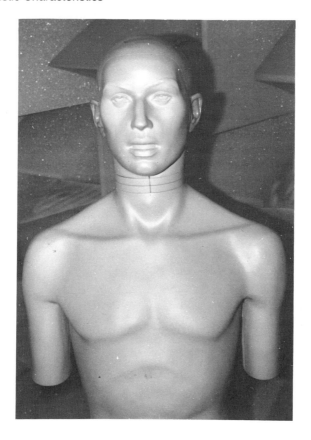

Fig. 2-32.   The KEMAR manikin

It can be referred to as *unaided ear gain*. In other words, to utilize the Zwislocki coupler in hearing aid measurements simulating use on a human ear, it is necessary to use the manikin to obtain the true gain of the instrument.

One of the difficulties involved in using KEMAR is the need for an anechoic chamber to eliminate sound reflections and standing wave problems as much as possible. If diffraction effects are to be measured, the chamber must be large enough so that the test point is at least one quarter wavelength distant from the nearest wedge tip. Therefore, if we want to make measurements to 150 Hz or below, the test point must be at least 22 in from the nearest wedge tip—yielding a chamber that is a minimum of a six foot cube. Unfortunately, most of us, clinically, have neither the space nor money for such a room, and must therefore depend on data from manufacturers and other research facilities. To date, relatively little of the published KEMAR research has had much clinical applicability. This will be discussed in greater depth below.

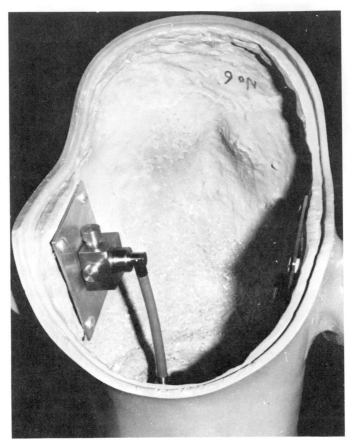

Fig. 2-33.   KEMAR with top of head removed to show Zwislocki coupler in place.

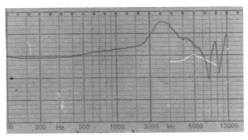

Fig. 2-34.   Frequency response of Zwislocki coupler in KEMAR

Another unresolved disagreement concerning KEMAR data is the actual measurement technique to be used. How far should the loudspeaker be from the manikin? Should a compressor control microphone be used during the actual measurements? If so, where should it be located—how far from the speaker and from KEMAR's ear? If not, and the test signal is prerecorded, where should the control microphone be located and should the manikin be present in the field during the recording? These are some of the technical problems relating to the set-up for KEMAR measurements. Other difficulties relating to hearing aid microphone placement and earmold configuration will be discussed below and in the next chapter.

It is generally agreed among those actively doing KEMAR measurements that the loudspeaker be located on a plane with the manikin ear and 1 m in front. The main area of disagreement relates to the control microphone. I have visited five manufacturer's laboratories using KEMAR and have contacted engineers in six others. Some have the compressor microphone present during measurements and some prerecord the sweep frequency signal.

Of those using the mike during measurements, it is variously placed immediately adjacent to the coupler ear of the manikin, between 3 in and 1 m above its head, half-way between the manikin and speaker, or up to 1 m to the side of the head. Figure 2-35 shows a series of unaided KEMAR response measurements made with different control microphone locations corresponding to those positions used in various laboratories. Figure 2-36 shows similar measurements with a hearing aid on the manikin. As you can see, the placement of the microphone substantially can alter the measured response because of differences in the sound level reaching the ear and the amount of diffraction effect. Since the sound field is kept constant at the compressor microphone, the closer it is to the head, the less will be the measured diffraction effect.

Other laboratories eliminate these considerations by removing the control microphone. In these cases, the signal is prerecorded using the compressor circuit, with or without the manikin present, to ensure a flat field, and replaying the tape for hearing aid measurements. Various terms have been used to describe such measurements: *insertion gain, etymotic gain, functional gain, orthotelephonic response,* and *substitution gain.* The scope of this chapter does not permit the thorough, lengthy discussion of these approaches. For those interested, I suggest reading Burkhard (1978).

Another question that has been raised is whether or not KEMAR should be clothed and wear a wig during measurments. To eliminate reflections from his shoulders, the manikin ought to wear at least a shirt. Figure 2-37 (top) shows some slight high frequency effects with and without clothing on the unaided KEMAR response. Most laboratories clothe the manikin. Figure 2-37 (bottom) shows little effect on KEMAR's response whether or not a wig is worn.

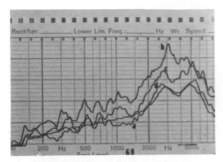

Fig. 2-35.   Effect of monitor microphone location on unaided KEMAR response: *A*, mike 3 cm from coupler; *b*, mike 1m from coupler ear; *c*, mike 60 cm above coupler ear; *d*, mike 3 cm above forehead.

Comparisons of Kemar and 2 cc Coupler Measurements

How different are response measurements made with KEMAR and with a 2 cc coupler? Figure 2-38 shows such comparisons with two different hearing aids. The upper pairs of curves are SSPL-90, while the lower pairs are reference test gain.

Studying these curves reveals one of the clinical problems with KEMAR— *variable results*. In the upper curves, KEMAR demonstrates more gain in the mid-frequency range. In the lower set, KEMAR shows greater gain across almost the entire range. Helle (1978) studied this and other questions and found no consistent degree pattern of differences for different hearing aid types, although he found the same direction pattern discussed above. Figure 2-39 shows KEMAR/2 cc comparisons for front mike (top curves) and bottom mike (lower

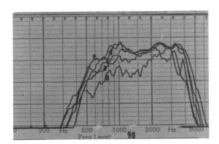

Fig. 2-36.   Effect of monitor microphone location on KEMAR response with aid: *a*, mike 3 cm from coupler ear; *b*, mike 1m from speaker, KEMAR 2 m from speaker; *c*, mike 1m behind KEMAR; *d*, mike 60 cm above coupler ear; *e*, mike 1m to side of coupler ear.

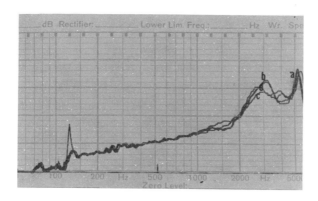

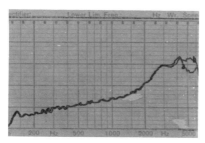

Fig. 2-37. Measuring KEMAR response. *Top,* effect of clothing on KEMAR response. *a,* shirt only; *b,* no clothing; *c,* sport coat; *d,* ski parka. *Bottom,* effect of wig on KEMAR response. *a,* with wig: *b,* without wig.

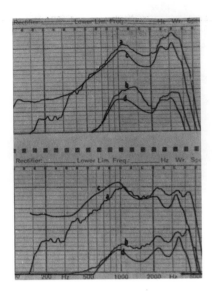

Fig. 2-38. Comparison of responses of two hearing aids on KEMAR and in a 2cm³ coupler: *a,* SSPL-90 on KEMAR; *b* RTG on KEMAR; *c,* SSPL-20 in 2cm³; *d,* RTG in 2cm³.

curves) hearing aids. We are only interested in the KEMAR and 2 cc curves. The third curve in each set can be ignored as they are not relevant to this discussion.

These and other comparative measurements lead to the safe conclusion that *2 cc coupler measurements can seriously underestimate hearing aid gain and output.* The problem, as can be seen from these figures, is that the *KEMAR/2 cc differences are not constant.* Depending on measurement set-up, microphone location, and receiver impedance, the degree of difference will vary. For this reason, *it may not be possible to generate a consistent correction curve, as some manufacturers have attempted, to convert 2 cc curves to KEMAR/real ear curves.*

Hearing Aid Directionality

In the late 1960s, so-called directional hearing aids came onto the American market. Manufacturer claims for this "revolutionary" innovation included a tremendous reduction of sound from behind the user due to the rear microphone port. When measuring hearing aid directionality in a sound box or in a sound field without a head, such effects can be seen. However, when measuring such phenomena on KEMAR, greatly different effects are seen. Figure 2-40 is the polar response of a nondirectional hearing aid and Figure 2-41 is the polar response of a directional aid on KEMAR and on a 2 cc coupler. In the 2 cc

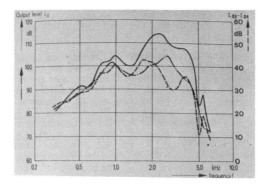

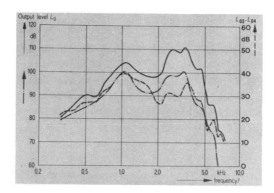

Fig. 2-39. Effect of microphone location on response of an ear-level aid. *Above,* front
mike; *below,* bottom mike.

— · — · = 2 cm³ coupler response.

_____ = KEMAR response

_ _ _ _ _ _ = Etymotic gain (aided KEMAR response minus unaided KEMAR
response. (Reproduced with permission from Burkhard, 1978.)

coupler, the omnidirectional or nondirectional microphone aid shows no directionality. However, on KEMAR, definite directional characteristics are seen due
to head shadow and diffraction. For the "directional" instrument, the KEMAR
response is very different from the 2 cc measurement. If you compare the two
KEMAR curves, you can see that both aids have substantial directionality, especially for sounds coming from the side of the head opposite the ear on which the

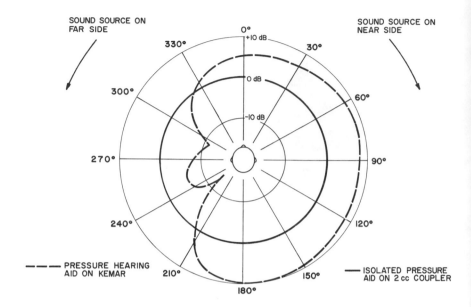

Fig 2-40.   Polar response at 2000 Hz for a nondirectional ear level aid in a free-field and on KEMAR. (Reproduced with permission from Burkhard, 1978.)

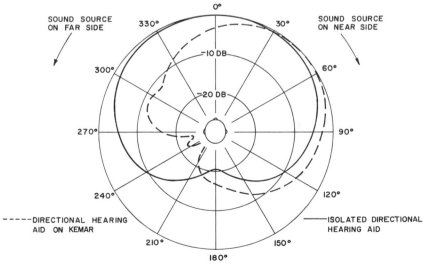

Fig. 2-41.   Polar response at 2000 Hz for a directional ear level hearing aid in a free-field and on KEMAR. (Reproduced with permission from Burkhard, 1978.)

82

aid is worn. The pattern for the directional instrument is somewhat more pronounced for sound sources between 150° and 210° than it is for the other aid.

The conclusion I draw from these data is that, *in use, any hearing aid worn
at the ear must be considered a directional instrument.* The "directional" microphones in some aids only alter the details of this directionality.

Zwislocki Coupler in a Test Box

*Most decisions about selections and fitting of a hearing aid are based on
earphone threshold measurements, which do not take into account head and
body diffraction effects.* Using data from 2 cc measurements for selecting hearing
aids, along with earphone threshold data, can, as has been demonstrated above,
result in less than optimal fittings. With the information now available about
KEMAR and its relation to real ear measurements, *the ideal situation would be
for each clinician to have a KEMAR set-up at his or her disposal.* Unfortunately,
spatial and fiscal realities make this an impossibility for most of us.

There is, however, an alternative that may prove viable for those of us
having hearing aid test boxes. It may be practical to replace the 2 cc coupler with
a Zwislocki coupler.

Comparing 2 cc and Zwislocki coupler data in a test box, Helle (1978)
found many of the differences reported above. Zwislocki measurements showed
a slight enhancement of low frequency response below 800 Hz due to the volume
differences of the two couplers. At the higher frequencies, the difference was
greater due to a decrease in the effective volume of the Zwislocki coupler.

Since all head and body diffraction effects would be eliminated, along with
the minimal pinna effects, the data obtained in a test box will not be as accurate
as on KEMAR.

I have made measurements comparing Zwislocki coupler data in KEMAR
and in a test box. Figure 2-42 shows the responses of the same coupler under the
two conditions without a hearing aid. Below 6000 Hz there is very little difference noted. The encouraging, yet disappointing, results were found when
measuring hearing aid responses under the two conditions. Figure 2-43 shows the
responses of three different aids measured on KEMAR and in a test box, using
the same Zwislocki coupler. As you can see, the results differ for the three aids,
although the differences are no greater than 6 or 7 dB at the most. The encouraging result is that the general shape of these reference test gain curves are the same
for each condition. Also encouraging is the fact that for two of the instruments,
the differences are not greater than about 4 dB.

The disappointing thing is the variability. While the direction of difference
is similar (somewhat less gain measured in the box than on the manikin), the

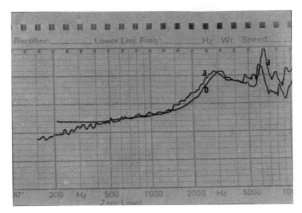

Fig. 2-42. Zwislocki coupler response on KEMAR and in test box—no aid: *a,* in box; *b,*
on KEMAR.

degree varies. However, our preliminary data suggest that it may be possible to
develop correction curves for aids with the same microphone location.

More research into this application of the Zwislocki coupler is needed and is
underway. The possibilities for such a use of the coupler seem very promising.

Cautions

While the Zwislocki coupler and KEMAR have given us much needed
information about hearing aid responses, almost as many problems and questions
have arisen as have been answered. Some of these, such as inconsistency in
degree of change, variables due to microphone placement and receiver impedance, the need for an anechoic chamber, and differences in measurement techniques, have already been discussed above. Only because of these factors, caution must be taken in applying KEMAR data to clinical work. Some of these
problems will be resolved if and when a set of standards for manikin measurements are developed and consistently used by all manufacturers.

In addition, there is a major caution that we need to consider. However
precise KEMAR measurements are and however similar to average real ear
measurements they are, such data are not absolute. *KEMAR is only an average
system* and there are many variables that need to be taken into account for each
patient, as there are no apparent constant factors among real people. Their ears
vary in volume, dimensions, impedance, pinna size, and head size (among other
differences) all of which will alter the response of the hearing aid on any one
particular person. Add to this the response changes possible with earmold modifications (Chapter 3) and many new questions should come to each of us.

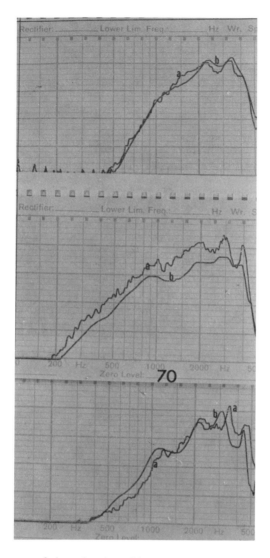

Fig. 2-43. Responses of three hearing aids measured with a Zwislocki coupler on KEMAR and in a test box: *a,* on KEMAR; *b,* in box.

At the present time, using KEMAR data we can, at best, begin to make more concrete general predictions about how the aid will function on the ear, up to the tympanic membrane. I hope that future research into meatus volume, pliability of meatus, and pinna tissues and their effect on aid response, along with answers to some of the other questions noted above, will give us data with which we can become much more accurate in our predictions and selections.

In the Meantime

Until researchers give us this much-needed information, I believe it is becoming highly incumbent upon hearing aid manufacturers to provide us with much more comprehensive technical data about each model they produce. Specifically, I would like to see the following.

1. KEMAR measurements at all aid control settings.
2. Specification of measurement procedures.
3. KEMAR versus 2 cc coupler measurements.
4. Comparative curves of the Zwislocki coupler in KEMAR and in a test box.
5. Comprehensive KEMAR curves demonstrating the effects of earmold modifications.
6. Complete data on the standard KEMAR/Zwislocki coupler configuration, as well as data on a modified system that would simulate smaller people, such as children.

Realistic Gain Measurements

In introductory Audiology courses we are told that SRT and Speech Discrimination measures are important because pure tone thresholds do not give a realistic indication of hearing handicap. After all, how often are we required to listen to and interpret pure tones in our everyday lives?

We can apply this logic to hearing aid measurements, especially acoustic gain. All measurement standards call for the use of pure tone input signals. I do not think this procedure is realistic in terms of how the aid performs under everyday listening conditions. Of course, running speech is acoustically too variable to be used as an input for electroacoustic measurements. However, couldn't a broadband random noise, such as "speech" noise or "pink" noise, serve a similar function? The Veterans Administration has been using such a random noise (200–5000 Hz) for evaluation of their contract aids for years. I would like to see research in this area.

Related to the input employed for gain measures is the setting of the volume control. All the standards require the control to be set at full-on. While this yields a nice number signifying maximum gain, it is also unrealistic. First of all, no hearing aid should be worn at full gain because, as I discussed earlier, distortion increases dramatically at gain control settings over about three-fourths rotation. Second, McCandless (1974) has reported on a study of 500 hearing aid users in which it was found that the average "use" gain setting was equal to about half the unaided SRT, i.e., if the unaided SRT was 50 dB, the "use" gain was about 25 dB.

While it would be impossible to measure gain at every "use" setting for purposes of specification sheet data, is it necessary to use full-on volume control settings? A more realistic approach would be to measure gain at a volume control setting below maximum, such as reference test level. The Veterans Administration measures gain and frequency response with the control set to give an output 12 dB below maximum. With this type of procedure, gain measures that more closely approximate the aid's performance at use settings would be obtained, and these data could be published on technical sheets.

In addition, it would be ideal if curves could be run on each aid at the individual listener's use settings. Then the actual electroacoustic performance of the aid at these everyday settings would be available. The advantages of this are obvious. Of course, this would require that every audiology clinic and hearing aid dispenser's office have a test box arrangement. With some thought and cooperation between audiologists and dispensers, perhaps a workable solution can be found.

RESEARCH NEEDS

Throughout this chapter I have alluded to numerous areas within the subject of electroacoustic characteristics that are in need of further extensive research. Rather than elaborate on each of them again, I have listed those that I consider the most important. Beside each is the page of the chapter on which it was first mentioned. In addition, on page 61 I have listed 11 areas generally ignored in the American standards. Each of them needs more investigation.

1. Tubing length and diameter effects on acoustic feedback (p. 35).
2. Feedback as a high frequency phenomenon (p. 38).
3. Utilization of external auditory meatus resonance characteristics for high frequency emphasis amplification (p. 38).
4. Use of "pink" noise and "speech" noise for electroacoustic measures (p. 86).
5. Gain and frequency response measures at use settings (p. 86).
6. Output-limiting standard measurements (p. 60).
7. Use of the Zwislocki coupler for hearing aid measurements (p. 72).
8. Interaction distortion effects (p. 54).

BIBLIOGRAPHY

American National Standards Institute: Electroacoustical characteristics of hearing aids. American Standard S3.3–1960, New York, ANSI, 1960
American National Standards Institute: Methods of expressing hearing aid performance. American Standard S3.8–1967, New York, ANSI, 1967

American National Standards Institute: Specification of hearing aid characteristics. American Standard S3.22−1976, New York, ANSI, 1976

Bell System pamphlet: The Bell System's Telephone Adapter, 1974

Berger KW: Hearing aid evaluative procedures. Natl Hear Aid J 21:6, 33−36, 1968

Berger KW: Prescription of Hearing aids: A Rationale. Kent State University, 1977

Berger KW: The Hearing Aid: Its Operation and Development (ed 2). Detroit, National Hearing Aid Society, 1974

Bode DL, Kasten RN: Hearing aid distortion and consonant identification. J Speech Hear Res 14:323−331, 1971

Bruel, Kjaer: "Cookbook" Operating Manual for B & K Hearing Aid Test System. Cleveland, B & K Instruments Co., 1973

Burkhard MD: KEMAR: A Manikin for Hearing Aid Tests. J Aud Tech 16:102−112, 1977

Burkhard, MD: Gain Terminology, in Burkhard MD (ed): Manikin Measurements. Knowles Electronics, Elk Grove Village, Ill, 1978

Burkhard MD: Protection against shock and vibration. Meeting of the Audio Engineering Society, New York City, 1965

Burkhard MD, Sachs RM: Anthropometric Manikin for Acoustic Research. JASA 58:214−222, 1975

Caraway BJ, Carhart R: Influence of compressor action on speech intelligibility. J Acoust Soc Am 41:1424−1433, 1967

Carlisle RW, Mundel AB: Practical hearing aid measurements. J Acoust Soc Am 16:45−51, 1944

Castle WE: A Conference on Hearing Aid Evaluation Procedures. ASHA Reports No 2, 1967

Curran JR: Harmonic distortion and intelligibility. Hear Aid J 27:12, 39, 1974

Curran JR, Ely WG: Clearing the compression jungle. Hear Dealer 24:16−17, 20, 33, 1973

Dalsgaard SC, Jensen OD: Measurement of the Insertion Gain of Hearing Aids. J Aud Tech 15:170−183, 1976

David H, Stevens SS, Nichols RH Jr, et al: Hearing Aids: An Experimental Study of Design Objectives. Cambridge, Harvard University Press, 1947

Ely WG: A Primer on Distortion in Hearing Aids. Hear Aid J 27:10−11, 34, 1974

Ely WG: Hearing Aid Battery Life. Hear Inst 29:12−14, 73, 1978

Erber NP: Body-baffle and real-ear effects in the selection of hearing aids for deaf children. J Speech Hear Disor 38:224−231, 1973

Harford E, Dodds E: Versions of the CROS hearing aid. Arch Otolaryngol 100:50−58, 1974

Harris JD, Haines H, Kelsey R, et al: The relation between speech intelligibility and the electroacoustic characteristics of low fidelity circuitry. J Audit Res 1:357−381, 1961

Hearing Aid Industry Conference: HAIC Standard Method of Expressing Hearing Aid Performance. New York, HAIC, 1961

Helle R: Frequency Response of Behind the Ear Hearing Aids Measured on KEMAR, in Burkhard MD (ed): Manikin Measurements. Knowles Electronics, Elk Grove Village, Ill, 1978

Hillman NS: Personal communication, 1974

Hudgins CV, Marquis RJ, Nichols RH Jr, et al: The comparative performance of an experimental hearing aid and two commercial instruments. J Acoust Soc Am 20:241−258, 1948

International Electrotechnical Commission Recommended Methods for Measurements of the Electroacoustical Characteristics of Hearing Aids, IEC Publication 118, Geneva IEC, 1959

Jeffers J, Behrens T, Rubin M, et al: Task force I: Standards for hearing aids. J Acad Rehab Audiol 6:13−19, 1973

Jerger J, Speaks C, Malmquist C: Hearing aid performance and hearing aid selection. J Speech Hear Res 9:136−149, 1966

Jirsa RE, Hodgson WR: Effects of harmonic distortion in hearing aids on speech intelligibility for normals and hypacusics J Audit Res 10: 213−217, 1970

Kasten RN, Lotterman SH: A longitudinal examination of harmonic distortion in hearing aids. J Speech Hear Res 10:777−781, 1967

Kasten RN, Lotterman SH: Influence of hearing aid gain control rotation on acoustic gain. J Audit Res 9:35−39, 1969

Kasten RN, Lotterman SH, Burnett ED: The influence of nonlinear distortion on hearing aid processed signals. Convention of the American Speech and Hearing Association, Chicago, 1967a

Kasten RN, Lotterman SH, Hinchman MJ: Head shadow and head baffle effects in ear level hearing aids. Acoustica 19:154−160, 1967b

Kasten RN, Lotterman SH, Revoile SG: Variability of gain versus frequency characteristics in hearing aids. J Speech Hear Res 10:377−383, 1967c

Knowles HS, Burkhard MD: Hearing Aids on KEMAR. Hear Inst 26:19−21, 41, 1975

Kranz FW: Tentative code for measurement of performance of hearing aids. J Acoust Soc Am 17:144−150, 1945

Lotterman SH, Farrar NR: Nonlinear distortion in wearable amplification. ASHA 7:364−365, 1965

Lotterman SH, Kasten RN: The influence of gain control rotation on nonlinear distortion in hearing aids. J Speech Hear Res 10:593−599, 1967

Lybarger SF: A new HAIC standard method of expressing hearing aid performance. Hear Dealer 11:16−17, 33, 1961a

Lybarger SF: Standardized hearing aid measurements. Audecibel 10:8−10, 24−25, 1961b

Lynne G, Carhart R: Influence of attack and release in compression amplification on understanding of speech by hypoacustics. J Speech Hear Dis 28:124−139, 1963

McCandless G: Hearing aids & loudness discomfort. Oticongress, Ill. Copenhagen, Denmark, 1974

McDonald FD, Studebaker G: Earmold alteration effects as measured in the human auditory meatus. JASA 48:1366−1371, 1970

Maxwell RJ, Burkhard MD: Vibration isolation of the BL microphone. Knowles Electronics Special Report, 1969a

Maxwell RJ, Burkhard MD: Vibration isolator design. Knowles Electronics Special Report, 1969b

Nordstrom D (Assistant Chief Engineer, Qualitone Hearing Aid Corp.): Personal communication, March 6, 1974

Nunley J: Automatic volume control instrumentation. Hear Dealer 24:22−24, 1973

Olsen WO: Peak clipping and speech intelligibility. Symposium on Amplification for Sensorineural Hearing Loss, Twin Peaks, California, 1971

Olsen WO, Carhart R: Development of test procedures for evaluation of binaural hearing aids. Bull Prosthet Res 10:22−49, 1967

Olsen WO, Wilbur SA: Hearing aid distortion and speech intelligibility. Presented at Convention of the American Speech and Hearing Association, Denver, 1968

Pascoe, DP: Frequency responses of hearing aids and their effects on the speech perception of hearing-impaired subjects. Ann Otol Rhinol Laryngol 84: suppl 23, 1975

Romanow FF: Methods for measuring the performance of hearing aids. J Acoust Soc Am 13:294, 1942

Sachs RM, Burkhard MD: Zwislocki coupler evaluation with insert earphones. Report 20022-1, Knowles Electronics, Inc, 1972a

Sachs RM, Burkhard MD: Earphone pressure response in ears and couplers. Eighty-third Meeting of the Acoustical Society of America, April, 1972b

Staab WJ: Hearing aid compression amplification: Fittings. Natl Hear Aid J 25:12, 34−35, 1972

Studebaker G, Zachman T: Investigation of the acoustics of earmold vents. JASA 47:1107−1115, 1970

Tonnison W: Measuring in-the-ear gain of hearing aids by the acoustic reflex method. J Speech Hear Res 18:17−30, 1975

Van Eysbergen HC, Groen JJ: The 2 ml coupler & the high frequency performance of hearing aids. Acoustica 9:381−386, 1959

Victoreen JA: Basic Principles of Otometry. Springfield, Ill, Charles C Thomas, 1973

Wanink A: Whistling in hearing aids. Fenestra 5:1968

Zwislocki JJ: An acoustic coupler for earphone calibration. Laboratory of Sensory Communication, Syracuse University. Special Report LSC-S-7, 1971a

Zwislocki JJ: An ear-like coupler for earphone calibration. Laboratory of Sensory Communication, Syracuse University Special Report LSC-S-9, 1971b

Michael C. Pollack
Ron Morgan

3
Earmold Technology and Acoustics

In the preceding chapter I described the various ways in which the electroacoustic characteristics of a hearing aid can affect user performance and satisfaction. This chapter considers delivery of the amplified signal from the hearing aid receiver to the tympanic membrane. Ron Morgan and I present a comprehensive overview of the importance of this coupling of aid and earmold and its effect on hearing aid performance. The most important concepts in this chapter are: (1) that a mechanical modification of the amplified signal can be made through alterations of the coupling system— earmold, tubing, canal length, bore size, and venting; (2) that data gathered from KEMAR measurements of earmold effects differ from classical views; (3) that the free-field earmold, which provides a true nonoccluding mold, can substantially effect user satisfaction; and (4) that coupling modification effects are not consistent for all aids, but are influenced by hearing aid electronics and mechanics. Everyone working with hearing aids should be thoroughly familiar with the manner in which aid flexibility can be increased, and the rather simple means available to mechanically solve many user complaints.

MCP

As was discussed in Chapter 2, hearing aids are designed and manufactured with specific electroacoustic characteristics in mind. Prior to the development of the transistor and the subsequent development of ear-level and eyeglass amplifiers, hearing aid output was delivered through an external receiver coupled to an earmold. This type of receiver is used today with body-style hearing aids and some ear-level hearing aids. Lybarger (1958) described the effects of the receiver type earmold. Berger (1974) overviews these and other data. Therefore, the discussion in this chapter will concentrate on coupling methods for hearing aids using internal receivers.

COUPLING METHODS

The earmold, sometimes called the earpiece, is a plastic or silicone insert designed to conduct the amplified sound from the hearing aid receiver into the ear canal and to the tympanic membrane. There are certain functions it performs that serve to make the earmold more than just a delivery system for the amplified sound. The flexibility of the earmold is very important to the user, as well as the fitter. First, the earmold is the component of the system that has intimate physical contact with the somewhat delicate tissues of the ear canal and concha. One of the user's primary concerns is that the earmold fit comfortably. Second, the earmold can acoustically affect the signal from the hearing aid, thus modifying it in either a positive or a negative way relative to user satisfaction. Therefore, the earmold must be mechanically and acoustically designed to deliver the amplified signal with controlled modifications. It is more than just a sound channel and must function as an integral part of the entire hearing aid system. As will be shown later in this chapter, an appropriately designed and modified earmold can rather drastically change the output signal of the hearing aid to suit the user's needs, in ways that the hearing aid itself cannot.

HISTORY OF EARMOLDS

Although the first earmolds appeared about the turn of the century, earmolds as we know them today did not begin to appear until the 1920s. It was about that time that Western Electric Laboratories patented a hearing aid earmold. It wasn't really a "custom" earmold, but rather a series of stock earmolds in various sizes. A dentist in New York initiated the idea that earmolds should be custom-made and subsequently began manufacturing custom earmolds. At that time, all earmolds were "regular," a style of earmold, described below, that is intended to snap onto an external receiver. It must be remembered that in those days there were no postauricular hearing aids.

With the development of the postauricular hearing aid in the 1950s, other styles of earmolds began to appear. These various styles will be described below. The skeleton and the shell earmolds were among the first styles to appear, soon followed by the canal molds. In those days, plaster of paris was the most common material used in making earmold impressions. During the late 1940s and early 1950s a soft pliable material became available for use in making impressions. This material was a substantial breakthrough since there were many problems inherent in the use of plaster of paris, the most common of which was difficulty in removing the impression from the ear once it hardened.

PURPOSES OF EARMOLDS

The primary function of an earmold is to provide a sound channel from the hearing aid receiver to the tympanic membrane. As will be demonstrated later in this chapter, the earmold can also serve to modify the acoustical signal after it is transduced by the receiver.

The third function is that the earmold serves as an anchor for ear-level hearing aids, affording retention of the aid to the ear. This is important in the event that the hearing aid falls off the ear. A properly fitted earmold will prevent the hearing aid from falling, under most circumstances. For body aids, the earmold provides a retainer for the receiver, as well as retention for the system in the ear.

EARMOLD STYLES

To readily understand the various styles of earmolds, as well as the many important considerations in earmold impression techniques, it is important that you familiarize yourself with the anatomy of the external ear. Figure 3-1A depicts the pinna and its various parts. Figure 3-1B shows a standard earmold. The same numbering system is used to identify the parts of both figures.

In 1962, the National Association of Earmold Laboratories (NAEL) was formed. Prior to that time there was no general agreement as to designations of earmold styles, tubing sizes, or earmold materials. In recent years, the NAEL has standardized tubing sizes, adopted standard nomenclature for earmold styles, and assisted in the development and introduction of new earmold materials as well as new styles of earmolds.

The following are the earmold styles in general use today, using the terminology standardized by NAEL in 1970.

Regular or Standard Mold

This receiver mold is a full, solid mold with a metal or plastic snap ring for the appropriate size nubbin to hold an external receiver directly to the earmold. It is designed to be used with body-style and some ear-level hearing aids that utilize an external receiver. It is designed to set as deeply into the ear as the diameter of the receiver will allow. Currently there are three retention ring sizes: standard, D-90, and the small 8080/4404 series.

It is also possible to utilize an ear-level aid with an internal receiver and

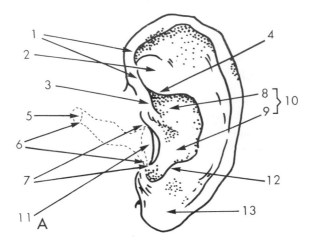

Fig. 3-1A. The pinna and its parts. 1. Helix. 2. Fosa. 3. Crus. 4. Anti-Helix. 5. Tympanic Membrane (Eardrum). 6. Auditory Meatus (Canal). 7. Aperture. 8. Canba. 9. Cavum. 10. Concha (Bow). 11. Tragus. 12. Anti-Tragus. 13. Lobule (Lobe).

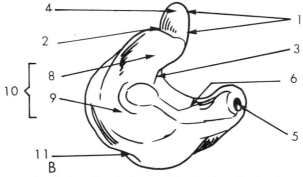

Fig. 3-1B.   Standard earmold with pinna landmarks.

regular earmold using a male adapter in the snap ring with a length of tubing attached between the adapter and the elbow of the hearing aid. The regular or standard mold is shown in Figure 3-2.

Shell Mold

This earmold is designed for use with behind-the-ear or eyeglass temple aids. It is, by design, the best earmold available in terms of acoustic seal. It fills the concha completely, yet has excellent cosmetic qualities and is used to great advantage in fitting more severe losses where higher levels of gain and output are needed. As was described in the preceeding chapter, one of the causes of acousti-cal feedback is the escape of amplified sound around a poor fitting earmold. The

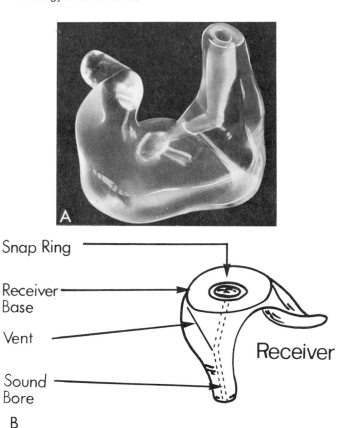

Fig. 3-2A,B.   Regular mold. (Courtesy of Westone Laboratories, Inc.)

shell mold has a full canal and a thin shell covering the bowl of the ear. It can be designed with or without a helix portion. Because it is used most often with high-gain postauricular hearing aids, it must provide a tight seal. Generally, thick-walled tubing is used to avoid feedback. This style is depicted in Figure 3-3.

Skeleton Mold

This is the same basic style as the shell mold with the center of the bowl portion removed, leaving instead a "ring" around the posterior perimeter of the concha for retention. It is used with mild and moderate gain instruments and is adaptable for short canal or open bore fittings, since the concha ring retains the mold in the ear. The skeleton mold and its variations are the most widely used earmolds today. Its primary variations are the "¾ skeleton," the "semiskele-

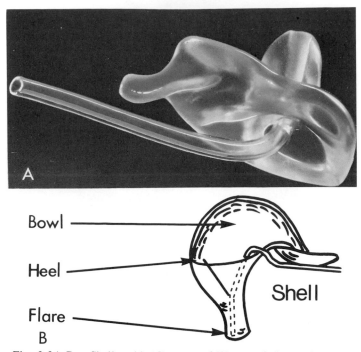

Fig. 3-3A,B.   Shell mold. (Courtesy of Westone Laboratories, Inc.)

ton,'' and the ''free-field mold.'' The skeleton, ¾ skeleton, and semiskeleton
molds are depicted in Figure 3-4.

¾ SKELETON

This is the same basic mold as the skeleton; however, the central portion of
the concha rim has been removed. Some ears have little or no undercuts in the
outer portion of the concha, thus affording no retentive features. The removal of
the concha rim is indicated both from a cosmetic and a utilitarian standpoint. This
allows maximum retention and maximum cosmetic requirements. The ¾ skeleton mold is also sometimes referred to as the ''phantom'' or ''phanto'' mold.

SEMISKELETON

This mold is a skeleton mold in which there is no concha rim. Other than the
canal portion of the mold itself, only the helix remains.

Half-Shell

The name of this mold denotes its style. The base of the mold covers only
about half of the concha bowl, that portion of the lower concha covering the
canal opening, filling the tragus and antitragus areas. This is a good mold for

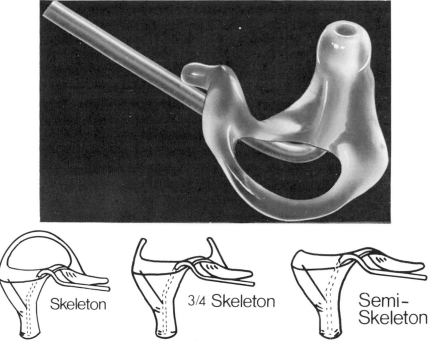

Fig. 3-4.   Skeleton mold and its variations. (Courtesy of Westone Laboratories, Inc.)

mild-to-moderate losses and is generally considered cosmetically acceptible. It is not a style of mold that is recommended for ''open'' or nonoccluding fittings. The half-shell mold is shown in Figure 3-5.

Canal Mold

This mold consists only of the canal portion and can be used for mild or moderate gain instruments. It is comfortable to wear, and has maximum cosmetic appeal. It should, however, be used only when the configuration of the external meatus will insure its retention. This mold is depicted in Figure 3-6.

Canal Lock

This mold, also referred to as the canal hook, is designed for mild-to-moderate losses. It affords reasonable acoustical properties with excellent concealment. In this context, the term ''reasonable'' refers to the fact that almost all of the acoustic seal is within the canal only; there is almost no seal in the concha area. For maximum retention, this type of mold should extend into the ear canal as much as one-half inch, if possible. Other than the canal portion of the mold

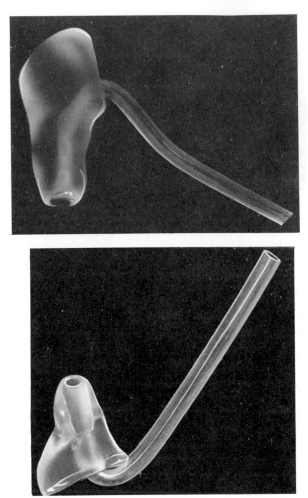

Fig. 3-5.   Half-shell mold. (Courtesy of Westone Laboratories, Inc.)

there is only the lower half of the conchal rim for retention. This partial rim can be an aid for many users in the insertion and removal of the mold from the ear. It is depicted in Figure 3-7.

All-in-the-Ear Mold

There are currently two styles of in-the-ear hearing aids. One style is designed with all instrumentation contained within the ear mold itself. The other is modular in that it inserts into a specially designed earmold. Figure 3-8 shows a modular all-in-the-ear mold.

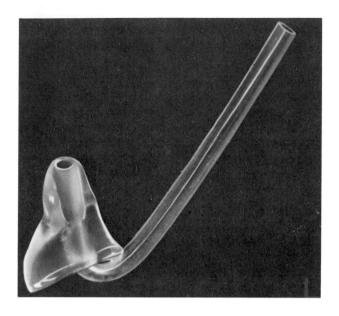

Figure 3-6.   Canal mold. (Courtesy of Westone Laboratories, Inc.)

Acoustic Modifier

A number of years ago, the Zenith Instrument Corporation designed an earmold they called the "acoustic modifier." Subsequently it was made available by many manufacturers under various names, such as, "discriminator," "word separator," "clarifier," etc. Generally, this mold has a very short canal and a large cavity hollowed out of the end of the canal, allowing as much volume of air as possible to remain between the end of the mold and the tympanic membrane. In addition to this, the mold is vented, either with one or two

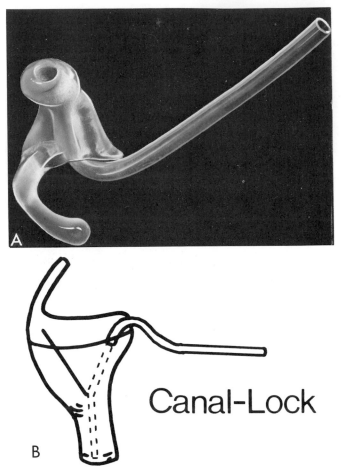

Fig. 3-7A,B.   Canal lock mold. (Courtesy of Westone Laboratories, Inc.)

one-eighth-inch vents, and the vents often contain a lamb's wool plug. Unfortunately, as will be described later in this chapter, the process of plugging a vent
with lamb's wool is not repeatable in terms of the effect it has on the response of
the hearing aid. However, by using a more repeatable venting system such as the
Positive Venting Valve (PVV), or Select-A-Vent (SAV), the hearing aid fitter
can selectively modify the venting on any earmold. Two types of acoustic modifier molds are shown in Figure 3-9.

    This type of earmold is most often used for fitting high frequency hearing
losses where a good deal of low frequency sound shunting is desired.

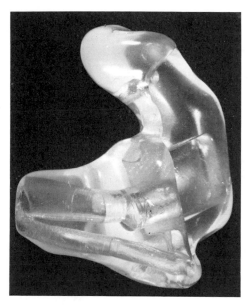

Fig. 3-8.   All-in-the-ear mold. (Courtesy of Westone Laboratories, Inc.)

Cros

The principles involved in the design and fitting of the CROS hearing aid, as described in Chapter 7, must employ an open or partially open coupler since feedback problems are minimized. Also, it is generally desirable for maximum amounts of unamplified sound to enter the ear naturally.

There are a number of styles of CROS-type molds, all performing these same basic functions (Fig. 3-10). The coupler may consist of nothing but a length of tubing projectinginto the ear canal or a skeleton mold designed to hold the tubing in place without blocking the ear canal. A third method, where greater retention of the hearing aid is required, is the use of the acoustic modifier type earmold.

Numerous studies have demonstrated improved speech intelligibility using an open coupler. Performance data were somewhat limited until recently as there was no standardized method of measuring the effects of an open mold fitting. However, the development of KEMAR, as described in the preceding chapter, has provided a means by which we can now obtain a more accurate approximation of the effects of open molds. At this point, it is important to understand that the open coupler acts as a high-pass filter with a cutoff at about 1500 Hz. Curran (1971) was one of the first to begin establishing a broad guideline for the dispenser in modifying the acoustic performance using "open" or "tube" fittings.

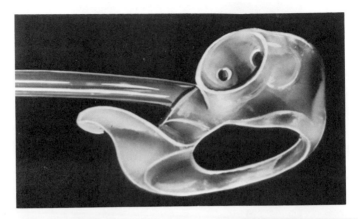

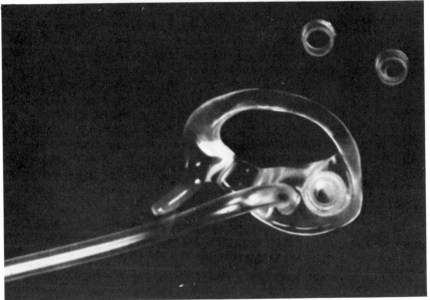

Fig. 3-9. Two types of acoustic modifier molds.

Generally the tubing is a heat-formed, heavy-walled, polyvinyl tube, and as it is moved closer to the tympanic membrane the cutoff of the response below 1500 Hz is shifted downward in frequency. The sharpest slope, cutoff frequency, and minimum gain characteristics occur when the tube is just barely inserted into the ear canal. This will be described in more depth below in the section on the ''free-field'' mold.

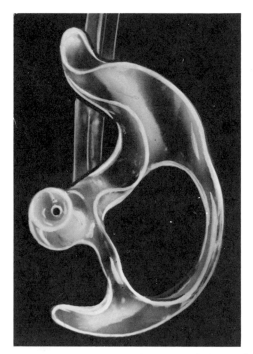

Fig. 3-10.   Cros mold (Courtesy of Westone Laboratories, Inc.)

Iros

The IROS or open mold was used for a number of recent years for subjects with bilateral, mild, high frequency hearing losses. In the past, individuals with this type of hearing loss were often not considered suitable hearing aid candidates because of the problem of overamplification of the low and mid frequency regions.

The primary problem with this type of IROS (ipsilateral routing of signals) coupler is feedback. Since there is no occlusion of the ear canal with a true open mold fitting, only a limited amount of gain can be provided.

Free-Field Mold

Although earlier CROS and IROS earmolds were called nonoccluding, all of them occluded the meatus to some extent. Until the development of the free-field earmold (Hewitt, 1977) there was no true nonoccluding earmold available. The free-field mold is shown in Figure 3-11. This mold is simply a plastic ring to hold the tube in the ear canal. As with other "open" molds, the free-field

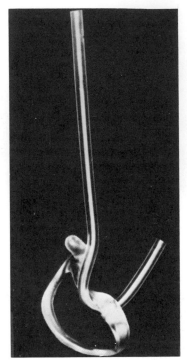

Fig. 3-11.   Free-field mold. (Courtesy of Westone, Inc.)

mold allows unamplified "natural" sound to enter the ear. This is important in light of the marked reduction in gain below 1500 Hz caused by the free-field mold. This also tends to reduce the "barrel" effect reported by many users, and greatly reduces low frequency electronic distortion. Another advantage of the mid and low frequency reduction is a decrease in amplified low frequency background noise.

Frequency response measurements with KEMAR have shown that the free-field mold yields a response almost identical to that obtained with only a tube inserted into the ear canal (Fig. 3-12).

Figure 3-13 shows the effects of an earmold on the response of the Zwis-locki coupler in a KEMAR manikin. The curve labeled "a" is the sound field Zwislocki coupler response with no ear mold. The curve labeled "b" is the KEMAR-Zwislocki response with a typical occluding earmold, in this case a skeleton mold. Hewitt (1977) has shown some of the effects of tube fittings (free-field mold) on hearing aid responses. These effects are also shown in Figures 3-14, 3-15, and 3-16. In all three of these cases the curve demonstrating the greater low frequency gain was obtained with a closed mold, while the curve with the greater high frequency gain was made with a free-field mold. In all three

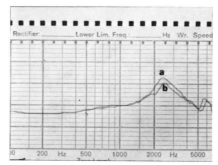

Fig. 3-12. Effect of free-field mold on KEMAR response: *a*, no mold; *b*, free-field mold.

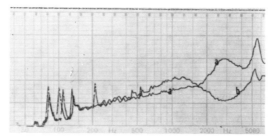

Fig. 3-13. Effect of closed mold on KEMAR response: *a*, no mold; *b*, closed mold.

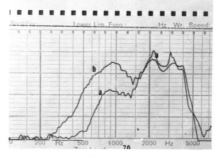

Fig. 3-14. Effect of tube fitting on KEMAR response of wide-band aid: *a*, tube fit; *b*, closed mold.

cases the two curves cross at or about 2000 Hz. You can see that there are two primary effects of the free-field mold. The first is a marked reduction of low frequency amplification below about 1500 Hz. The second is an emphasis of the high frequency gain of the instrument, in the range of 2000−4000 Hz. As was described in the preceding chapter, the specific effects of any specific modification will depend to some extent on the electronics of the hearing aid under investigation. As can be seen in these three sets of responses, the effects are not precisely the same. The general effects are, but the specific effects are not. Each

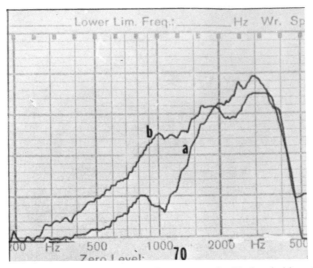

Fig. 3-15.   Effect of tube fitting on KEMAR response of wide-band aid: *a*, free-field; *b*, closed mold.

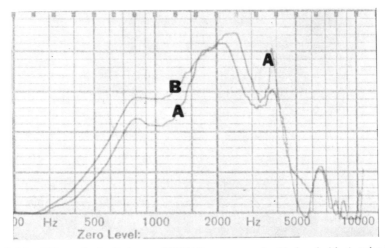

Fig. 3-16.   Effect of tube fitting on KEMAR response of wide-band aid: *A*, tube fit; *B*, closed mold.

of the three instruments has fairly substantial gain below 1500 Hz, so the low frequency effects of the free-field mold can be seen.

In contrast, Figure 3-17 shows the effects of the free-field mold on three "high frequency" hearing aids with little or no measurable gain below 1500 Hz. In these cases there is minimal low frequency shunting, because the low frequencies were not there to begin with. However, in each case the free-field mold does

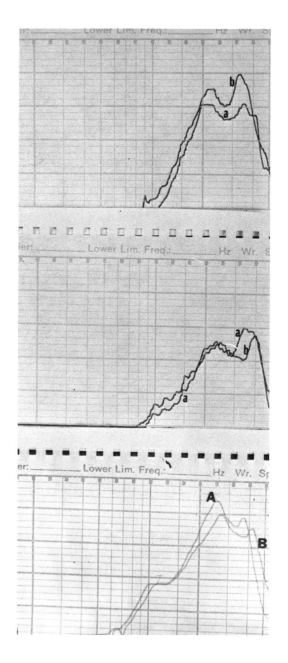

Fig. 3-17. Effect of tube fitting on three high frequency emphasis aids.
  Top: *a*, closed; *b*, tube
  Middle: *a*, tube; *b*, closed
  Bottom: *A*, tube; *B*, closed

result in an emphasizing of the high frequencies. This can be an important consideration in the fitting of many high frequency hearing losses, where little or no gain is desired below 1500 or 2000 Hz.

TUBE LENGTH

Another consideration in the use of the free-field earmold is the length to which the tubing is inserted into the ear canal. As mentioned above, the length of this tubing will have an important effect on the overall response of the instrument. Figure 3-18 shows the response of two instruments as measured on KEMAR with a free-field mold. In each case the tubing from the retainer ring of the free-field mold into the ear canal was set at four different lengths, 1.5 cm, 1.0

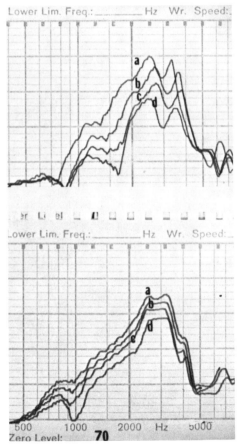

Fig. 3-18.   Effect of tube length on frequency response of two aids with free-field mold fittings as measured on KEMAR: *a*, 1.5cm; *b*, 1.0cm; *c*, 0.5cm; *d*, flush.

cm, 0.5 cm, and flush with the retainer ring. With both aids, the deeper the tubing was inserted, the greater the high frequency gain measured. Note that the effects of the tubing length differ on these two instruments. As noted in Chapter 2, KEMAR research has shown that we can not necessarily expect consistency in measurements with different hearing aids. This is especially true when investigating earmold acoustics. If you reexamine Figures 3-14—3-18, you will note that *while the direction of change caused by the modification is consistent, the degree of change is not.* With the free-field mold, for example, we can safely assume that there will be low frequency reduction and high frequency boost, but the amount of these changes and the frequency at which the crossover occurs is not consistent from and aid to aid. These differences apparently result from differences in receiver impedances and microphone locations.

EFFECT ON MPO

The graph shown in Figre 3-19 demonstrates the effect of the free-field mold on MPO. The curve showing the greater low frequency output was made utilizing a closed mold while the lower curve was made using a free-field mold. As can be seen, the effect of the free-field mold on the MPO of a hearing aid is similar to its effect on the gain. The MPO is markedly reduced below 2000 Hz.

Figure 3-20 shows a similar set of curves. In addition to the closed and free-field molds, a tracing was also made utilizing an acoustic modifier mold. As can be seen from the labeling, the more closed the mold, the greater the mid and low frequency output of the instrument. This particular instrument was a high frequency gain instrument with very little measurable gain below 750 Hz. This accounts for the rather rough tracings below that frequency.

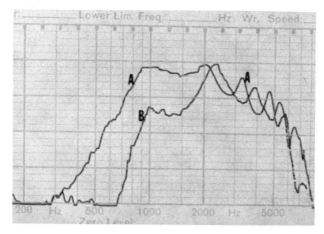

Fig. 3-19.   Effect of mold on MPO as measured on KEMAR: *A,* closed mold; *B,* free-field.

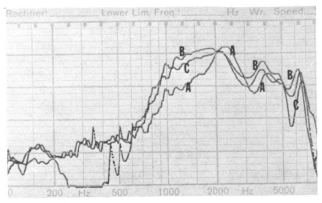

Fig. 3-20. Effect of mold on MPO as measured on KEMAR: *A,* free-field; *B,* closed mold; *C,* acoustic modifier.

Partial Closure of the Free-Field Mold

In some cases we found that a completely open free-field mold does not allow sufficient gain to be produced without the problem of acoustical feedback. For this reason we made various attempts to partially close the free-field mold, hoping that the response of the aid would not be greatly affected. The procedure for closing a free-field mold is relatively simple. A thin beeswax sheet is placed over the entire open portion of the mold. This can then be carefully trimmed back from either the anterior or posterior aspect of the mold. As each section of the wax is trimmed back, measurements can be made on the patient's ear until the point is reached where feedback becomes a problem. At this point a little wax can be added on to return to the point where feedback is not a problem.

We then mix an acrylic powder with a catalyst to make a thin acrylic paste. This is spread carefully over the wax and allowed to set until it is hard. The process is facilitated by placing the mold in hot water. During the hot water process, the wax will become disengaged from the mold. When the acrylic is firmly set it can be buffed and ground to remove any rough spots. Figure 3-21 shows one completely closed and two partially closed free-field molds.

As we mentioned above, the mold can be partially closed from either the anterior (tubing) side or the posterior (ring) aspect. The effects will be slightly different depending on how the mold is closed. Figure 3-22 shows the effect of partially closing a free-field mold from the posterior aspect on a high frequency emphasis instrument. The curve labeled ''A'' was made with the mold completely closed, and the other three curves were made with varying degrees of openness. As can be seen, once the mold is even slightly opened from the tubing, there is no further change in the response as it is opened more. On the contrary, Figure 3-23 shows measurements with the same instrument, closing the mold from the anterior aspect. In this case, as the mold is opened more and more from the back side, the response does change slightly. In all the curves made in the preceding two figures, the volume control was held constant.

Figure 3-24 shows four curves made with the same instrument as the preceding two figures; however, in each case the volume control was set to a point just below the setting at which feedback occurs. Curve "a" was made with the mold completely closed while curve "c" was made with the mold completely open. The curve labeled "b" was made with the mold partially open from the front while the curve labeled "d" was made with the mold partially open from the back. Results show there is very little change with this type of measurement, regardless of how the mold is partially opened. From these data you can see that the free-field mold can be partially closed from either the anterior or posterior aspects to reduce feedback without appreciably changing the response of the instrument.

This has proven to be a valuable tool, especially in cases where amplification below 1000 Hz is undesirable, yet feedback is a problem with a completely open free-field mold. Tracings similar to those of the preceding three figures have been made with wider response hearing aids, demonstrating similar results.

EARMOLD MATERIALS

An important consideration when ordering an earmold is determination of the type of material from which it will be made. The most commonly used material is lucite plastic, a hard, durable, clear material. The chemical name for this lucite material is methyl methacrylate. Besides being available in a clear material, it can be manufactured in various shades. Any style of earmold can be made out of lucite material. A number of other materials are also available from most earmold laboratories. These include ethyl methacrylate, a soft form of lucite. However, it is of generally poor quality, due to the absorption of body acids and other chemical materials. It tends to crack, break, and discolor more readily than the more commonly used soft material. Another soft material is known as PVC (polyvinylchloride) and is the leading soft material in use today. It has excellent acoustical properties. It is available in various degrees of softness. It resists discoloration and is very durable. It is available in clear or variations of skin tone. The PVC material is generally produced by high pressure injection molding process, providing a material of high density and minimum porosity.

Various silicone materials are also available from most earmold laboratories. They are generally softer than PVC and also provide the excellent acoustical seal and comfort. However, the silicone, unlike most other materials, does not readily lend itself to modification by the dispenser. Special equipment is required to make alterations. Even retubing a silicone earmold is difficult, as a special cement and "pretreated" tubing must be used. See details of this later in this chapter.

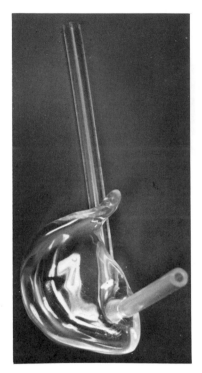 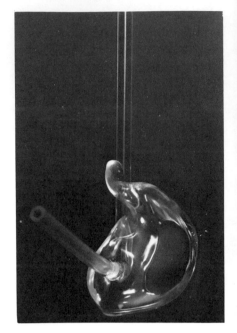

Fig. 3-21A,B,C.   Partially closing free-field mold. *A:* fully closed; *B:* open from rear; *C:*
open from tragus (see facing page).

Some hearing aid users tend to have allergic reactions to some of the
standard earmold materials. These reactions often take the form of itching,
irritation, or swelling in the canal and/or concha. Therefore, a nonallergenic
polyethylene has been developed for use with earmolds. It is not as soft as many
of the other materials, therefore not lending itself as well to acoustical sealing.

Lybarger (1958) reported that the type of material used for earmolds will not
have any appreciable effect on the response of the instrument. It can, however,
increase user comfort. The soft silicone or PVC materials are most often used in

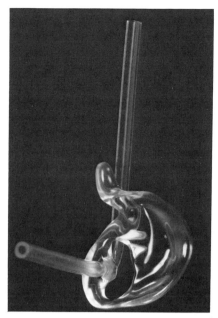

Fig. 3-21C. Legend continued from facing page.

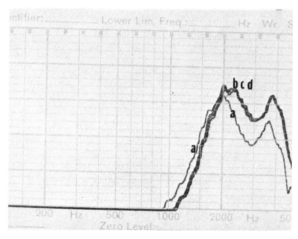

Fig. 3-22. Effect of closing free-field mold posteriorly as measured on KEMAR (open anteriorly): *a,* closed; *b,* ⅓ open; *c,* ⅔ open; *d,* fully open.

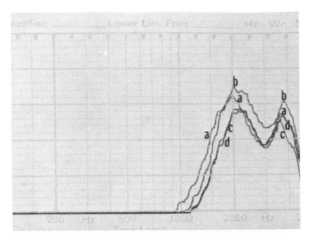

Fig. 3-23.   Effect of closing free-field mold anteriorly as measured on KEMAR (open posteriorly): *a,* closed; *b,* ⅓ open; *c,* ⅔ open; *d,* fully open.

cases where high gain and maximum acoustic seal is required, i.e., shell molds or high gain ear-level instruments. The soft materials are often used with children in order to protect the concha and meatus tissue in the event the child is hit on the ear containing the earmold.

TUBING

All ear-level and eyeglass hearing aids require a plastic tube from the receiver nozzle or elbow to the earmold. In 1970, the NAEL adopted standard tubing size designations. These are shown in Table 3-1. In addition to these

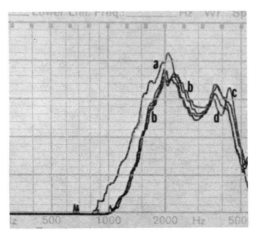

Fig. 3-24.   Composite effects of closing free-field mold: *a,* closed; *b,* open anterior; *c,* fully open; *d,* open posterior.

Table 3-1
Specifications for Tubing Sizes*

Number and Size	Inches ID	OD
12 Standard	0.085 × 0.125	
13 Standard	0.076 × 0.116	
13 Medium	0.076 × 0.122	
13 Thick	0.076 × 0.130	
14 Standard	0.066 × 0.116	
15 Standard	0.059 × 0.116	
16 Standard	0.053 × 0.116	
16 Thin	0.053 × 0.085	

*National Association of Earmold Laboratories.

standard sizes, a special heavy-walled tubing has been developed for use with the free-field mold. The specifications for this tubing are 0.062 × 0.125.

In Table 3-1, "ID" refers to the inside diameter in thousandths of an inch and "OD" is the outside diameter. The most common tubings are the #13 series. Presently both #13 STD and #13 MED are being used. Most earmold laboratories will provide one of these size tubes unless the dispenser requests a different size. Generally, the standard tubing can be used on mild gain hearing aids. The medium tubings are used on moderate gain instruments, and thick-walled tubing is an important consideration for high gain instruments in order to reduce feedback possibilities. As a helpful hint to the hearing aid dispenser, the #16 thin tubing will slip inside the #12 standard tubing, thus providing a "double-wall" tubing that will even further reduce feedback problems.

Effect of Tubing Length on Hearing Aid Response

The effects of the tubing length are shown in Figure 3-25. Note that the length of the tubing, in conjunction with the earmold, has minimal influence on the overall response of the hearing aid. There is some effect at the secondary peak, and almost no effect at the primary peak. In general, it can be stated that increasing the length will result in a minimal decrease in output above 1500 Hz. The length of tubing has minor effects on the output of ear-level instruments.

Effect of Tubing ID on Hearing Aid Response

Figure 3-26 shows that tubing sizes most often used with earmolds have little effect on the primary peak. When a hearing aid response curve has resonant peaks in the range of 2000−3000 Hz, a larger inside diameter tends to smooth them out. The aforementioned data were collected in a hearing aid test chamber utilizing a modified HA-1 coupler. As was pointed out in the preceding chapter, such measurements can differ appreciably from real ear measurements.

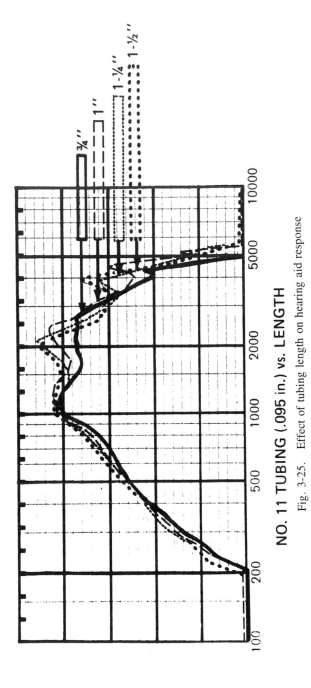

NO. 11 TUBING (.095 in.) vs. LENGTH

Fig. 3-25.   Effect of tubing length on hearing aid response

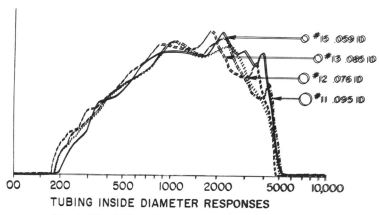

TUBING INSIDE DIAMETER RESPONSES

Fig. 3-26.   Effect of tubing ID on hearing aid response

Figure 3-27 demonstrates the effects of the tubing size on three different hearing aids, as measured on KEMAR utilizing a Zwislocki coupler. In all cases a #13 standard and a #16 standard tubing were compared. In all three cases shown, the #16, narrower, internal diameter tubing passed more of the low frequency amplification while reducing the high frequency amplification. Again note that the effects of the tubing size vary as a function of the instrument used. These effects are different than the traditional tubing size effects, as measured in a 2-cc coupler, and seen in most traditional literature.

Effect of Earmold Canal Length

Figure 3-28 shows the response of three different hearing aids measured with skeleton earmolds. The only difference between the molds was the length of canal, one being long and the other relatively short. The long canal extended 1 cm into KEMAR's meatus while the short canal extended less than 0.2 cm into the meatus. As can be seen from the three sets of curves, the short canal has the general effect of reducing low frequency amplification and somewhat enhancing high frequency amplification. Again, these measurements were made utilizing the Zwislocki coupler in the KEMAR mannequin, not in a 2-cc hard-walled coupler.

VENTING

A hole drilled from the face of an earmold to its sound input channel, or parallel to this channel, intentionally producing a sound leak, is called a vent. A vent, depending upon its length and diameter, can alter the response of a hearing

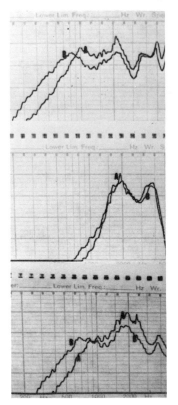

Fig. 3-27. Effect of tubing size of the response of three aids as measured on KEMAR: *a*, #13 tubing; *b*, #16 tubing.

aid. There are three primary reasons why an earmold might be vented. First, a small vent (0.020 inch) can increase the user's comfort by releasing sound pressure in the external auditory canal. Such a small vent will have very little effect on the basic response of the instrument. Second, venting can be utilized to improve the quality of sound heard by the user. This is often a subjective improvement and may be related to the release of sound pressure as described immediately above. Third, the size of the vent can change the response of the aid. This is often done by the fitter in order to obtain better speech discrimination and user comfort.

Figure 3-29 shows the effects of vent size on three different hearing aids. In each case the "a" curve was made with a closed mold. As can be seen, the general effect is reduction of low frequency amplification as the vent size is increased. However, again note that the overall effects are not consistent, but are dependent on the hearing aid electronics and mechanics.

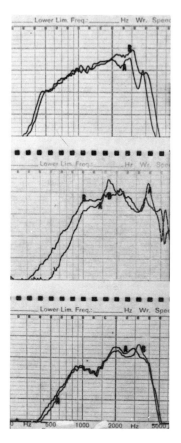

Fig. 3-28.   Effect of earmold canal length on the response of three aids as measured on KEMAR: *A*, short canal; *B*, long canal.

We encourage anyone working with hearing aids to use caution when anticipating the effects of venting or any other earmold modification. As has been shown numerous times in this chapter, the effects of a particular modification do depend to some extent upon the electronics of the hearing aid. The effects are not as standard as previous data obtained in hard-walled 2-cc couplers would lead us to believe.

Additionally, caution must be used in venting because of the possibility of inducing acoustic feedback. If too large a vent is utilized, feedback may become a problem. However, this can be reduced by inserting some lamb's wool into the vent, thereby reducing the feedback.

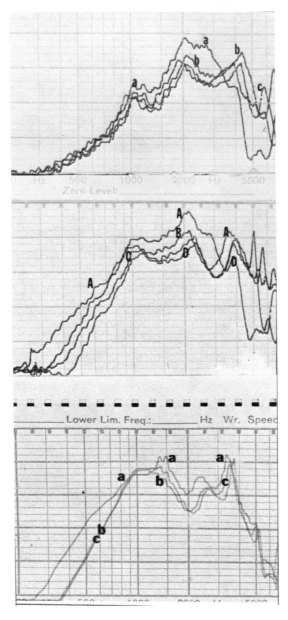

Fig. 3-29.   Effect of vent size on the response of three aids as measured on KEMAR: *a*, no vent; *b*, .020 in.; *c*, .062 in.; *d*, .125 in.

Location and Angle of Vent

Two types of earmold vents are the angled vent, which intersects the sound channel of the mold, and the parallel vent, which does not intersect this channel. These are shown in Figure 3-30. We recommend parallel venting for acoustical purposes whenever possible. As can be seen in the three sets of curves in Figure 3-31, the parallel vent (labeled "b") does not affect the response of the instrument as much as does the diagonal vent. The lower set of curves in this figure show that the parallel vent will reduce the low frequencies somewhat more than the diagonal vent. This reduction may be desirable. In many cases, the diagonal vent must be utilized rather than the parallel vent if there is insufficient space in the canal of the earpiece to drill the sound bore as well as a parallel vent. In all cases where the diagonal vent is used, the termination of the vent should be as

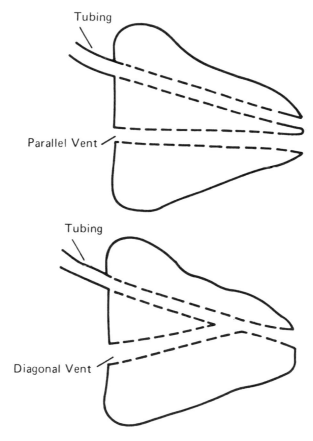

Fig. 3-30.   Schematic representation of parallel and diagonal vents

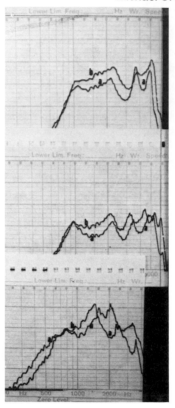

Fig. 3-31.   Effect of vent angle on the response of three aids as measured on KEMAR: *a*,
    diagonal; *b*, parallel.

near the end of the canal portion of the ear piece as possible. The further away
from the end of the sound channel the vent terminates, the greater will be the
overall change in the response and output of the instrument.

In many cases the direction of the vent is determined by the location of the
hearing aid microphone. Feedback can be a problem due to sound leakage
through the vent, picked up by the microphone. If the external opening of the
vent is directed at the microphone, feedback can be more of a problem. In
addition, location of the vent can also somewhat effect the response of the
instrument, as shown in Figure 3-32. In this figure, the effects of a parallel vent
in the superior aspect of the mold were compared to the effects of a parallel vent
in the inferior aspect of the mold. Both of these are compared to the response
without a vent.

An external vent can be used in some cases where it is physically impossible
to use either of the vents described above. The external vent is a groove drilled
along the external surface of the mold. It can also serve to ventilate the ear in
those cases where moisture and/or drainage is a problem. Generally, it is placed
along the inferior aspect of the mold.

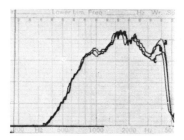

Fig. 3-32.   Effect of vent location as measured on KEMAR: *a,* no vent; *b,* top parallel; *c,* bottom parallel.

Variable Vents

In many cases, it is beneficial for the hearing aid dispenser to be able to vary the size of the vent to determine which will be most efficient for the user. Two variable venting systems are presently available from many earmold laboratories.

VARIABLE VENTING VALVE

Griffing and Shields (1972) reported on the Variable Venting Valve (VVV) as a method for easy adjustment of vents. This system utilizes a valve that has continuous action that can be adjusted by the user or dispenser to control the venting, relative to whatever the environmental needs may be. The VVV is shown in Figure 3-33. The valve is inserted permanently into the mold, and the degree of venting is controlled by a small plastic knob that can readily be adjusted by the user or dispenser. The primary rationale behind the use of this system is that the frequency response can thereby be altered to suit the individual's needs. Figure 3-34 demonstrates the effects of a typical ear level hearing aid system using the VVV. Note that from the closed to the full-open position, there is a considerable reduction in low frequencies, yet the high frequencies suffer minimal reduction. These data were obtained with a 2-cc coupler.

POSITIVE AND SELECTIVE VENTING SYSTEMS

The Positive Venting Valve (PVV) and Select-A-Vent (SAV) are two quick-change type venting systems offered today. They consist of a series of five small inserts, each of which has a different size vent hole, ranging from .020 to .125 inch, plus a plug insert for completely closing the vent. They may be changed in a matter of seconds by the dispenser by utilizing a tool to remove one plug and insert another. These systems offer a wide range of venting possibilities and are a worthwhile tool for the dispenser. Figure 3-35 shows the PVV system. Figure 3-36 demonstrates the effects of various vent sizes in these systems. It should be noted that the curves in this figure were obtained using a 2-cc coupler.

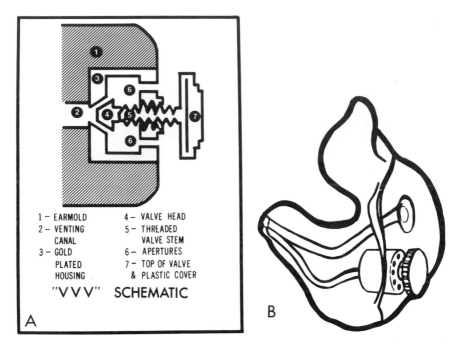

1 – EARMOLD   4 – VALVE HEAD
2 – VENTING   5 – THREADED
    CANAL   VALVE STEM
3 – GOLD   6 – APERTURES
    PLATED   7 – TOP OF VALVE
    HOUSING   & PLASTIC COVER

"V V V"   SCHEMATIC

A   B

Fig. 3-33A,B.   Schematic diagram of Variable Venting Valve (VVV). (Courtesy of HEDCO)

MECHANICAL INSERT FITTINGS

The previous discussion on altering the frequency response by venting is limited to ipsilateral (same side) fittings. When a user requires a considerable amount of amplification, the vented coupling system may cause feedback. It then becomes necessary for the dispenser to use a completely closed coupling system. When the need for altering the frequency response is dictated, mechanical means are employed.

Lamb's Wool

One mechanical method is the insertion of lamb's wool in the tubing or the mold itself. Lamb's wool can also be used to partially plug a vent. The degree to which responses change when lamb's wool is used is difficult to determine as the process is often not repeatable due to the density with which the material is placed into the tubing or vent or sound bore. It is strictly a trial and error process and the results are obtained subjectively from the user. The density of the packing determines the degree to which the response changes, as shown in Figure 3-37. The lower set of curves shows the effects of excessive damping with lamb's wool.

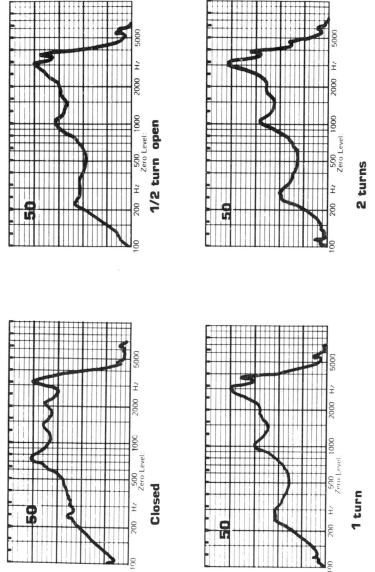

Fig. 3-34. Effects of VVV

125

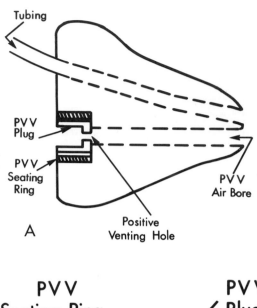

A

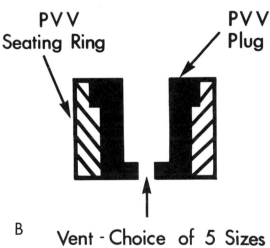

B   Vent - Choice of 5 Sizes

Fig. 3-35A,B.   Schematic diagram of Postive Venting Valve (PVV)

Sintered Filters

Another means of controlling the spectrum by mechanical means is to use Sintered Filters in the tubing. These are small cylinders of stainless-steel balls welded together in such a manner that predicted degrees of acoustical attentuation can result. Again, they are used to reduce the lower portion of the speech spectrum, the first two formats, with minimal effect on the third format of speech. Figure 3-38 demonstrates the response of one hearing aid in a 2-cc coupler using different sizes of Sintered Filters.

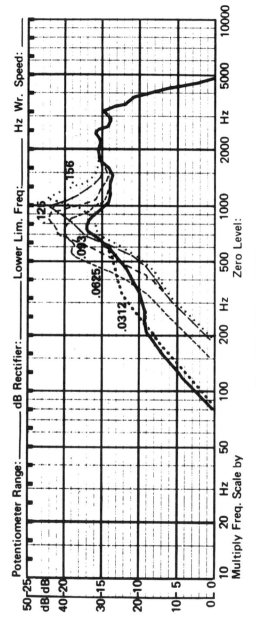

Fig. 3-36. Effects of PVV

127

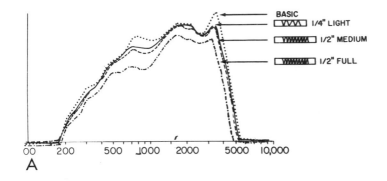

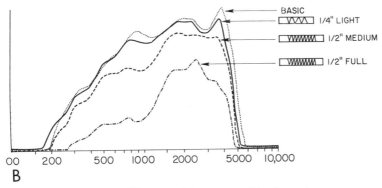

Fig. 3-37.   Effects on aid response of lamb wool

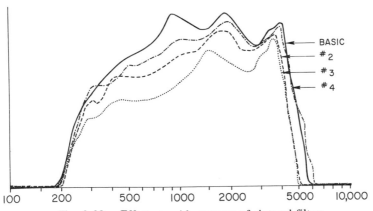

Fig. 3-38.   Effects on aid response of sintered filters

128

SUMMARY OF MODIFICATION EFFECTS

Table 3-2 summarizes the effects that can be achieved by various earmold modifications. Many of these alterations, as has already been noted, do not result in large changes in the response of the aid, but rather, can result in significant increase in subjective user comfort. For example, a very small vent (.020 inch), while not altering the frequency response appreciably, often does provide a release of sound pressure that can alleviate complaints of pressure or fullness in the ear.

In cases where even a small vent cannot be used because of feedback, a narrower earmold canal bore can have the same effect by providing extra displacement of the amplified sound away from the tympanic membrane.

User comfort can be improved, and complaints of fullness alleviated, by shortening the length of the canal. This can also reduce complaints of amplified sound being too reverberant or too loud. Lamb's wool or Sintered Filters will often reduce the "tinny" or "sharp" quality of amplified sound.

Above all, keep in mind the fact that while we can have a general idea of what the effects of a particular modification will be, the electronics of the hearing aid will be a major determinant. Therefore, it is important to utilize the subjective impressions of your user to determine the final modifications that will be made. This is a situation where use of the PVV and SAV can be beneficial in that various size vents can be tried until the user indicates the one that sounds best to him or her.

PROPER IMPRESSION TECHNIQUES

A properly fitted, comfortable, custom earmold is just as important as any other component in the successful fitting of a hearing aid. Since the finished earmold is a duplicate of the impression made, it is extremely important to understand and master the proper procedure for taking an ear impression.

Ear Impression Equipment and Materials

Otoscope or earlight
Cotton or foam block
Nylon thread or dental floss
Mixing bowl
Spatula
Tweezers
Impression powder
Catalyst
Syringe
Scissors

Table 3-2
Effect of Coupling Modifications on Hearing Aid Response

Modification	Effect on low frequencies (below 750 Hz)	Effect on primary peak (750–1500 Hz)	Effect on secondary peak (1500–3000 Hz)	Effect on high frequencies (above 3000 Hz)	Refer to figure
Longer tubing	Increases	Moves peak to lower frequency	Moves peak to lower frequency and decreases height	Negligible	3–18 and 25
Shorter tubing	Slightly decreases	Moves peak to higher frequency	Moves peak to higher frequency and increases height	Slightly increases	3–18 and 25
Larger I.D. tubing	Negligible	Moves peak to higher frequency	Moves peak to higher frequency and increases height	Negligible	3–26 and 25
Smaller I.D. tubing	May reduce below 1000 Hz	Moves peak to lower frequency	Moves peak to lower frequency and reduces height	Minimal	3–26 and 27
Large diameter bore	Negligible	Moves peak to higher frequency	Moves peak to higher frequency	Increases	
Smaller diameter bore	Negligible	Moves peak to lower frequency	Moves peak to lower frequency	Decreases	

Longer bore	Negligible	Moves peak to lower frequency	Moves peak to lower frequency and raises height	Negligible	3–28
Shorter bore	Negligible	Moves peak to higher frequency	Moves peak to higher frequency and decreases height	Negligible	3–28
Longer canal		Increases overall height of response curve			3–28
Shorter canal		Decreases overall height of response curve			
*Very small vent (.031 in)	Negligible	Negligible	Negligible	Negligible	3–29 and 17
Small vent (.042 in)	Decreases	Negligible	Negligible	Negligible	3–29 and 3–34
Medium vent (.064 in)	Decreases	Increases peak height	Negligible	Negligible	3–29 and 3–34
Large vent (.089 in)	Decreases	Increases peak height	Negligible	Negligible	3–29 and 3–34
Non-occluding mold (cros)	Eliminates	Moves peak to higher frequency and increases height	Increases peak height	Negligible	7–3 and 3–17
Open vented mold (high frequency)	Decreases	Reduces peak height	Negligible	Negligible	3–20
Sintered filter	Slightly decreases	Large reduction	Large reduction	Slightly decreases	3–38
Lamb's wool		Decreases overall height of response curve			3–37

*Primarily used for subject comfort by releasing sound pressure.

*Primarily used for subjective comfort by releasing sound pressure.

Examination of the Ear

A thorough examination of the ear should always be made with an otoscope before taking an impression. It is important in making this examination that the little finger and the ring finger are braced against the patient's cheek so that the speculum of the otoscope will move with any sudden movement of the head. The examination should include the following steps.

1. Inspect for any discharge or infection in the ear. Never take an impression of an ear when either of these conditions is present. In general, it is advisable to have clearance from a physician, preferably one specializing in diseases of the ear, before taking an earmold impression.
2. Inspect for excessive wax. If the canal is partially or entirely blocked by a heavy wall of firm, impacted wax, refer the patient to a physician before taking an impression.
3. Determine if the ear has undergone surgery and, if so, obtain medical clearance before taking an impression. This is also important in the case of the older mastoidectomy procedures in which a large mastoid bowl was often left. Special care will have to be taken to completely occlude this bowl before taking the impression.
4. Inspect for any malformations in the ear, such as moles or scar tissue. Be sure these irregularities are shown clearly on the finished impression and alert the earmold laboratory to them.
5. Inspect for a prolapsed canal. This condition is caused by a breakdown or sag of tissue around the canal, causing the canal to appear to be nearly or entirely closed. When this condition is present, a cotton or foam block large enough to hold the canal open to a normal size must be placed in it. If the ear has a heavy growth of hair, this should be snipped away before making the impression. Place a cotton or foam block in the canal to prevent the clippings from falling into the canal.
7. Finally, get a clear picture as to the size and direction of the canal. Also check the texture of the ear as to whether it is hard, medium, or very soft. Be careful when taking an impression of a soft ear so as not to stretch it out of shape. Many earmold problems can be traced to a dispenser pressing the material too hard into a soft ear, thus oversizing and misshaping the impression.

Each of the above items must be checked and noted before an impression is taken. If they are performed in a direct, professional manner, a great degree of confidence will be achieved. The information needed to make a perfect impression will also be gained.

Preparing the Subject

After completing the above examination, prepare a cotton block with a small pellet of cotton and nylon thread. The cotton should be flared. A handy item is the "pre-tied" one-size-fits-all foam blocks available from most laboratories. Place the cotton at the canal opening, and set it to the desired depth using an ear light. Normally the desired depth is a point just past the second bend of the canal. This is shown in Figure 3-39.

The cotton block is a must for taking a good impression. It protects the tympanic membrane. Additionally, without a block, the impression material will taper off and not give a true "picture" of the canal.

Making the Ear Impression

Anyone can make a near perfect impression every time by observing the rules described below.

Not all impression materials are the same. Some have a short working time, some long. Some are tough and can withstand changing temperatures, some cannot. A suggestion is to work with your earmold laboratory and find a material that you are satisfied with; one that is acceptible to your laboratory. We strongly recommend using a prepackaged impression material, i.e., individually measured units of powder and liquid. More poor impressions result from the improper balance of powder/liquid catalyst than any other one thing.

In mixing the material for an impression, pour the liquid into the mixing bowl first and then the powder. Using the spatula, mix the two materials vigorously until they are completely mixed. The use of a colored liquid catalyst will help in determining when the mixture is complete.

There are two approaches for inserting the material into the ear. One is to mix the material vigorously until it congeals, then work it in the palm of your hand and begin placing the material over the opening of the ear canal. Then press it firmly into the canal with the index finger, so the material reaches the cotton block and spreads out to occlude the canal. Then work the remaining material into the concha and helix curl of the ear. Be careful not to press too firmly less

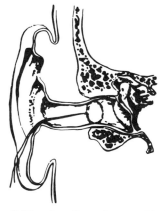

Fig. 3-39.   Insertion of cotton block

the ear be shoved out of shape. Too much pressure or continued working of the material in the outer part of the canal can and usually does create a misshaped impression.

The second is the syringe technique, which we recommend. The syringe offers an easy way to produce accurate ear impressions. After the impression powder and liquid are mixed, it must be put quickly into the syringe, using the spatula. Once this is done, push the plunger into the syringe until the material begins to come out the end of the nozzle. If the material falls over quickly when coming out of the nozzle, let it set a moment or two longer. When it is properly set, insert the end of the nozzle into the canal as deeply as possible and begin to inject the material. As the material begins to flow out the end of the nozzle, it will flow back and cover the top of the nozzle. This is good. Now, ease the nozzle out a bit and as the material begins to fill the ear, remember this: ALWAYS KEEP THE END OF THE NOZZLE IMBEDDED IN THE MATERIAL. This will avoid the entrapment of air and eliminate folds. As the canal is filled, move the tip to the lower concha and fill the bowl completely. Work the tip all the way up into the helix area and fill it also. Be sure to fill the bowl sufficiently to cover the tragus. After injecting the necessary amount of material into the ear for a good impression, discard the remaining material. You may use very light finger pressure to smoothe out the impression if necessary, but we do not recommend any hand pressure at all, as it can distort the shape of the ear and therefore the impression. Let the impression "set" in the ear for at least 15 min before removal.

To remove the impression, first move the ear away from the impression and then with the thumb and forefinger take hold of the impression at the center back and pull slightly forward. This will break the seal and help avoid distortion. Then pull out the top (helix) and pull straight out with a bit of upward and clockwise motion. The impression should release and come out easily.

Be sure to check the ear for any bits of material that might have remained. Be sure also that the cotton block came out with the impression. If not, pull on the string to remove the block. Never pull on string or thread to remove impression from the ear. To do so will distort the impression. Figure 3-40 shows a simple set of pictorial instructions for taking a good earmold impression.

Once removed from the ear, place the impression in open air for at least 30 min before packaging for shipment. This allows for final curing. Place the impression in the shipping box or on a cardboard platform in the box and cement it well so that it cannot move around during mailing. DO NOT USE WHITE GLUE. Model glue is good and is fast setting. White glue will not hold the mold to the cardboard as well. Finally, place the impression in the mailing box, fold the completed order form over the lower half of the box and close it.

Remember, nothing should touch the impression in transit to the laboratory. Figure 3-41 shows the proper packaging for an earmold prior to shipment to the earmold laboratory.

Preparing the Order Form

On the order form, be sure to include the patient's name and the specific information needed by the laboratory to make the mold you want. This should include mold style, material, severity of loss (preferably an audiogram), ear texture, tubing size, and venting. Incomplete order forms result in mistakes, delays, and costly phone calls to and from the laboratory. Any special instructions can be noted under "remarks" or entered on a separate piece of paper. It is also wise to write the individual's last name on the side of the impression in case it is separated from the order form in the laboratory. If a remake is requested, be sure to describe, in detail, the problem incurred with the original mold so the correction can be obtained.

SOME HINTS ON "IN HOUSE" VENTING, MODIFYING, BUFFING (POLISHING), AND TUBE CHANGING FOR BOTH HARD AND SOFT EAR MOLDS

A small electric motor with an "0 to ¼" chuck will suffice for venting and buffing; otherwise, one of the "Dremel" types with a variable speed attachment will do. The latter limits one to a specific size shank on drill, stone, etc. These sizes are $3/32$ and ⅛ inches, but a more versatile setup is preferred. Most earmold laboratories can furnish such a setup, including all tools necessary, such as drills, burrs, stones, polish wheels, and polish. The electric motor should be $1/6$ th HP and not more than ¼ th HP. It should have a double shaft; that is, a useable shaft on each end. It should be a two-speed 1725/3450 rpm motor. One end of the shaft is for mounting the buff wheel and the other one is for the chuck in using the drills, stones, etc. Have on hand some jewelers rouge (polish), a hood to contain the splatter and dust, and you're in business. Slow speed (1725 rpm) is recommended in venting and other modifying since the higher speed tends to "heat up" the plastic, resulting in poor quality work.

To vent a lucite earmold, choose the size drill bit for the needed vent. Remember, you can always enlarge a hole but it is difficult to make one smaller. If parallel venting is indicated, make sure there is sufficient space through the narrowest portion of the mold (usually the isthmus or at the very end of the canal). If the diameter is too small, then angle venting must be substituted. To produce a professional job, it is well to choose a drill bit slightly smaller than the intended vent. Drill the vent, then enlarge the vent to the proper size with a burr. The burr will give a clean, professional appearance to the vent. It can rarely be done as well with the drill bit only. Even at the 1725-rpm speed, the drill bit and the plastic will heat up, so it is suggested that a container of cool water (a small pan 6 × 8 inches, 1½-inches deep is just about right) be placed under the chuck or very nearby. Now, before drilling, have in mind the direction you plan to go.

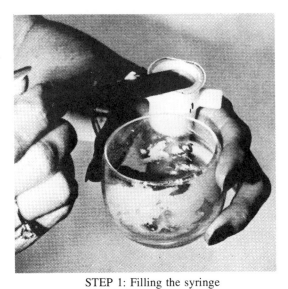

STEP 1: Filling the syringe

Fig. 3-40.   Proper earmold impression technique

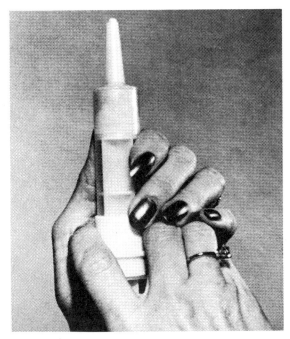

STEP 2: Eliminating air bubbles

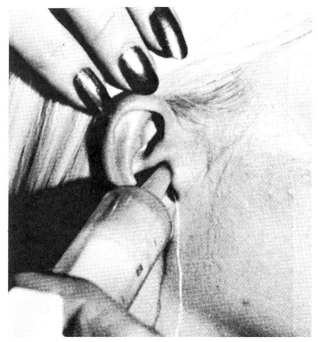

STEP 3: Filling the canal

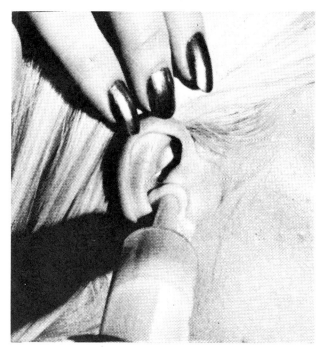

STEP 4: Filling the concha

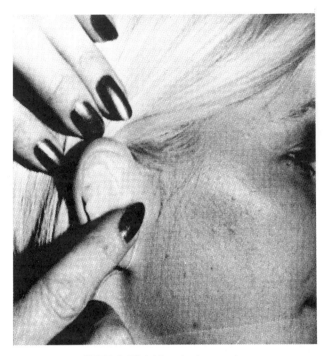

STEP 5: Finishing the impression

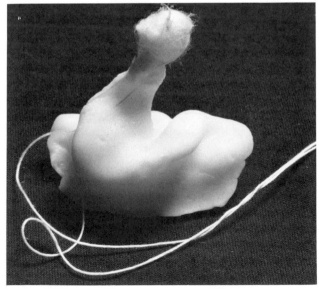

STEP 6: The finished impression

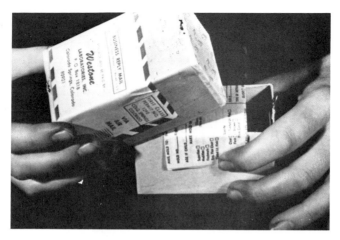

Fig. 3-41. Packing impression for mailing

Proceed to drill about ⅛ inch into the mold from the exterior of the mold. The beginning of the vent should be as far distant from the sound channel as possible but no closer than ⅛ inch to the edge of the earmold. This will help prevent accidental drilling through the mold to the outside or into the sound channel. Always try to maintain equal distance from the sound channel and the exterior of the canal portion of the mold. After the first ⅛ inch is drilled, cool the mold in water and dribble some water on the bit also. Check to see if the proper direction is being attained. By totally submerging the mold (if it is clear plastic) refraction will be eliminated and a clear view of the progress can be noted. All is well? Proceed another ⅛ inch and so on until you reach the bend in the canal or about halfway through the mold. Now start at the end of the canal using the same procedure and drill toward the point where the first hole stopped. Watch carefully and be sure you are "lined up" with the other point. When the two holes are about $1/16$ inch apart, stop and use a burr to finish. This will help straighten out any misalignment and of course, clean up the inside of the hole. Remember, you used a smaller drill bit and now you can enlarge the hole with the burr to the proper size quite easily. With the burr, go in small steps and use the same water procedure as outlined above. Angle venting should always be terminated as near the end of the canal as possible. A short angle vent will prevent proper tube insertion depth and, in many instances, the vent orifice into the sound channel has been occluded by the tubing being inserted to a depth beyond the vent entry into the sound channel.

Venting a soft (PVC) earmold is somewhat more difficult. A convenient tool is a "core drill," actually a steel tube of the proper size, sharpened to "core out" a plug. The core drill is hand-held and should be rotated in half turns clockwise and counter-clockwise. Follow the ⅛-inch method as with lucite molds, but, using needle nose pliers, pull out the ⅛-inch plug each time and continue. Caution should be observed as the core tends to get smaller if the drill is pressed too hard into the material or if deeper penetration is attempted without "pulling the plug." Again the use of a proper sized burr with cool water will give a smooth finish to the inside of the vent.

Two other methods of venting soft (PVC) molds can be used. First, a very high speed drill, above 3000 rpm, can be used. This will drill/burn a hole through the soft material. This is usually not the most successful method. Another method, an excellent one, is to freeze the mold in the freezing compartment of the office refrigerator for 10 min or more. This will harden the mold sufficiently to "slow speed" drill the vent.

Modifying an earmold can mean anything from simply buffing down a small offending area to shortening the canal or removing the helix. For lucite molds, with the aforementioned tools (a small one in difficult to reach areas) grind away the intended area using a large stone, then smooth and round out all surfaces to be refinished. After this is done and you have the modification complete, use some polish or the buff wheel and polish until the desired luster or finish is achieved. For PVC molds, use the same basic procedure, keeping in mind that large areas can be removed with a sharp knife or scissors prior to the work with the stone. Keep in mind also that PVC molds will heat up rapidly so take off small amounts of material at a time until the job is complete. Your finished work must be done with the stone since most PVC materials do not lend themselves to the dry polish procedures as do lucite ones. For the really professional touch to modifying PVC molds, a polish wheel and a slurry of pumice may be used. In this type of "wet" polishing the buff wheel should be soaked with water. Then, dipping the mold in the pumice slurry constantly, proceed to buff or polish with the pumice rather than with dry polish as on lucite molds. Always keep plenty of wet slurry on the area being polished.

Changing tubings in molds is quite simple. The only other "materials" needed are proper sized tubings, which can be purchased from your laboratory already preformed, and cement for both lucite and PVC molds. These tubing procedures apply to silicone earmolds as well as lucite and PVC; however, it is best to use especially treated tubes and silicone cement for silicone earmolds. Other tubing and tubing cements are not very successful. Your laboratory should be able to furnish you with these items.

Hot water (from the tap) will usually soften the cement holding the tube in the mold sufficiently so that it will pull out of either lucite or PVC molds. If it breaks off, the remaining tubing can be removed with a burr. Be sure the sound channel is clean and free of all foreign material such as bits of tubing, ear wax, or any other debris, and that the earmold is clean, inside and out, before installing a new tube. After selecting the proper-sized tube, you may cut the end to be inserted in the mold to such length as desired. Using a pipe cleaner or the brush applicator that comes with the cement, apply a very small amount of cement to the depth in the sound channel that you want the tubing to reach, and also dip the tube in the cement about the same distance. Shake off any excess cement on the tube and insert immediately. You may prefer to use the quilled type tubing and thread the tube all the way through the mold to a distance of ⅛ inch beyond where it is to be cut, cut it off, and then pull the tube back to a point ⅛ inch inside the mold. Very little cement is necessary using this method of replacing tubing. A bit of cement on the end of a toothpick pushed down between the tube and the sound channel will give all the retention necessary. There is no need to follow the procedure outlined in the preceeding paragraph except to remove the old tubing and clean the mold well before installing the new tubing.

The two methods above will work equally well on lucite, PVC, and silicone molds. Be sure to use proper-sized tubes, the proper cement, and in the case of silicone, properly treated tubings.

CONCLUSION

It is readily apparent that when you order an earmold you must give much thought to the many styles and variations of molds available. The decisions regarding these various choices will have a significant effect on the satisfaction of the user with his or her hearing aid. Remember, it is easier for the laboratory to modify the mold the way you want it than for you to do it. We do not mean to imply that the dispenser should not or cannot modify the mold. However, many office modifications would not be necessary if careful thought were given to the specifications of the mold when ordering it from the laboratory.

BIBLIOGRAPHY

Berger KW: The Hearing Aid: Its Operation and Development (ed 2). Detroit, National Hearing Aid Society, 1974

Curran JR: CROS Fittings and Open-Canal Amplification. Minneapolis, Dahlberg Electronics, 1971

Griffing TS, Shields J: Hearing aid performance and the earmold. Hear Dealer 23:6−9, 1972

Hewitt C: New ''free-field'' earmold for precipitous sensorineural losses. Hear Aid J Vol 30, #5 pp 10, 32, 1977

Lybarger SF: The Earmold as a Part of the Receiver Acoustic System. Radioear Corp, Cannonsburg, Pennsylvania, 1958

Joseph P. Millin

4
Practical and Philosophical Considerations

There are few areas within the field of audiology that generate more differences of opinion than the selection of hearing aids. Over the years a wide diversity of procedural options for hearing aid evaluations have been proposed. None has received universal acceptance. The next three chapters of this book relate to this very problem–how we select the appropriate amplification system for our patients.

In this chapter, Joe Millin discusses some of the controversies that have arisen and proposes solutions to many of them. This chapter is placed before the two on hearing aid selection in order to give you a greater foundation and insight into this complex area. Many "rules of thumb" have been used for years without much questioning on our part. They have been handed down, so to speak, from generation to generation. In this discussion, Joe looks at many of these "principles" with an objective eye and points out how many of them are no longer applicable.

MCP

There can be no justification for performing hearing aid evaluations unless we accept the premise that hearing-impaired listeners differ in their amplification requirements and the magnitude of these differences is not trivial. That such differences exist, however, has been difficult to substantiate in the laboratory. In 1960, Shore, Bilger and Hirsh stated that "there is no good evidence concerning a relation between the performance of an aid as measured through listening tests and the physical performance of an aid as measured through acoustical tests." A few such relationships have since been demonstrated, but only when electroacoustic differences among hearing aids were exaggerated to an order of magnitude not typically found among commercially available instruments (Harris et al. 1961, Jerger et al. 1966).

Failure to identify predictable relationships between hearing aid characteristics and measurable parameters of listener performance has left audiologists with an urgent need for valid procedures which will effectively identify the most appropriate amplifier for prospective hearing aid users. We are under fire because we have been unable to generate demonstrably valid selection procedures which can achieve universal acceptance among audiologists (ACO Statement, 1976). This failure to establish standard tests has resulted in a proliferation of widely differing individual methods of evaluation. It is probable that there are nearly as many procedures for selecting and recommending hearing aids as there are audiologists.

No matter how difficult it may prove to be, it is imperative, if continued participation in the hearing aid evaluation process is to be justified, that selection criteria demonstrably superior to the so-called *intuitive* and largely unscientific practices currently employed in many clinics be generated quickly. So long as evaluations are performed solely on rational grounds, unsupported by convincing experimental evidence, procedures used by audiologists are no more defensible than those of any other person, no matter how limited his training or suspect his motives. For years audiologists have been complaining about the minimal training given the hearing aid specialist, but when it comes to the critical clinical selection of an appropriate amplifier for the patient, the superiority of audiologic procedures cannot be demonstrated experimentally. Knowledge of such physical properties of hearing aids as the taper of the gain control or frequency response tells nothing of how this information can be used to optimize the patient's hearing. I have heard countless schemes for hearing aid selection proposed by audiologists, dispensers, physicians, and students. Many seemed to be "logical," yet the issue is not whether such schemes are logical but whether they do in fact identify the appropriate amplifier for the patient. In other words, logic does not insure validity.

TRADITIONAL HEARING AID EVALUATION AND SELECTION PROCEDURES

We have not always been so unsure of ourselves. Carhart (1946a, b, c, 1950), working in the World War II military hospital program, developed procedures based on experimental methodology. Often referred to as "traditional" or "conventional" procedures, they managed to achieve extensive but not universal acceptance. The logic of Carhart's procedures is compelling. The essential requirement is clinical comparison on prospective hearing aid users of the performance of several hearing aids selected for trial on the basis of predetermined criteria. An aid is sought which provides (1) the greatest improvement in SRT, (2) the best word discrimination score, (3) the widest dynamic range, and (4) the ability to maintain satisfactory speech discrimination in the highest level of noise.

Viewed in terms of experimental design, the traditional selection procedures are tests of the relationship between amplifier differences and the listening performance of the patient. Each of the four performance variables is tested separately. If, for example, the principal interest is the effect of trial aids on speech discrimination, the dependent variable is listener performance as reflected by word discrimination scores. Differences in the frequency responses of the aids is often chosen as the independent variable. The underlying ability of the patient to discriminate speech is assumed to be constant. Differences in performance are presumed to reflect changes, not in this underlying ability, but in the intelligibility of speech stimuli as influenced by the electroacoustic properties (in this example, the frequency response) of the trial hearing aids. The patient is thus treated as a constant effect, as are numerous other controlled variables, such as speech presentation level, test lists and, of course, the test environment. The hearing aid which produces the best word discrimination score is judged to be superior to the others in terms of how it enables the listener to discriminate speech sounds. Because they are based on experimental principles, these procedures have had great appeal, but, as we shall see, serious challenges to their validity have been made.

Modifications of Traditional Procedures

Obviously, if each of Carhart's four performance variables is tested separately, with three or four trial hearing aids, and each test is then repeated in noise, the total time of testing will be prohibitively long. Furthermore, one might argue that these trials should be performed in each ear as well as binaurally. It could also be necessary to test such additional factors as directional versus nondirectional microphones, head versus body placement, clipping versus linear versus nonlinear compression, CROS versus conventional placement, open versus standard coupling, and countless other modifications. Clearly, such extensive testing is not practical. The traditional procedures have, therefore, been modified on the basis of various theoretical and practical arguments. It is doubtful that they are now used anywhere exactly as Carhart described them.

Despite the many modifications of traditional procedures, the concept of clinical comparison of hearing aid performance on patients is still widely employed and as Ross (1972) points out, the continued use of Carhart's criteria in hearing aid research and in the clinic is a tribute to the ingenuity of his work.

Traditional Procedures Challenged

Anyone who has used the comparative procedures extensively must have been struck, at one time or another, by the fact that for many patients, differences in the effects of trial hearing aids are often surprisingly small, even when the electroacoustic differences among the aids are substantial. This observation led investigators to examine the reliability of traditional measures (Shore et al. 1960, McConnell et al. 1960). The study by Shore et al. (1960) had a major influence on subsequent research and clinical practice. They ranked the relative effectiveness of several hearing aids, which differed substantially in electroacoustic performance, on the basis of SRTs and word discrimination scores of hearing-impaired listeners. Unfortunately, these rankings were found to change when the subjects were retested, leading the authors to conclude "that the reliability of these measures is not good enough to warrant the investment of a large amount of clinical time with them in selecting hearing aids." They further concluded "that one does not find substantial or striking differences among the results of hearing tests obtained from patients using different hearing aids or different tone settings of hearing aids."

The Shore et al. (1960) study precipitated the abandonment of traditional evaluation procedures in two major clinics (Resnick and Becker 1963, Shore and Kramer 1965). Just how many other clinics or clinicians have followed suit has not been determined, but there is little doubt that the study seriously undermined confidence in traditional procedures and created an immediate need to generate workable alternatives for assessing the amplification needs of the hearing-impaired.

An alternative proposal by Resnick and Becker (1963) recommended that the audiologist give greater emphasis to patient counseling, particularly about the potential benefits and problems associated with hearing aid use. Since these functions were already part of traditional evaluation, the important departure from conventional practice was their recommendation that objective comparative tests of hearing aid performance be discontinued. The option of selecting specific hearing aids for clinic patients was transferred to reputable hearing aid dealers.

Assumptions Underlying Traditional Procedures

The merits of Resnick and Becker's clinical proposal have been argued elsewhere (Millin 1963, Jeffers and Smith 1964), but their important contribution to the understanding of traditional evaluation procedures was their identification and formulation of the three basic assumptions which constitute the rationale for hearing aid comparison. The assumptions are:

1. That there are significant differences among hearing aids in terms of how they enable the user to understand everyday speech.
2. That these differences change from one user to the next, that is, that there is an interaction between people and hearing aids.
3. That these differences can be demonstrated reliably by monosyllabic word (PB 50) intelligibility scores (Resnick and Becker 1963).

Students sometimes fail to differentiate between validity of these assumptions, which has not yet been determined, and the need to embrace the assumptions, valid or not, if traditional comparative evaluations are to be justified. If the first assumption is false and one hearing aid is as effective as any other, there can be no possible justification for performing comparative evaluations. While the notion that all hearing aids may be equally effective may be intuitively rejected, it is clearly one inference which can be drawn from the Shore et al. (1960) study, since they did not find "substantial or striking" differences among the effects of different hearing aids. The fact, however, that audiologists continue to perform selection procedures and to search for relationships between listeners and hearing aids strongly suggests a general conviction that significant differences among hearing aids do exist.

The second assumption, which is more subtle, requires the clinician to believe that the relative effectiveness of various hearing aids differs from patient to patient. One must assume that a hearing aid that has been found to be most effective for one patient may prove to be inferior to another instrument used by a different patient. Only if this kind of interaction between people and hearing aids exists can a need to compare several aids on every clinic patient be demonstrated. In the absence of such an interactive effect one would have to assume that the best hearing aid for any one patient would also be the best for all patients. Then it would only be necessary to identify the best hearing aid for any one patient and recommend this superior instrument for all patients. Paradoxically, the task of finding this "ideal" amplifier would presumably require a comparison of hearing aids on listeners, the same procedure Shore et al. (1960) found to be unreliable.

Even if there is a patient—hearing aid interaction, comparative evaluation of aids would be necessary only if the interaction is unpredictable. It is possible, for example, that all patients with steeply sloping audiograms will require a specifiable high frequency emphasis hearing aid frequency response, whereas patients with flat audiograms will do best with a flat frequency response. Because these two types of hearing losses would require different hearing aids for optimum performance, this would represent a hearing aid—listener interaction. If, however, we knew on the basis of empirical evidence precisely what hearing aids provide optimum performance for each group, we would not need to compare aids on these patients.

If, on the other hand, listeners with identical audiograms were found by research to perform best with greatly different hearing aids, and if the most appropriate aids for each of these listeners could not be predicted from audiometric data, then only a comparative procedure could identify the optimum aid for each patient. In order to justify comparative evaluation of aids on every patient, therefore, one must believe that precise prediction of patient amplification needs cannot, at the present state of the art, be predicted from unaided audiometric data. This premise finds support in the data of Pollack and Lipscomb (1979), which suggest that pure tone audiograms may not be providing an accurate picture of cochlear function.

Resnick and Becker (1963) rejected the second assumption, claiming to see no reason that an interaction effect should exist. Since this decision obviates the need for hearing aid comparisons, they recommend that patients be sent to cooperating dealers, chosen for each patient by rotation from an approved dealer list. The selection of an appropriate hearing aid is then made by the dealer. This system produces a wide distribution of different makes and models of hearing aids among patients—a proposition difficult to justify if you believe, as Resnick and Becker apparently do, that one aid may be superior to the others and should, therefore, be given to all patients.

There appear to be good theoretical reasons to support the assumption of an interaction between people and hearing aids, although audiologists would doubtless disagree on whether or not such interactions are precisely predictable. Suppose, for example, that a patient with moderate low-frequency hearing loss but no measurable hearing at or above 1000 Hz was fitted with a hearing aid that provides gain at only 1000 Hz and above. It is difficult to see how this amplifier could possibly benefit the patient, since all of its power is concentrated in the frequency region in which the patient has no residual hearing. This same aid, however, could prove to be of considerable benefit to other patients, such as those with moderate negative-sloping audiograms.

A major reason that the differential effects of hearing aids are so difficult to demonstrate relates to Resnick and Beckers' third assumption. The principal charge against traditional hearing aid evaluation procedures leveled by Shore et al. (1960) is that the performance of trial hearing aids cannot be reliably ranked by conventional speech discrimination measures. If differences in the effects of hearing aids are genuine but tests fail to reveal such differences, it is reasonable to infer that the intrinsic variability of these measures may produce greater differences among scores than those generated by the effects of hearing aids. This would, of course, obscure differences among hearing aids. Judging from the emphasis of recent research, most audiologists concur with this interpretation, thereby rejecting the third assumption that word discrimination scores will reliably differentiate among the effects of hearing aids.

THE SEARCH FOR IMPROVED TEST RELIABILITY AND SENSITIVITY

One way of interpreting the small differences in scores resulting from differences among hearing aids is to assume that speech discrimination tests are relatively insensitive to amplifier effects. If this is so, the usefulness of these tests is very limited in comparative hearing aid selection as well as in the broader search for predictable relationships between measurable parameters of hearing loss and electroacoustic properties of hearing aids. However, even a test of low sensitivity can be expected to detect differences in the level of variable if the magnitude of such differences is very large.

The thrust of recent research, therefore, has developed in two major directions. The first has been an attempt to generate new speech tests which have less variability (Jerger, Malmquist, and Speaks 1966, Campbell 1965, Margolis and Millin 1971). The potential value of such tests is obvious. With them, most of the questions confronting the audiologist can be answered readily, since even weak differences among instruments would exceed the variability inherent in the tests. Efforts to develop such tests, however, have been only modestly successful. The possible reasons that sensitive and reliable tests are so difficult to generate are critical to the entire concept of hearing aid evaluation and will be discussed fully under the topics "Reliability" and "Validity."

The second approach has been to employ traditional tests but to improve the chances of detecting the effects of instruments by increasing the magnitude of electroacoustic differences among experimental hearing aids (Harris et al. 1961, Jerger, Speaks, and Malmquist 1966), Jerger's group, for example, studied the effects of greatly differing levels of harmonic distortion on speech intelligibility. Not only did the authors succeed in discovering an inverse relationship between word discrimination scores and percentage of harmonic distortion, but they were able to demonstrate reliable intrasubject rankings of hearing aids as well. This study and others referenced above are of fundamental importance because they are among the first to demonstrate predictable relationships between listener and hearing aid performance, thus lending support to the first of the assumptions identified by Resnick and Becker (1963).

THE CONTROVERSY ON INTERACTIVE EFFECTS BETWEEN PEOPLE AND HEARING AIDS

It should be evident from the foregoing discussion that audiologists have, at best, limited solid scientific data on which to base their selection of appropriate hearing aids for their patients. Thus, the issue as to whether hearing aid comparisons need be performed on each patient remains unresolved. Furthermore, the strategy a clinician employs in recommending specific aids for his patients will depend in large measure on whether he accepts the assumption of an interaction between listeners and hearing aids.

Among those who reject the concept of interaction are certain advocates of selective amplification (see later discussion for definition of selective amplification). They assume that there are invariant relationships between audiometric pure-tone configuration and hearing aid frequency response, and that these relationships are the same for all patients with comparable audiograms. They reason, therefore, that research will ultimately discover and specify all such relationships precisely, after which it will be an easy matter to ascertain the optimum hearing aid frequency response for any patient simply by examining his audiogram. This group, therefore, can find no justification for comparison of trial hearing aids on every patient. Prescriptive selection formulas are based on the assumption that these invariant relationships are already well-developed enough to allow relatively precise specification of amplifier needs from a patient's unaided audiometric data. Fitting formulas are growing in popularity and are discussed in some detail later in this chapter.

Advocates of traditional hearing aid selection procedures, however, reject the assumption that the relationship between audiograms and frequency response are predictable from patient to patient. Instead, they believe that the relation between these variables is unique for each patient. They argue that since there is no present basis for predicting these interactions, the effects of a variety of frequency responses must be tested on every patient.

The tendency of audiologists to wholly accept or reject the concept of interactive effects between people and hearing aids seems to stem from the conviction that consistent and interactive effects must be mutually exclusive. There is, however, no particular reason why some amplifier effects might not be relatively consistent from listener to listener, while other effects are interactive. It is easily conceivable, for example, that frequency response requirements may vary among listeners even if their audiograms are identical, whereas power requirements may be a simple function of the severity of hearing loss. It is also possible that frequency response requirements may vary among one classification of patients, but not among others.

Whatever we may believe about interaction, there is—currently at least—only one known way to relate the effects of amplifiers to the behavior of listeners. One must systematically vary selected electroacoustic properties of hearing aids and measure their effects on the performance of listeners. This, like it or not, is comparative evaluation. Whether "real" hearing aids, master hearing aids, or special laboratory amplifiers are used, or individual or group performance is examined, the essential method will be comparative evaluation. If both reliable and valid data are successfully obtained on the relationships between these variables, the presence or absence of interactive effects will be resolved as a logical consequence of our efforts.

CONTRADICTIONS IN CLINIC PRACTICE

Before analyzing problems inherent in obtaining "good" data as to how amplifiers affect listening, a comment on the kinds of logical contradiction that occur when evaluative systems are used uncritically is in order. The rationale upon which many clinicians base the preselection of hearing aids for clinical trial appears to contradict the basis upon which the trials themselves are justified. Advocates of traditional procedures insist that each patient's amplification requirements are unique and unpredictable and must, therefore, be ascertained individually by comparative testing. Yet, in reducing trial aids to a practical number, three or four slightly differing aids are generally selected, with frequency responses falling within a range of contours believed by the clinician to approximate the listener's requirements. This judgment is usually based upon examination of the patient's audiogram and on the assumption that the clinician has some kind of foreknowledge, presumably based on experience, about the general kind of electroacoustic performance appropriate for the patient. The contradiction is obvious. The clinician claims that the patient's amplification needs are unpredictable and yet he depends on predictable relationships in selecting instruments for trial. To be logically consistent, the entire range of available frequency responses should be sampled on the patient, since any one response contour could prove to be as beneficial as another.

There appears to be another fallacy in this kind of preselection procedure. When the frequency responses of trial aids are deliberately restricted within a relatively narrow range of differences, it seems unreasonable to expect these relatively small differences to generate large and unambiguous differences in performance. It is also reasonable to speculate that this limiting process could account, in part, for the apparent instability of our tests, although Shore et al. (1960) got the same effect even when they deliberately used large amplifier differences.

The Harvard Report and Selective Amplification

With the introduction of electronic (vacuum tube) hearing aids, which permitted extensive manipulation of frequency response, major attention was given to using this adjustment capability to optimize hearing. An assumption was made that there is a unique pattern of hearing aid frequency response which will produce optimum speech intelligibility for each listener. This concept is called *selective amplification* or *audiogram fitting*.

The earliest form of selective amplification attempted to "restore" the patient's pure-tone thresholds to normal by providing gain equal to his hearing loss at all frequencies. There seemed to be an assumption that if the patient's aided thresholds were normal, his ability to understand speech would also be normal. The fact is, however, that hearing aids do not improve the listener's hearing; they improve the audibility of the stimulus. Furthermore, the level of conversational speech is always well above the threshold of normal hearing listeners and there appears to be no reason that the impaired listener need be able to understand speech close to the threshold level of normal ears.

A simple example will illustrate how complete compensation for hearing loss by frequency will generate intolerable levels at the listener's ear in the presence of modest speech levels. If a patient with a loss of 60 dB at 1000 Hz wears an aid with a gain of 60 dB in the presence of moderate speech levels around 60 dB SPL (re. 20 μN/m^2), the resultant pressure at the ear will be 120 dB. Even if the patient's ear does not recruit, this level will generally produce severe discomfort.

Such considerations led to other formulas for selective amplification. One was simply to provide gain proportional, but not equal, to the patient's hearing loss at each frequency. Here again, excessive loudness is sometimes experienced at frequencies in which the patient's loss is relatively great. A third modification of frequency response sought to solve the loudness problem by establishing a compensating hearing aid slope less steep than the slope of the patient's audiogram. Thus, a patient with a 15 dB drop in sensitivity per octave might be provided with a frequency response that rises only 4 or perhaps 8 dB per octave. Finally, a concept based on comfortable or "normal" loudness was recommended. Frequency response was to be adjusted so that the loudness of amplified speech at each of the speech frequencies is the same for hearing-impaired listeners as the loudness of ordinary speech is for normal listeners. Whether the criterion of comfort for tones will necessarily assure optimum hearing for speech, however, is not known. At least two research reports (Posner and Ventry 1977, Schmitz 1969) suggest that the most comfortable speech signal is often not the most intelligible.

All of these modifications, not to mention other proposed formulas, are based on manipulation of the relationship between the patient's pure-tone audiometric configuration and the frequency response of his hearing aid, always with the goal of optimizing speech understanding. While there were certain major differences in experimental methodology, the usefulness of selective amplification was analyzed in both the Harvard Report (Davis et al. 1946) during the vacuum tube aid era and in the Shore et al. (1960) study (discussed earlier) with transistorized instruments. Both studies suggested that the value of the selective amplification concept could not be verified with available performance measures. The Harvard Report concluded:

> The appropriate frequency characteristic for a hearing aid is not correctly indicated by current principles of "audiogram fitting" or "selective amplification." A uniform frequency characteristic that can be varied by a tone control between "flat" and a moderate accentuation of high tones will provide the most satisfactory performance for all or nearly all cases of hearing loss. . . . For the usual hard-of-hearing patient any detailed "fitting" is wasteful of time and effort. The differentials between instruments that are indicated by most current tests are largely illusory. (p. 5)

Despite the evidence against selective amplification, few other factors are really considered in comparative procedures. There is no problem, for example, in selecting values of distortion. Since it is inversely related to speech intelligibility, the solution is simply to minimize it. Similarly, the problem of tolerance is a matter of establishing a dynamic amplifier response that will maintain optimum speech sensation levels without permitting distracting, annoying, or uncomfortable levels. These are primarily engineering problems, not problems of selection or comparative evaluation.

Establishing appropriate hearing aid gain, i.e., the level the patient will use outside the clinic, is not the clinician's function. The patient will invariably make this decision. In my experience, instructing the patient to use higher or lower gain control adjustments is folly. In the first place, he will not do it, and in the second place, the level chosen by the listener is, in all likelihood, the best level for him, given a particular amplifier (Yantis et al. 1966). Any higher or lower level will probably result in reduced speech intelligibility. Furthermore, gain is a function of frequency response, since it is expressed in terms of the average of the gain at selected frequencies taken from the frequency response curve. It would appear, in fact, that the slope and smoothness of the frequency response are critical determiners of the amount of gain the listener will choose to employ (Jerger and Thelin 1973). In any event, the only problem with choosing gain is to assure that the overall gain of the amplifier is adequate and that at the listener's preferred setting, the instrument is not driven into saturation by input signal levels typically encountered by the patient.

Frequency Response Modification in Specialized Fitting Procedures

Published descriptions of specialized fitting techniques may not identify them as forms of selective amplification, but careful examination of their theoretical bases make it evident that they are, in fact, attempts to optimize performance by frequency response modification. CROS fitting is one example. While initial reports (Harford and Barry 1965, Harford 1966a, b) were largely concerned with overcoming the effects of the "dead" side of the head, it soon became apparent that the open mold provided drastic reduction of low-frequency response and thus was useful in fitting hearing losses with the greatest deficit in high frequencies and normal or near-normal sensitivity in the lower frequency range. An added benefit, of course, is that the open mold permits "natural" (undistorted) reception of low frequencies. The open mold, therefore, is used as a means of manipulating hearing aid frequency response (Dodds and Harford 1968, 1970), which is what selective amplification is all about. (See chapters 3 and 7 for discussion of CROS fitting.)

Similarly, low frequency emphasis aids for "deaf" children, whether based on an increase in the low frequency response of conventional hearing aid amplifiers or on frequency transposition (Erber 1971, Ling 1964, 1968) are based on frequency response manipulation and thus fall into the selective amplification category. They differ from traditional practice, however, in that they amplify speech in the frequency region where the patient's sensitivity is best, based on the assumption that the high-loss frequency region is essentially nonfunctional.

RELIABILITY

Traditional hearing aid evaluations are often tedious and time consuming. For this reason, few clinicians take time to repeat their tests. Until they do, however, they may never discover how variable speech tests really are, nor how this variability can mislead them in their clinical decisions.

Two students came to me recently, puzzled by a discrepancy of 16 percent between unaided sound-field word discrimination scores obtained from a single patient on two testing dates separated by about 4 months. One student argued that the patient's discrimination had, in fact, worsened, despite the fact that other audiometric measures had not changed significantly between tests. The second student attributed the discrepancy to possible procedural inconsistencies.

At my suggestion, four additional tests were made. The six scores were 84, 68, 80, 84, 72, and 80 percent. Nothing I might have said could possibly have so successfully engendered in those students the healthy suspicion every audiologist should have concerning speech discrimination tests. Needless to say, had the same scores been obtained with a series of trial hearing aids, the temptation to attribute the differences in scores to the effects of the hearing aids would have been irresistible. Obviously, therefore, score differences of this magnitude, which, by the way, are quite common, cast serious doubts on the validity of the data as an index of amplifier superiority.

Problems in Specifying Data

Analysis of major variables in comparative evaluation procedures suggests some of the sources of the instability of our tests. It is a relatively easy matter to achieve precise control of some kinds of simple physical variables. If, for example, the effect of selected volumes of water is to be tested on the growth of garden vegetables, it is an easy matter to measure desired volumes of water with great precision. When, however, attempts are made to specify the frequency response of trial hearing aids, it may be difficult to ascertain by examining the typically irregular, "squiggly" frequency response tracings obtained in the laboratory, just what response is represented by any particular hearing aid. Consider, for example, the curves in Figure 4-1.

Both of these curves could be roughly described as a straight line function of 6 dB rise per octave. I would hesitate, however, to assume that the effects of these two systems on speech intelligibility would be identical, nor am I sure which should be chosen to best represent the effects of a 6-dB rise per octave. It is conceivable, for example, that the peak in the response of aid number two will lead the listener to employ less gain with this instrument than he would with aid number one. Jerger and Thelin (1968) examined this problem.

The same difficulty is encountered in specifying harmonic distortion. The traditional formula (ANSI S3.3, 1960) provides a root mean square value of distortion. Like the frequency response slope, it is a second order derivation in which much of the original information is ignored. Suppose, for example, that using this formula, two aids were found to have 5 percent harmonic distortion, but the predominant distortion of one aid occurred at the second harmonic of the test frequences, while the distortion of the second aid was more evenly distributed over several harmonics. I doubt if the audiologist would be willing to predict with confidence that the influence of both aids on speech intelligibility would be the same. Again, we are faced with the need to decide which aid will best sample or represent the effect of 5 percent harmonic distortion (See Pollack, Chapter 2).

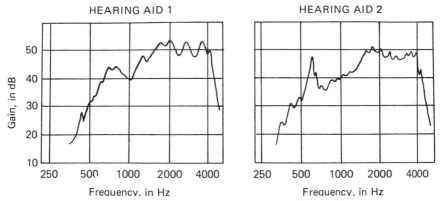

Fig. 4-1. Frequency response of two commercially available behind-the-ear hearing aids.

Maximum gain and maximum output data, the two remaining standard measures of hearing aid performance, are also averaged data obtained at three arbitrary points on an irregular curve. As such, they too are subject to uncertain interpretation, as are other nonstandard measures, such as intermodulation distortion or noise floor levels (See Pollack, Chapter 2).

Ideally, two general conditions should be met in order to compare the effects of amplification on a listener. The first is that any independent variable, such as frequency response, should be specified very precisely. To do this properly, amplifiers with smooth, unambiguous response curves would be needed. Three slopes could then be chosen to test on the listener, perhaps one with a negative slope of 8 dB per octave, one with a flat response and one with an 8 dB rising response.

The second requisite condition, virtually impossible to achieve, is that all other performance variables of the trial aids should be held constant. That is, each aid should have equivalent maximum gain, distortion, transient response, noise floor, and maximum output, to name only a few measurable parameters. The problem is that frequency response is not really independent of these other parameters and thus cannot literally operate as an independent variable (Chial and Hayes 1974, Bode and Kasten 1971). As frequency response is changed, some of the other properties will also change, and until changes in all but the independent variable can be minimized, changes in a patient's scores may or may not be largely dependent upon differences in frequency responses among aids rather than upon uncontrolled differences among other factors.

Macrovariables

Clearly then, our independent variable, which we call hearing aids, is not a single variable at all but is instead a conglomerate set of variables whose effects are sometimes additive, sometimes in opposition to one another, and sometimes largely independent. Such gross conglomerates are often referred to as macrovariables. It is my feeling that these relatively uncontrollable and unspecifiable collective macrovariables, with their interactive internal effects, are not likely ever to be cleanly related to listening behavior. Until the effects of these internal variables can be controlled, there will be little hope of establishing invariant relationships between hearing aid and listener performance.

Stimulus Macrovariables

In like manner, speech discrimination is a macrovariable. Word discrimination tests attempt to assess a listener capability which is made up of a complex set of interdependent factors. Developers of these tests have attempted to eliminate or stabilize the effects of such factors as word familiarity, talker differences, phonetic balance, presentation level, and transmission system fidelity. Each of these factors can generate excessive test variability if these effects are not controlled across listeners. Furthermore, it is becoming apparent that we have only begun to identify the seemingly endless number of factors which influence speech intelligibility.

Equivalent Test Forms

A very troublesome source of variability in traditional hearing aid comparisons results from attempts to employ "equivalent" test forms. It is important to have several test lists, each of which, if used to test the same patient under identical conditions, will produce nearly identical scores. These lists are necessary when performing successive tests of several hearing aids on a patient in order to avoid, among other things, the learning effect that results from repeating a single list. A problem emerges, however, from the fact that this equivalency has been established on the basis of group or averaged data. While the lists may produce identical average scores when tested on large groups, they tend not to be equivalent for individuals, as is apparent from the six scores obtained from the patient discussed earlier. The result is that the effects of nonequivalency of lists cannot be differentiated from the effects of differences in amplifiers.

This equivalency problem is one of the major barriers to the effective use of traditional procedures in hearing aid comparisons. It so happens that if the same list is repeated over and over, the patient's scores will be quite stable. When, however, different hearing aids are used, this "lock-in" or consistency effect appears to be stronger than the effects of the hearing aids. Thus, it will frequently happen that scores will not vary when the same list is used, even if variables other than hearing aids are altered substantially. I found, for example (Millin 1968), that room reverberation produced varying effects on discrimination where equivalent lists were used, but prior to the experiment, when I tried to repeat the same list, changes were infrequent. Therefore, I was forced to use equivalent lists despite their inherent intrasubject instability.

I have heard arguments that certain speech discrimination tests are satisfactory for clinical use but lack either the precision or the stability necessary for use in research (Elpern 1960). Actually, in most applications the reverse is true. If a decision must be based on a single comparison (which of two amplifier circuits provides superior performance for a listener) it is imperative that measures be used that are relatively precise and invariant. If the sampling distributions of scores obtained from the two aids overlap greatly, the region of uncertainty is so wide that it is often impossible to decide which of the two distributions is the source of a single test score. Thus, the audiologist will have little confidence in his decisions. In research, on the other hand, one can afford the luxury of making repeated measures. Therefore, differences in the effects of amplifiers will emerge eventually, even if the stability of the measures is relatively poor.

Clinically, the important factor is not simply whether the reliability of a procedure is good, but whether it will differentiate between the effects of hearing aids unambiguously. Only if the effects of aids are larger than the inherent variability of the test employed to detect them will it be possible to make correct, unambiguous decisions. Present tests appear to lack the kind of precision necessary to make clear-cut decisions within a reasonable period of time. Thus, the search for stable, practical tests continues.

VALIDITY

If, by virtue of some good fortune, a speech discrimination test, with reliability good enough to permit stable ranking of hearing aids, was suddenly available, a critical question would still remain. Will the hearing aid that is found to provide the best performance for a patient in the clinical setting maintain its superiority when used by the patient outside the clinic in everyday life?

The clinical environment differs dramatically from typical conditions of everyday listening, since it is carefully controlled in order to prevent the operation of certain variables that may, in unpredictable and sometimes almost random fashion, generate spurious variability that is not only unrelated to but can totally obscure the effects of trial hearing aids. This phenomenon can be illustrated by what might be called the "slamming door principal." If two persons were talking in a room in which a storm door was randomly slamming in the wind, the intelligibility of their speech would depend a great measure on the correlation between the slamming and the occurrence of key words in their conversation. If the key words of one talker unintentionally coincided with the slammings, but occurred at less critical times during the speech of the second talker, one could be misled into believing that the first talker was inherently less intelligible than the second. Although numerous kinds of masking or interfering events, such as the slamming door, occur more or less continuously in everyday listening, they are frequently eliminated in the clinic since the randomness of their occurrence makes it impossible to isolate their effects from those of the hearing aids. In eliminating such effects, of course, salient features of everyday listening are prevented from operating in the clinic.

To what extent the audiologist can control or eliminate extraneous kinds of noise and interference without invalidating the test data is not clear. Historically, of course, noise and competing speech have been introduced into the sound room, but often under conditions of control that negate many of the effects of real-world noises. White noise noise, for example, simply does not have the same effect on speech intelligibility as the staccato and unpredictable noises of the factory or office. Thus far, these kinds of noises seem to defy meaningful representation in the test room. Nonetheless, they are so common that they should probably be represented in the test room, no matter how they affect performance.

The Distinction between Diagnostic and Predictive Tests

When the audiologist uses diagnostic tests only to measure the present status of a patient's hearing, the validity of the tests has been established by relating measures obtained in the test room to external criteria, such as otologic diagnosis. In this manner, norms have been developed which provide information about the patient's auditory system without reference to his everyday listening performance.

The goal of hearing aid evaluation, however, is not to establish present function, but to predict the patient's future performance under amplification in the many communicative environments he will encounter. While it is sometimes conveniently assumed that the correspondence between test-room and everyday performance will be high, this relationship has not been established experimentally. The validity of hearing aid selection procedures seems, therefore, to be based solely on the apparent resemblance between test room and common listening tasks in the "outside world." This kind of dependency on face validity is always questionable, particularly in procedures like hearing aid comparison, where monosyllabic word lists and sound-treated rooms are rarely, if ever, encountered in the nonclinical environments about which predictions are to be made.

The Need to Improve Face Validity

High face validity is considered important only when empirical validation is lacking. Simply because test conditions may appear to resemble conditions in the real world does not assure that test performance will predict real-world performance. Therefore, until such time as test validity can be demonstrated empirically, it would seem to be imperative to control test variables in a manner that retains, as much as possible, the salient features likely to operate in the anticipated conditions in which the hearing aid will be used. This is apparently why Senturia et al. (1943), in the early days of hearing aid evaluation, recommended that clinics construct "typical living rooms" for use in testing the relative effectiveness of hearing aids. Improved face validity is also one of the purposes of recent attempts to generate sentence tests of speech discrimination (Berger 1967, Jerger, Malmquist, Speaks 1966) in which speech stimuli more nearly resemble ordinary conversation. Attempts to assess the effects of competing speech (Tillman et al. 1970, Carhart 1965) and room reverberation (Millin 1968) have been made for the same reason.

To ascertain validity experimentally, it is necessary to relate predictions of the relative performance of trial aids in the clinic on a suitable sample of patients to the relative performance of the same aids on the same patients outside the clinic. Simple as this may sound, the problems of validity testing are so formidable that, to my knowledge, no serious effort to ascertain the predictive validity of any selection procedure has ever been made.

Problems in Establishing the Validity of Selection Procedures

The most imposing problem is generating criteria that will adequately estimate the patient's aided performance in the many environments he will typically encounter. Like our clinical measures, the reliability of such criteria must be established, after which their validity as appropriate indicators of performance must also be determined. The problem of developing reliable measures of real-world performance is even more complex than the development of clinical tests because there are many uncontrollable sources of variability in everyday environments. Unfortunately, any attempt to manipulate these variables artificially represents an intrusion into the natural events that influence listening and thus tends to contaminate the validity of the measures. In fact, it appears that the mere act of observing the listener's behavior represents such an intrusion, particularly if the listener is aware that he is being observed. Problems of this kind discourage investigations of test validity.

Report of an Experiment with Improved Face Validity

Millin and Glaser (1971) reported a study in which Carhart's procedure for testing the effects of trial hearing aids on word discrimination in quiet was compared with a procedure that differed only in terms of the level at which speech was presented to the listener. The study demonstrated how a change in a single control variable, made for the purpose of improving face validity, can improve the audiologist's ability to draw inferences from test data.

Carhart's procedure requires that the patient set the gain of each trial aid for comfortable listening in response to ordinary speech presented in the field at 40 dB HL (about 60 dB SPL). Discrimiination scores are then determined by presenting monosyllabic word lists at a level 25 dB above the SRT obtained with each aid. This use of a constant sensation level for word presentation presumably serves the purpose of stabilizing the stimulus level at the listener's ear, thus permitting only the effect of electronic circuit differences among trial aids to influence test scores. This concept may, however, be fallacious. Since aid differences do, in fact, generate differences in the patient's threshold for speech, these differences would be expected to have important effects on performance in everyday listening. It would seem, therefore, that the effects of the various aids on SRT should be permitted to operate during discrimination testing.

When a constant sensation level is used to control the stimulus level reaching each trial aid, however, the differential effects of the aids on speech threshold are largely counteracted. By this device, an aid that produces highly effective gain for the patient will be handicapped by the use of a very low speech presentation level for discrimination testing. In contrast, an aid that produces a poor SRT will be given the advantage of a high word list presentation level. Since no such compensatory adjustment of stimulus intensity is possible in everyday listening, it seems inappropriate to permit it to occur in the test room. This amounts, in effect, to permitting the listener to "turn up" or "turn down" the volume of the talker. If he could do this, it is difficult to understand why he would need a hearing aid. A further confusion can result from this procedure, since with aids that produce relatively large differences in SRT one aid would be compared at soft-speech input with another with average- or loud-speech input. Furthermore, when the poor sensitivity of an aid is compensated for by increasing the level of speech with the audiometer, in effect the speech audiometer is being used to generate power the aid failed to provide.

Another effect results from manipulation of the stimulus level across aids. Often the open ear has a relatively good threshold, since it is common practice to leave the better ear open so that it can contribute to aided performance. Thus, when an aid produces a poor SRT, the practice of elevating the intensity of the speech signal not only increases the input to the hearing aid but elevates the sensation level to the open ear as well.

Such considerations led to comparisons of word discrimination scores obtained with Carhart's procedure with those obtained using a constant speech presentation level of 60 dB SPL. This level was chosen because it is commonly encountered and frequently presents problems for listeners. Two aids, one with a flat response and one with a rising response of 8 dB per octave were tested on 10 subjects with mild sensorineural impairment. The mean performance of the two aids was almost identical under both procedures, but the conventional procedure produced only two aid preferences when score differences of 6 percent or less were ignored. Under the constant stimulus level method, however, seven patients showed aid preferences generally of a magnitude over twice those obtained by the conventional method. Furthermore, retesting by the modified method produced the same seven preferences, whereas only one held up by the conventional procedure. It was relatively easy, therefore, to make unambiguous decisions by the modified (constant stimulus level) procedure. I cannot help but speculate that the constant stimulus level, because it permits the aid to function more as it would in everyday use, increases the sensitivity of word discrimination tests to differences in hearing aid frequency response effects.

It is not suggested that this study solves the problem of hearing aid selection. However, it does demonstrate that greater sensitivity may result from efforts to improve the rationale of test procedures. Also, it is worth noting that this is the only known study in which Carhart's procedure was followed precisely. The Shore et al. (1960) study employed a method of setting hearing aid gain which, in my opinion, produced gain levels far exceeding those patients would choose for themselves. It is interesting that they purported to test the value of Carhart's method, when the method they employed was not Carhart's but their own.

UNTESTED AXIOMS AND HYPOTHESES

I alluded earlier to the "intuitive and largely unscientific" practices employed by some audiologists. I have no wish whatever to disparage the importance of clinical judgment or experience. On the other hand, there are numerous clinical rules of thumb or general principles accorded wide acceptance without critical evaluation, even though they appear to lend themselves readily to experimental validation. Examples are numerous. Among them are, roughly paraphrased:

1. Fit the ear with the best discrimination.
2. Fit the ear with the flattest audiometric curve.
3. Fit the ear with the highest tolerance level.
4. All other things being equal, fit the ear with the poorest pure tone thresholds.
5. If monaural testing cannot be achieved with a very young child, use a Y cord or binaural fitting.

I take issue with these principles, not because they are not reasonable but because they are untested hypotheses. If their validity is ever tested, some of them may prove to be fallacious. I have seen patients with mild hearing losses, for example, who insist that they hear better with amplification in the ear that has better pure-tone thresholds, despite the fact that audiometric tests showed no significant differences in discrimination or tolerance.

There are other "axioms" that have found acceptance both within our own profession and with professionals from other fields. Some of them persist despite evidence against them. Others are simply so farfetched that it is sometimes difficult to believe they are taken seriously. I have no wish to insult anyone, so I will omit references here, but I would like to give some examples. There are those who hold that "marginal" or mild hearing losses cannot benefit from amplification. Having fitted a judge who had a loss of only about 20 dB in the speech range (this was many years ago, I might add) and who feels that his hearing aid literally saved his job, I am convinced of the fallacy of this concept. While there are doubtless marginal losses that will not benefit from amplification, there are a significant number that will. CROS fittings, incidentally, have proved particularly useful for some of these cases, primarily, I think, because of the open mold and its usefulness in giving a slight boost to the high frequencies, while permitting undistorted sound in the lower frequencies to reach the ear directly.

The strangest claim of all, perhaps, is that hearing aids are of no value to patients with "nerve" loss. It is hard to believe that many professionals are unaware that the overwhelming majority of hearing aid users have sensorineural impairment, and that most conductively impaired patients seek medical remediation rather than hearing aids. Nonetheless, patients still insist that they were advised not to wear aids because they have nerve loss.

Another often-heard claim is that amplification is of no value for patients with poor discrimination for speech. It is quite possible, of course, that even with amplification many patients will have a very difficult time understanding speech. The question is, however, whether they can understand anything at all without a hearing aid. Any improvement in the ability to understand speech at ordinary conversational levels will be welcomed by the patient who understands little or nothing without amplification. If aided discrimination is superior to unaided discrimination in response to speech presented at conversational levels, the patient is a likely candidate for amplication.

There are still audiologists who insist on body-worn hearing aids for patients whose hearing losses are severe. It is now clear, however, that patients rarely employ gain levels exceeding two-thirds of their hearing loss for speech. Some use even less than 50 percent (Millin 1965, McCandless 1974). Thus, head-worn hearing aids with maximum gain approaching 50 dB may prove quite adequate for selected patients with losses as high as 70 or 80 dB.

Another source of concern to me is the clinician who advocates some pet hearing aid evaluation theory with fanatic zeal. The more strongly he defends his theory, the less convinced I am of his objectivity or his competency. When an audiologist strongly advocates a particular evaluative system, knowing full well that no system enjoys scientific verification, his motives as well as his objectivity must be questioned.

THE FUTURE

If we are ever to have procedures that will unambiguously differentiate among the effects of hearing aids, I think new test strategies as well as new test materials must be generated. The search for novel approaches to evalution has, in fact, already begun (Bode and Carhart 1973). Before discussing potential solutions to the evaluation problem, however, assumptions underlying evaluative procedures require further consideration.

Despite the bleak picture I have drawn of the present state of the art, I have little doubt that effective procedures for detecting significant amplifier effects will soon be developed. When these procedures arrive, providing the criterion measure required in Resnick and Beckers' third assumption, the critical first and second assumptions may then be tested. I suspect that both of them will prove to be valid. The interactive assumption, however, will likely prove to be not a random interaction between individual listeners and hearing aids, but rather an interaction between definable subgroups of hearing loss and hearing aids. In other words, homogeneous groupings, such as patients with similar pure-tone and speech audiograms, common site of lesion, similar linguistic competencies, and similar physical and emotional health are likely to have similar amplification requirements. Some groups, however, like postmeningitis may show dissimilar performance. These latter patients may require individual selection procedures, while the more homogeneous groups will not. Needless to say, these predictions are speculative, but evidence supporting them is beginning to accumulate (Glaser 1974, Millin and Glaser 1971).

The Effect of Time on Performance

Chial and Hayes (1974) have raised the issue of the time dependency of listener and hearing aid interaction effects, suggesting that these are time-variant and thus cannot be sampled adequately at a single point in time. While this speculation has merit, I am not convinced that performance variation of significant magnitude continues indefinitely within a given environment. During my several years as a hearing aid dispenser, I had the opportunity to develop continuing relationships with nearly 1500 hearing aid wearers. It was clear to me that most of them exhibited listening performance remarkably stable over time, once the initial adjustment to amplification was completed. Variations in performance were seen in differing acoustic environments, but rarely within a single environment.

The issue seems to be, therefore, not whether tests at a single point in time can predict future aided performance, but whether some minimal period of experience is required before performance stabilizes sufficiently to make such predictions. There is the further question of whether tests will need to be performed in a number of environments typical of those encountered by the patient. I suspect that research will demonstrate that performance in varied environments can be predicted with acceptable precision from measures obtained in one or possibly two clinical environments. I also suspect that successful comparative evaluations will require sufficient listening practice to stabilize the patient's performance with each trial hearing aid.

The Chial and Hayes statement "that the assumptions about hearing aids and hearing-aid assessment given by Resnick and Becker (1963) are somewhat superficial, if not actually misleading'' is a glaring inconsistency in an otherwise illuminating article. It should be remembered that Resnick and Becker were speaking specifically of the Carhart procedures. They did not say that other procedures may not ultimately prove to be more useful. Obviously, the third assumption will play no part in a procedure that does not employ PB 50 word lists. The first assumption, however, is likely to hold true in any hearing-aid assessment system. I cannot possibly imagine why anyone, Chial and Hayes included, need concern themselves with hearing aids at all if we do not assume that ''there are significant differences among hearing aids in terms of how they enable the user to understand everyday speech.'' No assessment strategy can have any meaning if there is nothing to assess. As for the second assumption, its validity will determine whether the amplification requirements of every patient must be assessed individually or whether the needs of all patients can be predicted from data obtained from a single representative sample. This can hardly be considered a superficial question.

Directions for Future Research

Although such schemes seldom materialize, a national or even an international task force to identify promising research strategies and to coordinate and interrelate research activities would probably offer the best chance of solving the problems of hearing aid evaluation. There is little relation or continuity among research activities in amplification.

One of the first moves should be to abandon the preoccupation with present commercially available hearing aids. Existing hardware is not the concern; desirable electroacoustic characteristics are. We seem to approach hearing aid selection as though the ideal amplifiers for patients are already on the dispenser's shelves, and our principle task is simply to locate them. The fact is, however, that current instruments are far from ideal. I have always been impressed by the superior performance claimed by those who use television induction loops with their hearing aids. They invariably insist that the device dramatically improves their ability to understand speech and to enjoy music. Since the induction coil transformer couples the TV audio amplifier directly to the hearing aid amplifier without the intervention of distortion-producing transducers, it is not surprising that the listener can hear better. The point is, however, that the success of this device emphasizes how standard hearing aids fall short of providing optimum hearing for the hearing-impaired listener.

This suggests that research should employ amplifiers of high quality, the performance of which can be controlled with high precision. Once having identified desirable acoustic characteristics, one of the important functions of the audiologist should be to recommend to manufacturers that these characteristics be made available to the buyer. Little has been done to give direction to the manufacturer. This is unfortunate, since knowledge of the hearing process and the strategies and devices necessary to improve hearing are features that pressumably separate the audiologist from others who recommend or dispense hearing aids.

Stimulus Materials

There have been two traditional forms of speech-testing materials. The first are those in which redundancy has been reduced to a minimum, such as monosyllablic word lists. Other examples might be materials made up of distinctive feature differences, phonetic differences, or even contrasting nonsense syllables. The theory is that if the information in the stimulus is minimal, it will be difficult enough to discriminate that superior amplification systems will enable the listener to identify more items than inferior systems. It is assumed that if the listener can identify minimum information-bearing items readily, he will have even less difficulty with information-rich sentences.

The second class of test items has been sentence tests or tests in which redundancy is high and in which syntactical structure more nearly resembles genuine conversational content. The attempt here is to introduce more "realistic" or meaningful test items. In other words, face validity is improved. Furthermore, by introducing meaningful materials or common grammatical and syntactical forms, some underlying linguistic sufficiency is presumably sampled by the test. The greatest problem with this concept is that the test items are almost invariably too easy. Scores tend to hover near perfect performance and differentiation among hearing aids is actually reduced. There is the further formidable problem that the redundancy of meaningful material is dependent on the experience of the listener, and thus the effects of experience and amplifiers are confounded.

There appears to be merit in both approaches. The low redundancy tests, however, seem to offer the best short-term payoff for resolving the hearing aid evaluation problem.

Test Strategies

I hope I have already made a case for the use of a constant problem level for presentation of speech materials. The audiologist is really not very interested in how a listener responds to very high levels. He needs to know how the patient performs when listening to speech that ordinarily gives him difficulty. While I tend to prefer 60 dB (re. 20 μN/m^2), any problem level can be justified if it is a frequent problem level for the patient. What is critical, however, is that once a level is chosen, it should be held constant across trials of hearing aids. For a review of this problem, reread the section called "Report of an Experiment with Improved Face Validity."

One promising strategy is to literally train patients with each trial hearing aid before obtaining a performance measure. Short sets of test items can then be given continuously, with each set scored until improvement in performance stabilizes. The stabilized level will be taken as the performance measure for the hearing aid under test. The training and testing procedures are then repeated for subsequent trial aids and the superior performer selected for fitting. Of course, test materials will need development, but I suspect that randomly selected nonsense materials will suffice so long as a reasonably broad representation of phonetic elements is present in each subset. As few as 10 items per set may prove to be adequate. The critical element in this strategy is to provide the listener with substantial practice with each trial hearing aid.

Another variant of this concept employing similar stimuli may have potential value. This is the "constant effect" concept of Ebbinghaus (1913). The time required to attain a predetermined level of performance is employed as the dependent variable. The patient is trained to the predetermined performance level and the time required to attain the level is carefully measured. The hearing aid that enables the patient to reach the criterion level in the shortest period of time is assumed to be superior to the others in terms of how it enables the patient to process speech. This method offers an opportunity to drastically reduce testing time, which is always an important clinical consideration.

These suggestions by no means exhaust possible experimental approaches, nor do they address the problem of validity, which will not be effectively resolved until stable clinical measures are available. There is an additional approach to selection that has received limited attention but may prove to be among the most important, once superior tests are available. I am speaking of quality judgments and listener preferences (Jeffers 1960, Zerlin 1962). Success with this concept has again been limited by the instability of traditional measures. (Thompson and Lassman 1970). If, however, use of a constant speech presentation level effectively stabilizes hearing aid performance measures, correlation between these measures and listener preferences can then be tested. This was done recently by Weldele (1973), who found good agreement between the two sets of data. This suggests that preferences may yet prove to be a useful basis for hearing aid selection. The proposition that patients may reject an aid that is superior for them because the perceived quality of speech differs greatly from that to which they have grown accustomed was not borne out by Weldele's study.

PRESCRIPTIVE OR FORMULA FITTING

As noted earlier, the concept of selective amplification has persisted ever since the development of the electronic hearing aid (see Carhart, Introduction). There is compelling logic in the simple notion that a patient's gain requirements should be greater at frequencies where hearing loss is great than at frequencies where hearing loss is slight. Beyond this vague generalization we have no good idea as to how hearing aid gain and hearing loss should be related. As Carhart points out, "Clinical audiology has not yet formulated any systematic general theory as to the role and proper applications of selective amplification" (see Introduction).

Numerous systems for specifying appropriate hearing aid performance characteristics for clinic patients have been proposed (Lybarger 1963, Markle and Zaner 1966, Reddel and Calvert 1966, Gengel et al. 1971, Kee 1972, Butts and Creech 1972, Byrne and Tonnison 1976, Shapiro 1976, Berger et al. 1977). All such formulas or prescriptive techniques are based in great part on selective amplification.

Each of these systems provides some method for calculating specific hearing aid performance data by specifying mathematical operations to be performed on each patient's pure-tone data to arrive at a "gain-frequency response" presumably appropriate for the listener. Some systems also provide a means for specifying hearing aid saturation sound pressure levels, usually from UCL data. There seems to be a growing conviction that specification of output limitation is of major importance, primarily for the purpose of compressing the wide variation in speech intensities within the restricted dynamic range of comfort for individual patients.

One of the more recent of these systems, that of Berger, et al. (1977), seems to have been adopted in many clinics nationwide. This system specifies different divisors to be divided into the patient's thresholds at each speech frequency. The resultant values plus a reserve of 10 or 15 dB are then sent to a manufacturer to be built into an aid for the patient. Specific SSPL levels by frequency are also built into the hearing aid.

Since each formula generates a different set of amplifier characteristics for a given patient, the audiologist is faced with the task of deciding which system is likely to produce optimum speech intelligibility for the listener. This can be difficult, since the various schemes are backed by widely differing arguments, some largely speculative, others using available hearing aid research to varying degrees. The Berger et al. (1977) system, for example, makes substantial use of research on typical habits of instrument usage by "successful" hearing aid wearers. One can question, of course, whether typical behavior is necessarily optimum behavior, especially since most aid users do not have unlimited opportunity to try other fitting options. No matter how well satisfied a patient may be, we have no way of knowing whether he might be even better satisfied with a different aid. Despite this limitation of dependence on typical behavior, it is at present the most convincing data we have and, of the many formulas, I find that of Berger, et al. (1977) to be the best reasoned. Other audiologists may disagree.

A slightly different concept is described by Victoreen (1973), in which free-field responses of patients wearing a calibrated hearing aid are used to ascertain the coupler gain required to generate a comfortable equal loudness contour across the speech frequencies. The resulting loudness response presumably corresponds closely to speech comfort level and, as far as I can judge, is supposedly close to the loudness level perceived by normal hearing listeners. It is assumed that a flat loudness contour resembling that of normal ears will be optimum for hearing-impaired listeners. Frankly, I am not convinced that normal loudness response is even optimum for normal hearing listeners in certain listening environments.

Before considering practical and theoretical aspects of formulas, I hasten to point out that they all lack experimental validation at this time. It is true that the levels recommended by the various formulas can be verified by coupler or field measurement and that these measures have good repeatability. This "objectivity" is often touted as a major virtue of formulas. While these are indeed useful features, the greater issue is whether the formula derived measures do in fact represent appropriate fitting levels for hearing aid candidates.

While it is possible to show that patients are satisfied with results obtained by them, it has not been demonstrated that one formula produces better results than others or that any formula clearly identifies optimum or near-optimum hearing aid performance characteristics. The problems of establishing the real-world validity of these prescriptive procedures are as formidable as those of validating comparative procedures.

One objection raised by formula critics is that the manufacturer achieves the prescribed values by generating them in a standard 2-cm^3 coupler. It is argued that this does not accurately replicate the sound pressures which will occur in the patient's ear and that a Zwislocki coupler should be used instead. In my judgment this argument is trivial for two reasons. In the first place, differences among formulas are often larger than the differences produced by the couplers. Since there is no evidence that the levels produced by any formula are highly critical, it would be difficult to argue that slight differences between specified and obtained values are all that meaningful. Finally, both couplers represent an attempt to duplicate the impedance of the average adult ear. Since the individual ears of clinic patients vary greatly from average, neither coupler will accurately predict the levels that hearing aids will generate in specific patients. This is particularly true of children. Only real-ear measurements of some kind will determine what pressures will actually occur in a given patient's ear.

The Berger group recommends that aided free-field measures be obtained when the aid is returned from the manufacturer, with due attention given to the problems of field testing. The resulting thresholds are then compared to those which can be predicted by subtracting the recommended gain values from the patient's unaided thresholds in the aided ear. If they differ by more than a few decibels, Berger recommends that the instrument be returned to the manufacturer for readjustment. Since this requires only relative changes, the choice of coupler is no longer critical.

Practical and Theoretical Issues in Prescriptive Fitting

The efficiency and convenience of formula fitting are substantial. Only threshold and UCL data are needed. Children without speech or adults who, for one reason or another, cannot be tested with speech tests can be fitted quickly without need for a second appointment or lengthy evaluation. Furthermore, the formula provides a clear goal, and success in achieving it can be objectively measured by free-field testing. These are important advantages. If formulas could be shown to be as effective as traditional procedures, an important advance in clinical selection would be achieved. I know of no evidence favoring either strategy.

Prescriptive fitting raises many questions. One must believe that appropriate amplification for speech can be predicted solely from pure-tone or other non-speech data and, further, that all persons with identical audiograms should have identical hearing aids, no matter how speech scores or other data might differ among patients. The formulas also imply that thresholds for tones and tolerance levels are the most important features for predicting speech understanding and that the critical objectives in fitting hearing aids are to establish optimum frequency response, adequate intensity, and normal loudness response. This, I suggest, is an overpreoccupation with the purely intensive aspects of audition. Ward (1978) states the concept nicely:

> Even though you may get to the point where your loudness sensation is normal, this does not mean that you are hearing the same thing that you would hear if you had a normal cochlea. I think this is the issue we want to address here; just how sophisticated an approach is it feasible to use in processing speech in such a way that we both minimize the undesirable distortion produced by the instrument itself, and also do something to the speech that will allow it to be more easily perceived by this particular faulty cochlea.

Clearly, by concerning ourselves solely with loudness and intensity, we may be overlooking parameters which are more critical to successful function of the faulty auditory mechanism. We are just beginning to examine other potential strategies (Yanick 1978). With the growing sophistication in microcircuitry, for example, we can begin to examine how speech might be recoded into unconventional units which may be better perceived by impaired ears.

As for frequency response, I think it unlikely that a single response will serve a patient equally well in all environments. It is likely that several options should be available to patients as they move from one acoustic condition to another. There is evidence, for example, that listeners hear better in noise with dramatic low-frequency suppression but that they prefer restoration of the lows in quiet (Harford and Fox, 1978). During my dispensing years I attempted to solve listener problems by studying particular environments which gave them difficulty. In addition to frequency response modification, solutions often required switching the aid to the opposite ear, binaural fitting, CROS-type variations (see Chapter 7), special microphone placement, and other strategies related to the effects of environmental noise, head shadow, reverberation, or weak signals.

These experiences suggest that factors other than frequency response are of critical importance in aid selection and fitting. Formulas do not, for example, generally deal with extension of the upper frequency range (Triantos and McCandless 1974) or reduction of low frequencies in noise. One of the virtues of the evaluation method described by Jerger and Hayes (1976) is that it permits testing of positional effects and as such broadens the scope of hearing aid evaluation to take cognizance of factors other than frequency response, which has been the major preoccupation of formulas. These and countless other issues must be understood before true sophistication in specifying hearing aids can be achieved. The greatest danger in adopting any universal selection strategy at this time, when we know so little about a number of factors which may be important, is that we may retard the search for better methods. Students in particular, often seek "cookbook" solutions to complex problems and tend to accept uncritically schemes promoted by teachers or other authority figures. At present, formulas should be regarded as useful interim strategies representing hypotheses to be tested and revised as research and experience dictate.

Speech Testing and Formulas

Despite uncertainties surrounding formulas, I have found the Berger et al. (1977) procedures to be useful. I do not see substantial differences between fittings recommended by this formula and those arrived at by comparative procedures. This fact more than any other makes it difficult to justify the tedious comparative process. On the other hand, I am bothered by the lack of any dependence on speech tests. Until such time that I am convinced that nonspeech stimuli can unerringly predict a patient's hearing for speech I feel compelled to use speech measures to test the adequacy of formula recommendations. I feel it is mandatory to evaluate in some manner how the patient performs using a real hearing aid and listening to real speech.

Certain free-field comparative measures seem to me to be of particular value. I view the free-field PB max score as a rough estimate of the patient's optimum ability to discriminate speech, even though the audiometer has a flat frequency response which may not be ideal for the listener. This score serves as an approximate goal to be reached with a hearing aid when speech is presented at conversation level (60 to 65 dB SPL). Unaided WDS in the field at conversation level serves as an estimate of discrimination under typical listening conditions. The difference between this score and PB max is a useful estimate of the amount of improvement an appropriate hearing aid should provide. If the unaided score at conversation level approximates unaided PB max, it is doubtful that amplification will be successful.

After years of using these measures to compare hearing aid frequency response effects, I am convinced that frequency response differences produce dramatic performance differences for only a few listeners who appear to be particularly sensitive to slope variations. Only speech testing will identify such persons. A very few listeners, however, actually do more poorly aided than unaided. Alteration of frequency response generally does little to improve the performance of such persons and they are rarely good hearing aid candidates.

The Controversy

There is an emotional controversy between advocates of comparative evaluation and advocates of prescriptive formulas. The comparative evaluation group sees formulas as arbitrary and oversimplified. They want to know why 2 is the precisely correct divisor at 500 Hz or why 2.5 wouldn't do as well. They ask how to be sure that the listener will, during his daily pursuits, adjust the gain to the levels specified in the formulas. Formula advocates, on the other hand, are not convinced that comparative procedures do, in fact, detect differences among trial aids in view of the demonstrated excessive variability of speech measures. Neither do they see a reasonable basis for trial aid preselection, in view of the almost unlimited number of parameters that could be compared, or the formidable problems in specifying performance characteristics cleanly.

Neither group seems to realize that its major challenge is to the validity of the other's method. There simply is no convincing evidence that either system clearly identifies optimum hearing aids for listeners. Neither has it been shown that clear differences in general recommendations result between methods. All this uncertainty could lead us to believe that neither method is of value. My belief is that, given the limitations of current hardware, both produce satisfactory recommendations for the most part, which is why we do not see startling differences between results obtained by either method. I suspect that small differences in mid-range frequency response may prove to be less critical to success than other performance parameters, once research begins to isolate the critical variables.

DISPENSING BY AUDIOLOGISTS

Dispensing is extensively discussed elsewhere in this book, so I will make only a few observations and predictions. Most audiologists will soon be dispensing and even those who will not will need to be informed on the subject. The emphasis of your practice will change in many ways as, for the first time, you will have a long and continuing relationship with your patients and will come to know most of them as individuals. This experience will help us to better understand the patient's problems and requirements, but it will also generate new duties and responsibilities.

I expect audiologists to adopt the optometric practice of selling hearing aids for a reasonable profit. The cost of hearing aid sales is surprisingly high if done ethically and with quality service to the patient. This will require additional administrative personnel; new record-keeping and accounting procedures; efficient business machines; additional space; high telephone and postal expense; an inventory of batteries, accessories, and hearing aids; new and unexpected tools; vendor's licenses; repair services or facilities; an advertising budget; occasional evening hours; and numerous other costly extras. It is inconceivable to me that these requirements can be supported from any anticipated increase in caseload. It will soon become evident that these costs of sales must be absorbed in the hearing aid selling price (Millin 1972).

There will also be temptations. I have had enough private conversations with clinic directors to know that at least some see hearing aid dispensing as a potential source of added income. I hasten to point out that there is ample evidence that hearing aid sales are not very profitable (Kefauver Report 1962). The two major advantages I see in dispensing are the opportunity to provide a complete and continuing service to the patient including postfitting training, which was largely discouraged by traditional dispensers, and the opportunity to research and refine rehabilitative techniques.

The distinction between dealer and audiologist will slowly vanish along with the friction between them as more and more audiologists take on this responsibility. The level of training and competence among dispensers will rise sharply and the availability of rehabilitative services within the same establishment will improve service to the public. If we approach dispensing with a determination to upgrade the quality of our product, to resist temptations to sell unnecessary frills, and to maintain our efforts in research and development, the hearing-impaired public will be the great benefactor.

THE STATUS OF AUDIOLOGY

Recent attacks on audiology from traditional dispensers and, unexpectedly, from otology are probably the best evidence that audiology has come of age. The academic and practicum requirements, the high ethical standards, and the voluminous research of audiologists have made them easily the most knowledgeable hearing aid rehabilitationists in the world.

Problems with dispensers will be resolved by the gradual infusion of audiologists into dispensing. To the competent and ethical traditional dispenser this will pose no threat. Many have been employing trained audiologists for years. The only real threat is to the untrained and unethical dispenser. No one will mourn his passing.

The relationship with otolaryngology is another matter. Audiologists and otolaryngologists have worked together harmoniously for nearly 40 years, each publishing research in the other's journals. It is a rare ear specialist today who does not have one or more audiologists on his staff. An attempt has been made by the National Hearing Aid Society to convince physicians that audiologists plan to compete with them in medical diagnosis and treatment of hearing disorders. Perhaps a few mindless audiologists somewhere may have such intentions. It is clear that the profession itself does not, nor has our professional organization ever permitted or advocated such activity. We are interested in diagnostic auditory tests only to the extent that they can add useful information to that obtained by physicians to aid them in diagnosis. We have no interest in medical treatment whatever. The perceived threat to medicine is a fiction.

Working together, audiologists and otolaryngologists can provide a complete service to the hearing-impaired that neither can accomplish alone. If audiologists have any concern, it is that some physicians feel compelled to manage and control nonmedical aspects of audition that deal with communicative problems, whether or not they have any training or expertise in this area. Historically, few physicians have shown great interest or undergone extensive training in rehabilitative audiology. I cannot imagine why they would want to waste time in relatively unprofitable activities in a field outside their preparation. In the most successful institutions I have seen, both medical and audiologic services are offered, each practitioner leaving the other to pursue his own specialty. The current crisis will pass quickly as more and more physicians come to appreciate how well we complement each other. In the meantime, it is incumbent upon audiology to continue to pursue the highest possible academic clinical and research standards.

ACKNOWLEDGMENT

I am extremely appreciative of the invaluable critical review or technical assistance in the preparation of this paper by the following persons: Martin R. Adams, Kenneth W. Berger, Cheryl Croskey, Jennybel Millin, Mary Ann Reiser, and Martin Schultz.

BIBLIOGRAPHY

ACO: Report of ACO Subcommittee on Hearing Aids. Newsletter of the American Council of Otolaryngology, September, 1977

Berger KW: The KSU speech discrimination test. Kent State University, Kent, Ohio, 1967. Tape recorded tests available from Audiotone, Inc.

Berger KW, Hagberg EN, Rane RL: Prescription of Hearing Aids: Rationale, Procedure, and Results. Kent, Ohio, Herald Publishing House, 1977

Berger KW, Millin JP: Hearing aids, in Rose DE (ed) Audiological Assessment. Englewood Cliffs, Prentice-Hall, 1971

Bode DL, Carhart R: Measurement of articulation functions using adaptive test procedures. IEEE Trans Audio Electroacoust 21:196−20, 1973

Bode DL, Kasten RN: Hearing aid distortion and consonant identification. J. Speech Hear Res 14:323−331, 1971

Butts FM, Creech HB: Tracing the MCL: An approach to hearing aid selection. Paper presented at the Convention of the American Speech and Hearing Association, 1972

Byrne D, Tonnison W: Selecting the gain of hearing aids for persons with sensorineural hearing impairments. Scand Aud 5:51−59, 1976

Campbell RA: Discrimination test word difficulty. J Speech Hear Disor 8:13−22, 1965

Carhart R: Selection of hearing aids. Arch Otolaryngol 44:1−18, 1946a

Carhart R: Volume control adjustment in hearing aid selection. Laryngoscope 56:510−526, 1946b

Carhart R: Tests for the selection of hearing aids. Laryngoscope 56:780−794, 1946c

Carhart R: Hearing aid selection by university clinics. J Speech Hear Disor 15:106−113, 1950

Carhart R: Monaural and binaural discrimination against competing sentences. Int Audiol 5−10, 1965

Chial MR, Hayes CS: Hearing aid evaluation methods: Some underlying assumptions. J Speech Hear Disor 39:270−279, 1974

Davis H, Hudgins CV, Marquis RJ, et al: The selection of hearing aids. Laryngoscope 56:85−115, 135−163, 1946

Dodds E, Harford E: Modified earpieces and CROS for high-frequency hearing losses. J Speech Hear Res 11:204−218, 1968

Dodds E, Harford E: Follow-up report on modified earpieces and CROS for high-frequency hearing losses. J Speech Hear Res 13:41−43, 1970

Ebbinghaus H: Memory: A contribution to experimental psychology. 1885. HA Ruger, CE Bussenius (Tr), New York, Teacher's College, Columbia University, 1913

Elpern BS: Differences in difficulty among CID W-22 auditory test. Laryngoscope 70:1560−1565, 1960

Erber NP: Evaluation of special hearing aids for deaf children. J Speech Hear Disor 36:527−537, 1971

Gengel RW, Pascoe D, Shore I: A frequency response procedure for evaluating and selecting hearing aids for severely hearing impaired children. J Speech Hear Dis 36:341−353, 1971

Glaser R: Hearing aid evaluations using spectral density classified word lists, doctoral dissertation, Kent State University, Kent, Ohio, 1974

Harford ER: The clinical application of CROS, Arch Otolaryngol 83:455−464, 1966

Harford ER: Bilateral CROS. Arch Otolaryngol 84:426−432, 1966

Harford E, Barry J: A rehabilitative approach to the problem of unilateral hearing impairments. The contralateral routing of signals (CROS). J Speech Hear Disor 30:121−138, 1965

Harford ER, Fox J: The use of high-pass amplification for broad-frequency sensorineural hearing loss. Audiology J Audit Comm 17:10−26, 1978

Harris JD, Haines HL, Kelsey PA, et al: The relation between speech intelligibility and the electroacoustic characteristics of low fidelity circuitry. J Audit Res 5:357−381, 1961

Jeffers J: Quality judgment in hearing aid selection. J Speech Hear Disor 25:259−266, 1960

Jeffers J, Smith C: On hearing aid selection, in part a reply to Resnick and Becker. ASHA 6:504−506, 1964

Jerger J, Speaks C, Malmquist C: Hearing aid performance and hearing aid selection. J Speech Hear Res 9:136−149, 1966

Jerger J, Malmquist C, Speaks C: Comparison of some speech intelligibility tests in the evaluation of hearing aid performance. J Speech Hear Res 9:253−258, 1966

Jerger J, Thelin J: Effects of electroacoustic characteristics of hearing aids on speech understanding. Bull Prosthet Res 159−197, 1968

Jerger, J, Hayes, D: Hearing aid evaluation: Clinical experience with a new philosophy. Arch Otolaryngol 102:214−225, 1976

Kee WR: Use of pure tone measurement in hearing aid fittings. Audecibel 9−15, Winter 1972

Kefauver Report: Prices of hearing aids. Hearings, Subcommittee on Antitrust and Monopoly, Committee on the Judiciary, United States Senate, 1962

Ling d: Implications of hearing aid amplification below 300 cps. Volta Rev 66:723−729, 1964

Ling D, Maretic H: Frequency transposition in the teaching of speech to deaf children. J Speech Hear Res 14:37−46, 1971

Lybarger SF: Simplified fitting system for hearing aids. Radioear Specifications and Fitting Manual, 1963 1−8

Margolis R, Millin J: An item-difficulty based speech discrimination test. J Speech Hear Res 14:865−873, 1971

Markle DM, Zaner A: The determination of gain requirements of hearing aids: a new method. J Audit Res 6:371−377, 1966

McCandless GA: High frequency hearing loss and hearing aid selection. International Hearing Aid Seminar, San Diego, 1974

McConnell F, Silber EF, McDonald D: Test-retest consistency of clinical hearing aid tests. J Speech Hear Disor 25:273−280, 1960

Millin JP: Speech discrimination as a function of hearing aid gain: Implications in hearing aid evaluation, masters thesis. Western Reserve University, Cleveland, Ohio, 1965

Millin JP: The effect of small room reverberation on discrimination tests, doctoral dissertation. Case-Western Reserve University, Cleveland, Ohio, 1968

Millin JP: Conventional hearing aid selection. ASHA 5:880−881, 1963

Millin JP: A review of specific tasks involved in hearing aid dispensing. Paper presented at the Convention of the American Speech and Hearing Association, 1972

Millin JP, Glaser R: Comparison of a traditional and modified hearing aid selection procedure. Seminar: Amplification for Sensorineural Hearing Loss, Audiology Center of Redlands, Twin Peaks, California, 1971

Pollack M, Lipscomb, D: Implications of hair cell-pure tone discrepancies for oto-audiologic practice. Aud Hear Educ 5:16−23, 36, 1979

Posner J, Ventry IM: Relationships between comfortable loudness levels for speech and speech discrimination in sensorineural hearing loss. J Speech Hear Disor 42:370−375, 1977

Reddell RC, Calvert DR: Selecting a hearing aid by interpreting audiologic data. J Audit Res 6:445−452, 1966

Resnick DM, Becker M: Hearing aid evaluation—a new approach. ASHA 5:695−699, 1963

Ross M: Hearing aid evaluation, in J Katz (ed): Handbook of Clinical Audiology. Baltimore, Williams & Wilkins, 1972

Schmitz HD: Loudness discomfort level modification: J Speech Hear Res 12:807−817, 1969

Senturia B, Silverman SR, Harrison CE: A hearing aid clinic. J Speech Hear Disor 8:215−226, 1943

Shapiro I: Hearing aid fitting by prescription. Audiol 15:163−173, 1976

Shore I, Bilger RC, Hirsh IJ: Hearing aid evaluation: reliability of repeated measurements. J Speech Hear Disor 25:152−170, 1960

Shore I, Kramer J: A comparison of two procedures for hearing aid evaluation. J Speech Hear Disor 28:159–170, 1965

Thompson G, Lassman F: Listener Preference for Selective vs. Flat Amplification for a High Frequency Hearing Loss Population, J Speech Hear Res 13:670–672, 1970

Tillman T, Carhart R, Olsen W: Hearing aid efficiency in a competing speech situation. J Speech Hear Res 13:789–811, 1970

Triantos TJ, McCandless, GA: High frequency distortion. Hearing Aid: June, 1974

Victoreen JA: Basic principles of otometry, Springfield, Ill, Charles C. Thomas, 1973

Ward WD: The effects of noise on speech communication, in Yanich P (ed): The Application of Signal Processing Concepts to Hearing Aids (chap 2). New York, Grune & Stratton, 1978

Weldele FJ: The usefulness of psychophysical listener judgments in hearing aid evaluation, masters thesis. Kent State University, Kent, Ohio, 1973

Yanich P Jr: The Application of Signal Processing Concepts to Hearing Aids. New York, Grune & Stratton, 1978

Yantis PA, Millin JP, Shapiro I: Speech discrimination in sensorineural hearing loss: Two experiments on the role of intensity. J Speech Hear Res 9:178–193, 1966

Zerlin S: A new approach to hearing aid selection. J Speech Hear Res 5:370–376, 1962

Henry D. Schmitz

5

Hearing Aid Selection For Adults

As of this writing, there is no general agreement among audiologists as to what is the best procedure for selecting and evaluating hearing aids for adults. For the most part, many of the approaches which have been presented over the years appear to be defensible. Unfortunately, with the present state of the art and the availability of clinical tools, no one procedure can be proven to be superior to the others.

In this chapter, Henry Schmitz examines some of the classic and current approaches to hearing aid selection and evaluation. He brings many years of theoretical and clinical background to this endeavor, and its content should stimulate a good deal of thought and discussion among the hearing-health community.

MCP

The audiologist's hearing aid selection procedures are intended to provide a hearing aid that allows the patient to obtain optimum acoustic compensation and meet practical needs. Traditionally, the measures that demonstrate such performance, compared to the unaided conditions, have been improved speech reception threshold and speech discrimination in quiet, competing noise, or in competing speech. Theoretically, the hearing aid should satisfy all of the patient's practical problems. It should be dependable, manageable, rugged, unaffected by temperature variations and moisture, and have minimal harmonic and transient distortion and subaudible feedback. Good signal reproduction, efficient output limiting, and long battery life are also important. As desirable as these goals are, they are impossible to meet totally at this time.

Nevertheless, far from abandoning the responsibility to demonstrate and assure such difficult-to-attain goals, the audiologist is now using more imaginative and sophisticated approaches to evaluate hearing aid procedures. Rather than being less involved in hearing aid evaluation and in recommending auditory rehabilitation, the audiologist appears to be more involved. This is exemplified by his utilization of technologic advances, new stimuli that create a more realistic listening situation, competing speech and noise, and rating scales for understanding the subjective behavioral effectiveness of amplification.

This chapter reviews some current and recommended approaches to hearing aid selection. Potential problem areas involving stimuli, presentation levels, acoustic environments, and special instrumentation are presented.

In addition, this chapter suggests a reconsideration of comfortable, habitual, clinical viewpoints. For example, it is suggested that expanding beyond the traditional procedures, through experimentation and new approaches, may help the clinician to create a supportable series of tools that will assure optimum acoustic compensation for the hearing-impaired adult. Such tools depend initially on accurate determination of candidacy and preselection of hearing aids. Assessing the benefits of amplification through functional measures, such as nonspeech-based stimuli, appears to be predictive of differences between hearing aids.

Hearing loss previously regarded as unsatisfactory for amplification purposes includes the following: namely, mild losses, high frequency and mid-frequency basin-shaped losses and profound losses requiring body-type amplification, all of which can be aided satisfactorily by ear-level hearing aids. In addition, the introduction of KEMAR allows measurement of absolute hearing aid performance. Such new information demonstrates problems with a master hearing aid approach. It is also instrumental in removing more of the previously unknown, which has been excused as the "art" of the hearing aid selection process.

Despite these advances, the clinician must recognize the functional limitations imposed by anatomical and physiologic changes in the auditory system. Neural pathway degeneration in presbycusis, central processing problems, cochlear degeneration due to ototoxic effects, or trauma to the ear, are problems that require special efforts by the clinician. Reality counseling, changing expectations, and proper motivation of the patient assure that the true benefits of amplification will not be obscured. If unrealistic expectations are not properly managed, the patient may be dissatisfied with amplification. Alpiner's (1973) survey of 119 patients showed that 33 percent did not receive the benefits that they expected. Seventeen percent wished to know more about the difficulties rather than the advantages they would encounter with a hearing aid. Family members and friends frequently have the greatest expectations for aided communicative function. Often they do not understand the difficulties that an elderly patient or a stroke victim has at a dinner-table conversation. Modifying the communicative expectations and habits of those with normal hearing is frequently the most difficult task, and is the only guarantee that the hearing-impaired individual will have some modicum of communicative success.

Therefore, assessing the patient's communicative complaints and needs is critical prior to any type of hearing aid evaluation. Such an approach is not limited to merely providing a hearing aid, but focuses on solving as many of a patient's communicative difficulties as possible. As the audiologist dispenses the hearing aid and determines its benefits, he must also accept responsibility for total aural rehabilitation of the patient.

Once the audiologist performs the necessary analysis and recommends or dispenses an aid, he can no longer only be content with generated data. He must relate that data to the patient's adjustment needs and communicative satisfaction. *If this is not done successfully, then perhaps the audiologist should function solely within the legally safe sanctitude of academia.*

This chapter is written from the viewpoint of the audiologist as a dispenser of hearing aids. Consequently, the focus is on making the audiologist's recommendations clinically defensible and valid. This chapter emphasizes that *there is no single standard of hearing aid selection; no valid predictor of a hearing aid's performance for all possible acoustic conditions that an individual may encounter.* One approach for the professional to consider is to eliminate the concern of discovering the "best hearing aid for a person" and to focus, as Ross (1976) has suggested, on the electroacoustic dimensions that relate positively to intelligibility, and to select those aids for evaluation that embody the desired design characteristics.

CANDIDACY FOR AMPLIFICATION

Hearing loss by itself cannot determine candidacy for amplification per se. The individual's communicative requirements become the primary determining factor. An additional consideration is the age of the individual. Hearing impairment increases markedly as age increases. Solving the communicative complaints of the aged is a major activity of the clinical audiologist. The Federal Trade Commission (1978) estimates that 30% of the 20 million Americans over the age of 65 have significant hearing impairments. The elderly, then, constitute nearly half of the more than 14.5 million people in the United States who have hearing problems.

In the past, a considerable number of potentially successful hearing aid users have been denied the benefits of amplification because of strict application of assumptions about communicative abilities described solely by pure tone hearing loss, speech reception thresholds, or speech discrimination. Furthermore, as Berger (1979) has suggested, the patient's lifestyle also is an important consideration for candidacy for amplification. An inactive lifestyle (and nondemanding communication) in fact may not require the use of a hearing aid unless the hearing threshold loss in the region of 1,000−4,000 Hz in the better ear is worse than 30 dB. However, applying such rules about hearing aid candidacy may not be in the best interests of the hearing-impaired. *Candidacy is more properly determined by the patient's communicative difficulty, not by an average hearing loss expressed in dB HL.* Therefore, table guides matching dB hearing levels with possible communicative needs (Hodgson, 1977) are not reviewed here.

Sanders (1978) gives examples of how the old rules about hearing aid candidacy simply do not apply today. One of his examples is of the frequently encountered high frequency hearing loss with normal low frequency hearing sensitivity. Another example is of the patient with an unaided speech discrimination score of 60% who may have been advised that a hearing aid will be of little benefit. That 60% score changes to 90% in quiet, and 88% in noise, with the use of a hearing aid. It is not uncommon that high frequency hearing losses make a substantial gain in speech discrimination, as much as 30% or more, in the presence of competing noise. *The criterion measure is aided speech discrimination in sound field in the presence of competing noise, rather than speech discrimination in quiet, either under earphones or in sound field without a hearing aid.*

Predicting hearing aid performance solely on the basis of responses to stimuli under earphones should be avoided. For example, a patient with a severe hearing loss in each ear in excess of 70−80 dB, and with poor monaural speech discrimination, has usually been regarded as a poor candidate for amplification. However, the binaural speech discrimination cannot be predicted from the monaural speech discrimination score under earphones, nor can monaural aided speech discrimination be predicted from the earphone measurement. The earphone measurement may show that the patient has an insufficient sensation level to achieve maximum speech discrimination. The insufficiency can be overcome with the use of a hearing aid, and the patient's monaural speech discrimination may be markedly improved.

The clinician should keep in mind the patient's needs as they relate to gain requirements: the aid's maximum output and frequency response, the presence of a telephone switch, the location of the microphone, the output-limiting characteristics, and the ease of manipulation and location of the volume control. Equally as important are questions asked of the patient regarding his needs for amplification:

1. Is there a need within his social environment and his vocational setting to hear and understand speech better?
2. Is he having personal problems in communication of which he is aware, and is he willing to confront and solve these problems?
3. Is he aware of the potential advantages of amplification?
4. Is he aware of the limitations of amplification?
5. What demands are being placed on him currently for communication with which he is not satisfied?
6. What is his family's attitude and their willingness to assist him?

7. Does he have physical limitations that make the manipulation of a hearing aid volume control difficult?
8. What is his honest attitude toward the use of a hearing aid?

Hopefully, the patient will answer these questions honestly. His feelings and his problems can then be explored further. The use of inventories of communicative disabilities and the various scales discussed later in this chapter may provide additional information. However, candidacy for amplification is usually not determined by these scales. The scales do provide information about the effectiveness of the hearing aid related to specific communication problems. Lamb's (1974) Speech Discrimination Assessment Scale, for example, focuses on the potential hearing aid user's ability to understand speech in a number of different social and vocational contents, in quiet and in competing noise. A revised 90-item form is now available. The use of inventories and scales are helpful because the patient is frequently unaware of his communication problems. It is the family and friends who often motivate the individual to seek help. Only after the hearing evaluation does the patient begin to gain insight into his communication problems. Then Griffing's (1978) suggestion can be applied ". . . solutions must be arrived at by letting the client identify and describe his problems and concerns."

TYPE OF HEARING AID

The type of hearing aid for a patient is determined by his/her needs, desires, and factors of physical comfort, such as the ease of adjusting the volume control. Most of the hearing aids worn by patients today are postauricular hearing aids (see Chapter 2). The all-in-the-ear hearing aid has increased in application. Eyeglass and body type hearing aids are utilized only for special patient preferences and needs.

The type of instrument to be considered for evaluation is usually dictated by the patient's preference. Despite the patient's preference, however, clinical judgment may have to prevail. If the hearing loss is severe, and satisfactory gain cannot be achieved with an all-in-the-ear hearing aid, then the use of such a hearing aid should be discouraged. Likewise, even though the patient would like the practical appeal of an eyeglass type hearing aid, such an aid is not in his best interest if he does not wear eyeglasses consistently throughout the day. Nevertheless, unless the patient has a very clear understanding of why his preferences cannot be satisfied, he will sooner or later usually acquire the hearing aid that he wants, with or without an audiologist's involvement. If the audiologist's persuasion is ineffective, then practical experience or a trial period with such amplification may be instrumental in convincing the patient to modify his viewpoint.

Although all-in-the-ear aids constitute more and more of the hearing aid market, feedback problems and venting techniques do create definite limitations.

When these problems become unsolvable, then the use of an ear-level instrument must be recommended. The use of the power CROS (see Chapter 7), may be helpful for this kind of a problem. Power CROS will allow postauricular amplification in many cases of severe hearing loss that, due to feedback problems, cannot be corrected either with an ear-level or an all-in-the-ear hearing aid.

In turn, if physical manipulation is a problem with ear-level instrumentation, then a body type hearing aid must be considered. This is especially true for severely arthritic individuals who cannot manipulate the insertion and control of an ear-level hearing aid. The success of amplification is much greater when the patient uses a larger unit with more easily adjustable volume controls. The body type hearing aid is also applicable to hearing losses that exceed gain abilities of ear-level hearing aids.

Bone conduction body aids are still utilized today for certain conditions that do not allow the use of an earmold, power CROS, or ear level amplification. Anatomical problems of the pinna and external ear canal that are nonsurgically reversible may require the use of bone conduction amplification. Some manufacturers still produce an eyeglass temple vibrator that can be used for bone conduction amplification. However, such eyeglass vibrators usually do not provide consistent or optimal pressure of the vibrator against the skull. The best results with bone conduction hearing aids appear to be achieved with those having broad frequency, high gain, and low distortion. A conventional headband mounted bone conduction transducer is used with either a body or post-auricular aid.

In general, the best candidate for amplification is the patient who experiences the least distortion of incoming speech signals, the widest dynamic range, and the greatest loss of sensitivity. If the poorer ear cannot be considered a candidate for amplification, then the better ear is selected. An attempt is always made to achieve equivalency between the ears by balancing the hearing levels.

Unfortunately, the individuals who frequently need amplification the most, namely, those with severe deterioration of the central auditory system and with temporal problems of speech intelligibility and auditory memory (Konkle et al., 1977), are also the ones who are the most poorly motivated and who give up hope.

PRESELECTION

Determination of Needed Amplification Characteristics

The selection of hearing aids to be used in the hearing aid evaluation process is determined by the monaural unaided functions of:

1. The severity of hearing loss.
2. The frequency configuration of the hearing loss.

3. Speech discrimination.
4. Most comfortable loudness level (MCL).
5. Loudness discomfort level (LDL).

The configuration of the hearing loss, speech discrimination ability for each ear, the MCL of each ear, and the loudness discomfort level (LDL), together comprise the hearing aid's functional chracteristics of frequency response, gain characteristics, and maximum output limitations.

It is imperative that preselection of the hearing aid is made on the basis of pure tone thresholds that lie within the frequency range of the hearing aid. However, the patient may complain of sharpness or metallic quality. High frequency emphasis amplification for high frequency hearing losses may then have to be modified. The patient may, in fact, do better with a flat frequency response that is modified by the earmold (see Chapter 3).

Berger's (1979) gain-frequency response formula (presented later in this chapter) is an interesting approach to hearing aid selection. The formula is for an ear-level hearing aid with a front microphone, closed earmold, and sensorineural hearing loss. Changing any of these factors forces a change in the response formula. The formula seeks to establish maximum gain on the basis of air conduction threshold sensitivity. It provides excessive gain for mild and moderate losses at 500 Hz and reduced gain for threshold levels of 50 dB or more at 500 Hz. Berger's (1979) approach recognizes that reducing the gain for low frequencies facilitates the reception of speech in most situations.

Piminow (1963) recommends reducing the gain of amplification for those patients whose hearing loss exceeds 60 dB HL. He suggests that since the dynamic range will be restricted, the potential for internal distortion is great. This approach is similar to Huizing's et al., (1960) "Triplet" audiometry. Both authors suggest using filtered speech discrimination materials. In their tests, if speech discrimination was poor for any one of the three band pass conditions, then this region would not be amplified. Consideration was given to decreasing the gain of an instrument for those regions that had the greatest hearing loss. In the preselection process the subtleties of reducing gain in those areas where the hearing loss is actually greatest may be difficult to predict. Hence, the classic mirroring approach may be the most efficient for the clinician to use initially. Later, if the clinician is alert, modifications of the hearing aid's responses can be made.

A strict mirroring approach can lead to over-fitting a patient's loss—a frequent criticism heard by audiologists. The error is committed because the gain characteristics required by a hearing aid user are related exactly to the pure tone hearing loss. Describing the requirements of the hearing aid's gain in terms of dB sound pressure has the same potential problems.

Shapiro's (1978) approach reduces the risk of over-fitting. To arrive at the gain characteristic of an instrument, he suggests the use of a formula of one-half of the patient's hearing threshold level for narrow bands of noise. Another approach is to predict the gain requirements of a hearing aid. This is done by taking the speech reception threshold and dividing it by two. Clinical experience suggests that a hearing aid user will generally set the gain control of his hearing aid to a midpoint of his most comfortable loudness level. This level may also approximate the point at which the speech discrimination is maximum (Yantis et al., 1966).

The most comfortable loudness level (MCL) can be established with speech stimuli for each ear to determine the most comfortable hearing level above the SRT. The MCL's importance for purposes of hearing selection is not accepted by everyone. Berger et al. (1979) believe that the MCL has too much test-retest variability and that it is a difficult psychoacoustic task influenced by background noise. They feel that the MCL affects maximum speech discrimination scores only.

The loudness discomfort level (LDL) test determines which ear has the best dynamic range for loudness. The LDL may also reflect near normal or better hearing sensitivity within the hearing loss range for certain frequencies. As Kamm et al. (1978) have demonstrated, there is considerable variation in the sound pressure level over which LDLs occur for individuals with the same hearing thresholds. Thirty of their subjects had LDLs that exceeded 124 dBSPL. These subjects were assumed to have cochlear pathology. When used for hearing aid preselection and/or hearing aid evaluation procedures, LDL, as MCL, must be measured directly. Predicting an LDL from hearing threshold measures should be avoided (Kamm et al., 1978). Such a procedure is highly inaccurate.

LDL can be established using either pure tones or spondees. Since the dynamic range of loudness is most appropriately determined with speech, speech stimuli, such as nonsense syllables or running speech, should be used.

LDL can be assessed with an up-down adaptive procedure applied to both LDL and MCL measurements as described by Kamm et al. (1978). Ten dB steps in an up-down procedure are utilized ascending from 20 dB SPL until two consecutive positive judgments are established. Then, 2 dB steps are utilized until six reversals are obtained. The initial two reversals are discarded. The midpoints of the last four runs are then averaged to provide a 50% estimate of the LDL.

Matching the LDL to the output limitations of the hearing aid assures that the maximum sound pressure is delivered to the ear, without exceeding tolerance capabilities. Supposedly, the normal nonpathologic ear can hear and understand at sound pressure levels above 100 dB SPL. It is possible that the determination of the LDL is so much a function of instructions that any specific, valid internal criteria for such a stimulus cannot be assessed adequately. McCandless (1973) suggests asking the patient what he is experiencing at LDL levels. McCandless feels that the LDL level is 95 or 90 dB SPL for many mild losses.

The use of stapedial reflex thresholds has been suggested as an indicator of loudness tolerance levels. In cases where a hearing loss is less than 70 dB, it may be useful to plot reflex thresholds for the nonaided ear at different frequencies for narrow bands of noise and speech babble. However, as McCandless (1973) has pointed out, reflexes occur in only about half of the cases with losses above 70 dB. The relationship between LDL and acoustic reflex thresholds (ART) is controversial. Ritter et al. (1978) have shown that LDL and acoustic reflex threshold patterns are not necessarily the same. LDLs ". . . do not occur at the same SPLs necessary for elicitation of the acoustic reflex threshold." They also point out that the proximity of the SPLs for LDLs and ARTs depends upon instructions, stimuli, and hearing sensitivity of the subject.

LDLs can also be established using narrow bands of noise centered at 250, 500, 1000, 2000, 3000, and 4000 Hz. These data are then translated to the required maximum power output limits of a preselected hearing aid. Shapiro (1976) suggests that the use of narrow bands of noise will require less time than conventional hearing aid evaluation procedures, and will provide measures of audition that are directly related to hearing aid function.

The clinician should remember that a reduced LDL does not always relate to a recruiting ear. The assumption that a truly recruiting ear always has a tolerance problem for all patients is not valid based on clinical experience.

Furthermore, the frequent assumption that the LDL can be modified, i.e., that tolerance can be expanded or developed, is not supported by research on patients with bilateral, sensorineural hearing loss (Schmitz, 1969). A physiologic basis for modification of LDL has not been demonstrated. If a modification of tolerance does take place, then it must involve the psychologic aspects of the patient, such as his or her anxiety level and general level of contact and comfort with the world of sound. The assumption by Silverman and Pascoe (1978) that "sounds that are uncomfortably loud at first become tolerable with a little practice" is not supported by research (Schmitz, 1969) or clinical experience. Many patients do not modify their LDL's with the use of an aid. Those for whom loud sounds become tolerable represent a re-entry into a world of sound after a period of relative silence. The previously sharp, unexpected, short-time duration sounds that were surprising, uncomfortable, and undesirable, now become acceptable as a function of desensitization.

If the aid is equipped with a telecoil, its value should be assessed once the LDL, frequency response, gain characteristics, and maximum output levels of an aid have been determined. In certain parts of the country, the telecoil may become a special problem to a patient. General telephone receivers in 17 states do not have enough magnetic flux field to operate a hearing aid telecoil effectively. A gain of 30 dB or more is needed to activate the telecoil. The national Bell system has installed a blue grommet in the hand-set of pay phones to designate those receivers that will work with a telecoil. The audiologist needs to know the effectiveness of telecoils with phones within his or her geographic area, and should counsel patients about potential problems with different phones.

ASSESSING THE EFFECTIVENESS OF AMPLIFICATION

Traditional Hearing Aid Evaluation Procedures

In the past, the audiologist has functioned as an independent evaluator of the benefits of amplification and, subsequently, as a referral source for hearing aid dispensers.

The audiologist traditionally has tried to differentiate the performance of one hearing aid from another. He also considers the functional differences of hearing aids as they reflect electroacoustic systems. Assuming that hearing aids generate different patterns of gain by frequency when applied to the individual, we study the loss and then relate the instrument's electroacoustic characteristic to that loss. Subsequently, we measure the benefits of that instrumentation relative to the patient's satisfaction with the amplification. The traditional comparative—evaluative procedure assumes that there are differences among amplifying systems. With the components of advanced electronics such as millifilm, chip technology, circuit boards, and new microphones and amplifiers, differences become more difficult to define. In addition, modifications provided by the coupling system (earmolds, see Chapter 3) also result in differences that previously have not been recognized.

As the ASHA Conference On Hearing Aid Evaluation Procedures (1967) concluded, ''If all of the procedural problems could be solved, the characteristics of the aid needed would be known, and a prescription could be used. The manufacturer would have specifications that would enable him to supply that particular hearing aid. . . .'' Unfortunately, 12 years later the challenge is still present.

The "Throw-The-Hearing-Aid-On" Approach

One way of assessing the benefits of amplification is a proposed system that is termed ''customer selection.'' This approach operates without the benefit of professional audiologic advice or diagnostic apparatus. The customer merely chooses the one aid he prefers from a variety of makes and models of instruments. How he makes this decision is not clear. It is assumed that he is a sophisticated listener able to make quality judgments of sound, perception of pitch differences in frequency responses, and comfort settings. The approach ignores the effects of a long-standing partial hearing loss. The ''customer'' has no baseline of what social hearing used to be when his hearing was normal. The crucial question is whether he can overcome his concept of comfort of sound and quality and opt instead for the improvement in speech intelligibility.

Silverman and Pascoe (1978) suggest that ''. . . with the help of a friend, it is not difficult to come to a useful opinion . . .'' on performance features. The authors suggest a trial period at home and in everyday listening situations ". . . under same conditions and in the same place . . ." When home testing is not possible, it is suggested that the friend carry out tests under ". . . as nearly the same conditions as possible." "The friend must have a good, normal voice and be willing to practice the trick of speaking test words and reading some selected passage from a book or a magazine . . ." at the same tone and loudness. "If he can standardize three different voices—average, faint, and loud—so much the better." It is suggested that with the help of the friend, speech intelligibility is assessed with materials from a book or newspaper using monosyllabic words under the same conditions.

Another nonevaluative, perhaps less adventuresome approach to providing a hearing aid is suggested by a friend of mine who is a successful and respected hearing aid dispenser. He stated, I suspect in jest, that what he does when fitting a hearing aid is "You look in the drawer and you find what's been in there the longest and you use that." In response to my question, "how do you make it work when it's not appropriate for the patient?" he states, "that's where willpower comes in—namely counseling." Undoubtedly, some sort of system like this, with subjective evaluation of comfort of speech and quality of sound, is used by many individuals who are dispensing hearing aids. Apparently, it is successful to some degree as people do use their hearing aids without open hostility toward dispensers. However, whether the patient is being provided with optimum amplification is questionable. These approaches come perilously close to the old method of shopping for corrective devices (such as glasses), by going out on the street to a pushcart and picking one out. Most consumer agencies and professional individuals discourage the patient from such an approach.

The Master Hearing Aid Approach

Many hearing aids are sold on the basis of data provided by a "master" hearing aid. Master hearing aids, utilized by the hearing aid industry, are referred to as "consultant" audiometers. Such equipment evaluates a person's residual hearing response through amplification and seeks to determine the gain response characteristics and output limits of an individual's hearing aid. The master hearing aid utilizes live voice and an assorted myriad of recorded and unrecorded speech samples (see Chapter 9.) The deception here is that the customer will hear with the hearing aid as well as he hears through the master hearing aid. As the FTC (1978) Staff Report Summary indicates,

This is deceptive because the master hearing aid almost certainly is technologically different from or superior to the actual hearing aid that will be purchased. In addition, the listening experience with the master hearing aid is an unrealistic approximation of the real world.

The contention is that the filtering characteristics of the master unit "approximate" the response characteristics of the subsequently manufactured aid. The hearing aid user is "sold" a concept of "custom" or "prescription" fitting. The customer is told that since it is custom-made or follows a specific prescription, it is, in fact, perfect for him and beyond reproach. There is an implied positive relationship in the interaction between the manufactured hearing aid and the user's hearing loss with the implication that the hearer is now receiving the maximum, optimal benefits.

In reality, the prescription or custom-fitting of different hearing losses is probably one of the greatest misrepresentations perpetrated against the consuming public. Available filtering circuits in the master hearing aid are not individually reproducible. There are only a number of available circuit boards, amplifiers, and microphones that in combination will produce a limited number of frequency responses. These frequencies may or may not represent the patient's hearing loss and the necessary gain and output limitations of the aid as specified by the subjective evaluation. Manufacturers approximate the requirements of such descriptive information, and cannot exactly customize the response of the instrument in all cases. This is especially true for basin-shaped, low frequency, and very steeply falling high frequency hearing losses.

The master hearing aid is, in fact, a unit that often has little in common with the acoustic and electromechanical properties of the actual hearing aid when the aid leaves the manufacturer's mail room. It is also questionable whether a patient who has not had complete contact with sound is able to make sophisticated judgments of pitch preference, comfortable loudness levels, and loudness discomfort levels. Furthermore, studies to investigate the reliability of such responses have not enjoyed publication.

The honest manufacturer will admit that the sound pressure device known as the master hearing aid provides only trend information. Nevertheless, the use of such a master hearing aid has appeal due to its potential simplicity and ease of application.

Since 1974, a wearable master hearing aid has been produced (Levitt et al., 1976). The aid measures $5.5 \times 3.25 \times 1$ inches and is equipped with conventional hearing aid receivers. A variety of plug-in units allows changing the frequency response, compression, gain characteristics, and maximum power output.

A pool of 300 hearing-impaired individuals is currently being assessed with this wearable master hearing aid. The purpose is to determine the best estimate of optimum hearing aid selection. The aid is worn for 1 week. The subject then returns for reassessment and a systematic alteration of the hearing aid's performance characteristics until optimum performance has been reached. This approach may have promising clinical application in the future, especially since it utilizes earmolds and hearing aid receivers as well as ongoing modification in the patient's listening environment.

Traditional Hearing Aid "Selective" Evaluation Procedures

Carhart's (1946) comparative hearing aid evaluation procedures have been reviewed extensively (Hodgson et al., 1977, Berger et al. 1971, Rose, 1978) and will be only briefly outlined here. The outgrowth of Carhart's methodology is a selective evaluation procedure that usually consists of evaluating three or more hearing aids while holding stimuli conditions and head positions constant. The speech reception thresholds are obtained at a comfort setting determined by the patient's manipulation of the hearing aid's volume control. Continuous discourse is presented at 40 or 50 dB HL. The hearing aid's volume control should be set, ideally, at the half-volume position. As a rule of thumb, if the instrument's volume control is barely on, then the hearing aid is too powerful. If the volume control is set all the way up, then the aid is not powerful enough for the patient's needs.

Traditionally, the patient responds to stimuli by repeating the words he or she hears. Valid criticisms of this approach are numerous. Written responses are recommended, especially when competing noise is utilized. Furthermore, recorded stimuli should be employed to eliminate differences among speakers and to standardize the procedure within one clinical setting. Theoretically, intelligibility scores obtained in this fashion will then be comparable. Clinically, such an approach may not be realistic, and live voice is often utilized to conserve time.

The inherent question of the comparative procedure is whether the differences between amplification systems truly warrant the attention and expense involved in the evaluation and comparison approach. The question specifically is: "Why not just find the best constructed hearing aid in the frequency and gain category and recommend that for all patients within that category?" Such an approach, of course, is based on the assumption that there is no interaction between a hearing aid's function and an individual's hearing loss.

Beattie and Edgerton's (1976) investigations have demonstrated that there is, in fact, an interaction between the hearing aid's function and an individual's hearing loss. These findings are in contrast to Jerger's (1967) findings. Jerger concluded that ". . . the best aid for anyone appeared to be the best aid for everyone." Similarly, Olsen and Carhart (1967) also did not find an interaction between hearing loss and hearing aids. One of the reasons that major differences between hearing aids' performances are not recognized is that the stimuli have not been demanding enough.

Selective amplification has additionally consisted of ". . . tailoring the frequency response to fit the individual audiogram" (Hodgson, 1977). Strictly applied, this consists of the frequency response of the aid being the exact reverse image of the hearing loss plotted on the audiogram. Although "selective" amplification has not appeared to perform better than a general flat response system, there is now considerable clinical, and some research, evidence to suggest otherwise. For example, Redell and Calvert (1966), working with patients having sloping sensorineural hearing losses, found that better speech discrimination was obtained with hearing aids that had frequency responses that fit their hearing losses. Important to note, however, is that some of the differences did not show up until noise was used in conjunction with speech discrimination stimuli. This has also been demonstrated by Thompson and Lassman (1969), who thought selective amplification to be helpful for ears functioning at low distortion levels. Likewise, Zerlin (1962) showed that additional word discrimination test techniques did not reveal differences between hearing aids. Subjects could, however, differentiate among aids by rating them according to which produced the most intelligible speech. The key factor is that conversational speech was imbedded in a background of cafeteria noise.

Hodgson (1977) suggested that the approach to hearing aid selection need not be one of finding the "best hearing aid" but rather to ". . . assess aided performance of the patient's response to amplification."

Assessing the patient's reactions to amplification should be part of the evaluation process. The patients' reports, such as surprise at the sound or the volume of their voice, and recognition of noise within their immediate environment, should be noted. The patient will either hear more than expected or not enough. The patient may comment that understanding of speech is good in quiet but much more difficult in the presence of background conversation and competing noise. For the patient, the individual experience in these situations is unique. It is of little comfort to the patient that most other hearing aid users have exactly the same problem and report the same experiences. Nevertheless, the reports of patients should suggest to the critical professional that a more demanding and realistic approach to evaluating amplification is needed.

Stimuli other than monosyllabic words presented in a noncompeting environment should be employed in the evaluation. Although most audiologists utilize monosyllabic words (Burney, 1972), the approach has been criticized by numerous authors including Shore et al. (1960), Resnick et al. (1963), and Jerger (1967). The question is whether or not the aided test-retest speech discrimination scores are reliable. According to McConnell et al. (1960), and Carhart et al. (1972), test-retest reliability of aided speech discrimination was good at 85%. Likewise, Olsen et al. (1967) used signal-to-noise ratios with presbycusic patients and found significant correlation coefficients of 85%.

STIMULI CONSIDERATIONS AND THE EVALUATIVE– COMPARATIVE HEARING AID PROCEDURE

Use of 25-Word Lists Compared to 50-Word Lists

Edgerton et al. (1978) raised two questions in their experimentations: (1) whether 25-word speech discrimination tests were as reliable as 50-word tests for differentiating behavior performances among hearing aids, and (2) when full-lists are divided into half-lists, are the dervied half-lists equivalent in respect to intelligibility? They used the NU6 materials with competing noise at signal-to-noise ratios of +20dB. Half-list reliability coefficients were not as high as the full-lists, reducing the speech discrimination score consistency of test-retest rank order of hearing aids by 50%.

Edgerton et al. (1978) suggests ". . . that both the half-list/full-list correlation coefficients and the corrected half-list/full-list correlation coefficients are misleading indicies of half-list reliability." Furthermore, the authors suggest that "the differences between half-lists' speech discrimination materials . . . were of sufficient magnitude to contra-indicate the use of different half-lists for the evaluation of hearing aids." This is in agreement with Shore et al. (1960), who found that the Rush-Hughes recordings of PB50's half-lists were insensitive to differences between hearing aids, whereas full 50-word lists appeared to differentiate hearing aid performance, especially in the presence of white noise. These findings are in direct contrast to those of Elpern (1961), Resnick (1962), Schumaier et al. (1974), and Manning et al. (1975), who reported that half-lists can be substituted for full-lists.

The prediction of speech discrimination problems for a patient's environment based on performance with phonetically balanced words (especially half-lists) is, at best, risky. While it is generally true that lower speech discrimination scores lessen the understanding of speech, it is not possible to determine from unaided scores what the person's speech intelligibility will be with an instrument. Unaided speech discrimination scores are a function of sensation level. If the sensation level is inadequate, then speech discrimination will be poor. This is especially true when high frequency residual hearing is limited to 80−90 dB HL. The SRT, reflects the contribution of low and mid frequency hearing sensitivity. Speech discrimination based only on the SRT may not be maximum because a sensation level of 10−20 dB may be insufficient. Furthermore, speech discrimination in quiet does not reflect the electroacoustic performance of the hearing aid in the presence of competing noise and background speech.

The popularity of half-list speech discrimination stimuli in hearing aid evaluation procedures continues not so much because clinicians are unable to break from tradition, but because of the constraints of time when different hearing aids must be evaluated. Until half-lists are truly equivalent, differences between instruments are the reflection of differences in test materials. It would, therefore, be advisable to abandon the use of half-list stimuli.

Use of Competing Noise

The logic of using competing noise when assessing the performance of a hearing aid is compelling, since the hearing aid user never listens in a pure acoustic environment such as found in the sound room. The use of a combination of a noise background in conjunction with speech audiometry (Niemeyer, 1976) represents an approach that allows some realistic predictions about a person's functioning in a usual noisy communicative situation. Not only is this approach more realistic, but it also serves to separate hearing aid performance.

Beattie et al. (1976) have examined the value of such an approach. Using 24 subjects with mild to moderate senorineural loss, they presented Northwestern University's Auditory Test #6 at MCL, in conjunction with white noise at a signal-to-noise ratio of +20 dB. Four hearing aids were assessed, three of which had essentially high frequency emphasis. Significant differences were defined by a score difference of 12%. Although a single aid could not be reliably identified by monosyllabic words in a background of noise, the procedure did consistently eliminate inferior aids in 50% of the subjects. The authors concluded that, "The best aid for one person is not the best aid for all individuals." Learning effects were not demonstrated for monosyllabic speech intelligibility in a background of noise. This is in contrast with previous research by Shore et al. (1960), and Jerger et al. (1966 b), who showed a learning effect associated with test-retest speech discrimination in noise. Beattie et al. (1976) conclude that monosyllabic discrimination in the presence of white noise can, nevertheless, differentiate among commercially available hearing aids. They suggest 14% as a criterion for significant differences. Another important finding of their research is that the smoothness of a hearing aid's frequency response is not a good predictor of speech intelligibility for sensorineural subjects with sloping hearing losses.

Based on the results of this research, it is clear that *speech intelligibility should be assessed in a background of noise*. The type of noise can be either white noise, speech noise, or competing speech. Since we do not know how well intelligibility tests assess communicative ability in everyday listening situations, it is reasonable to attempt to duplicate, as closely as possible, the competing speech background noise in which most listening occurs.

Nonspeech Stimuli

Among the nonspeech stimuli for hearing aid evaluation purposes are: (1) pulsed pure tones or warbled tones, and (2) narrow bands of noise presented at the centering frequencies and narrow bands of noise presented in a sweep frequency mode.

Pulsed pure tones are more desirable as a stimulus than are continuous pure tones because standing waves break up in sound field. Warbled tones in turn are better than pulsed pure tones. Narrow bands of noise, however, are considered ideal by many researchers and clinicians.

Berger et al. (1979) suggest that gain by frequency be established with narrow bands of noise. Like pure tones, bands of noise are relatively stable, easily obtainable with conventional clinical equipment, and repeatable and uncomplicated (Berger et al., 1979). These stimuli are also sensitive to changes in the earmold and frequency emphasis.

Gengel et al. (1971) also suggest using narrow bands of noise to determine both the maximum output of a hearing aid and the requirements for volume setting. Similarly, Garsteki et al. (1976) have shown a close relationship between hearing aid acoustic gain and changes in aided narrow band thresholds. They recommend the use of narrow bands of noise when traditional measures (such as speech stimuli) cannot be employed.

Rather than regarding narrow bands of noise as a substitute stimuli, many clinicians favor employing the stimulus to directly reflect requirements for the effective functional gain and output limits of the hearing aid. The frequency response of the ear is felt to be well reflected by the use of such stimuli.

Berger's Formula Approach to Specification of Hearing Aid Performance

Berger et al. (1979) describe a prescriptive procedure that requires 5 min or less, assures uniformity of approach from clinician to clinician to clinician, and avoids the use of variable speech stimuli.

Berger's formula is:

$$\frac{\text{HTL at 500 Hz}}{2} + 10 \qquad \frac{\text{HTL at 1000 Hz}}{1.6} + 10$$

$$\frac{\text{HTL at 2000 Hz}}{1.5} + 10 \qquad \frac{\text{HTL at 3000 Hz}}{1.7} + 10$$

$$\frac{\text{HTL at 4000 Hz}}{2} + 10$$

The denominators (2, 1.6, 1.5, 1.7, and 2) were selected to provide gain in an instrument that is slightly more than half of the hearing threshold level. The formula is applicable irrespective of the type of hearing aid. Whether an earmold is open or closed is also irrelevant. The 10 dB represents a reserve gain. Berger et al. (1979) feel that this reserve gain is desirable for the high frequencies of 2000 and 3000 Hz. A manufacturer may be asked to supply the maximum gain desired, or the clinician can match the frequency response of his consignment aids to these requirements.

Using Berger et al.'s (1979) example of the application of the formula to an actual hearing loss:

$$
\begin{aligned}
&\text{500 Hz: } 55 \text{ dB} \div 2 &= 28 \\
&\text{1000 Hz: } 55 \text{ dB} \div 1.6 &= 21 \\
&\text{2000 Hz: } 60 \text{ dB} \div 1.5 &= 20 \\
&\text{3000 Hz: } 65 \text{ dB} \div 1.7 &= 27 \\
&\text{4000 Hz: } 70 \text{ dB} \div 2 &= 35
\end{aligned}
$$

These levels are plotted on the audiogram and constitute the predicted levels of the actual hearing aid's performance.*

After the hearing aid has been provided for the patient, the patient's responses are evaluated in reference to the predicted levels. If small differences are noted, then Berger et al. (1979) suggest that the earmold be modified, and the tone control be altered, or that filters be employed. Large differences, of course, would necessitate a new fitting.

According to Berger et al. (1979) ". . . considerable documentation exists to show that the closer the obtained aided thresholds are to the predicted, the better the aided speech discrimination will be." Actual experimental and clinical data still need to be supplied to completely substantiate this statement.

Berger's formula allows reserve gain in each frequency of 10 dB (about the predicted operating gain). Maximum gain is defined as operating gain plus reserve gain. This correction is applicable to both hearing thresholds or SPL levels.

The formula gives a gain by frequency response, the SSPL to be satisfied, and assures that the patient's electroacoustic requirements are satisfied. The formula, however, does not utilize any speech-like stimuli to which the patient can relate.

Berger's (1979) formula for LDLs to be assessed with pure tones rather than speech. He suggests a conversion of HL to SPL for tones by adding 11 dB to 500, 7 dB to 100, and 9 dB to 2000/4000 Hz hearing threshold levels. It is suggested that 115 dB be specified as a saturation sound pressure level (SSPL) at 500. Berger et al. (1979) believe that this will limit the spread of upward masking. They summarize these recommendations:

Maximum Permissible SSPL

---

500 Hz:UCL in HL + 11 dB or 115 dB SPL
1000 Hz:UCL in HL + 7 dB
2000 Hz:UCL in HL + 9 dB
4000 Hz:UCL in HL + 9 dB

Minimum Desirable SSPL

Og + 75 dB
Og + 75 dB
Og + 72 dB
Og + 70 dB

---

*The formula is printed on a slide rule that is available through Associated Hearing Instruments, 6796 Market Street, Upper Darby, Pa. 19082.

Utilizing the concept of SSPL is more accurate than referring to maximum power output (MPO), since the actual measurements do not employ power, but pressure.

Sentence Stimuli

Berger et al. (1968) recommend the use of synthetic sentences in the hearing aid evaluation process. The scoring procedure allows randomization of sentences, and is not dependent on the listener's criterion of a correct or incorrect spoken response by the patient. A sentence is also more apt to measure the integrity of the peripheral hearing system and the patient's cognitive potential.

Gerstman's (1976) approach is to control the effects of word familiarity and levels of semantic predictability. His test contains target words in the final position of sentences. Monosyllabic nouns serve as key words. Sentences are recorded in lists of 41 items each in the presence of speech babble created by 12 voices speaking simultaneously. This creates an unintelligible, and as he says, a "rather aversive" signal. The final test version will consist of predictably low and predictably high sentences (low: "I will never say the word 'clock;' " high: "we heard the ticking of the clock.") The test is currently being evaluated on a clinical population. The author's objective is to develop a measure of sentence discrimination that describes hearing impairment and is useful for hearing aid evaluations procedures.

A sentence approach to hearing aid evaluation holds much logical merit. The stimuli are more like everyday speech than are word lists, and they are simple to administer. Message competition ratios can be applied.

Kalikow et al. (1977) have developed a one key word sentence test for speech intelligibility in babble-type noise. The last word in the sentence, a monosyllabic noun, has either high or low predictability (high: "the little girl cuddled her doll," low: "Miss Brown can't discuss the slot.") The 50-item forms are balanced for: intelligibility, familiarity, predictability, phonetic content and length.

Bekesy Audiometry in Sound Field

Bekesy sweep frequency audiometry can be applied to hearing performance in a variety of ways. Tracking procedures can be used to obtain aided and unaided thresholds of intelligibility for continuous discourse, as suggested by Rubin et al. (1972), or to establish most intelligible listening levels. Tracking procedures in sound field have been suggested by Fournier et al. (1967) and Green et al. (1968). These authors concluded that the technique was reliable for the assessment of hearing aid performance. Schmitz et al. (1971) have suggested, however, that although such tracking procedures may show improvements in the aided condition, the improvements are functionally invalid. Their research demonstrates that Bekesy Sound Field tracking procedures may be helpful in assessing hearing aid performance for someone without functional speech or language. Small and potentially critical differences between hearing aids may be evident from such trackings, but will not be reflected in comparable differences for speech reception or speech discrimination. Conversely, significant differences between aids reflected in speech discrimination scores for CID W 22 stimuli were unaccompanied by tracking differences. Using 20 monaural and 12 binaural hearing aid users, Schmitz et al. (1971) found that a four frequency average of monaural-and binaural-aided pure tone thresholds was not predictive of either the SRT or speech discrimination. The pure tone stimuli, however, could have been affected by the room conditions, speaker calibration, head position, and listening distance.

Bekesy Sound Field using narrow hands of noise, however, can reflect differences in hearing aid gain if these differences are greater than 10 dB.

Bekesy Sound Field is also applicable to the measurement of LDL. The technique appears to be less variable than words or narrow bands of noise for continuous discourse. However, gain and frequency response differences of hearing aids must be substantial (10 dB or more) before they become evident in the tracking procedures. Bekesy Sound Field may also not be related to SRT and speech discrimination. Based on their preliminary research, Schmitz et al. (1971) felt that Bekesy Sound Field data for pure tones, narrow bands of noise, or connected discourse, are not definitive enough at this time to warrant the conclusion that the procedure is reliable, valid, or useful as an indication of differences in aided performance.

Conventional speech discrimination materials are not sensitive enough to differences in high frequency sensitivity. A high frequency hearing loss with normal, low, and mid frequency sensitivity will not show a difference in the aided speech reception threshold. Bekesy Sound Field can, however, be helpful in demonstrating the effects of high frequency emphasis amplification. Bekesy Sound Field audiometry, using pulsed tones or narrow bands of noise, can demonstrate differences in gain between unaided and aided hearing thresholds. Although large gain differences are obvious (Fig. 5-1), the tracking procedure is unable to differentiate between hearing aids whose frequency responses are substantially different from one another. Nevertheless, more research should be directed towards the application of this procedure. Bekesy Sound Field audiometry is easy to instrument and to control, and is simple to execute by the patient. It provides an effective counseling tool for explaining the demonstrated benefits to the patient.

An additional use of Bekesy Sound Field audiometry is to determine the existence of possible islands of normal or significantly better hearing that may not be visible by conventional octave-step, pure tone threshold audiometry unless 1500 and 3000 Hz are used consistently. Schmitz (1970) has shown that patients

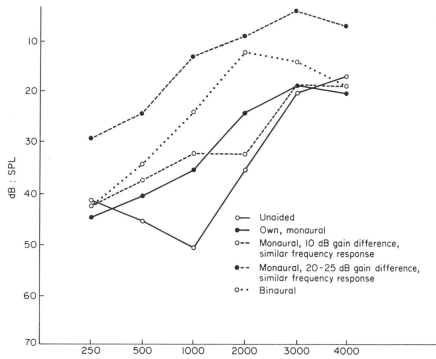

Fig. 5-1. Bekesy narrow band noise thresholds for a patient with unaided, monaural and binaural aids of different gain and similar frequency response.

associate such sensitivity peaks with subjective complaints of: (1) unpleasant, metallic, sharp quality of sounds and speech; (2) better monaural speech discrimination ability in bilateral, symmetrical, severe senorineural hearing loss; and (3) an inability to tolerate amplification. As Figure 5-2 shows, the sensitivity peaks are not always completely described by octave-step frequency thresholds. It is also possible that irregularities in aided frequency responses could be visualized this way. In order to apply this technique, pulsed pure tones should be used since they tend to yield greater threshold sensitivity, less intratest variability, and smaller amplitude of excursions (McCommons et al., 1969).

The Most Comfortable Loudness Level

MCL serves as a predictor of the gain required for a selected hearing aid. As Cox et al. (1978) have pointed out, two assumptions underly this practice: (1) that the MCL when wearing a hearing aid can be predicted from the unaided MCL, and (2) that the patient will set the aid's volume control to achieve MCL for input signals. Cox et al. (1978a) investigated MCL at several frequencies for aided and unaided subjects and assessed the extent to which the aided MCLs

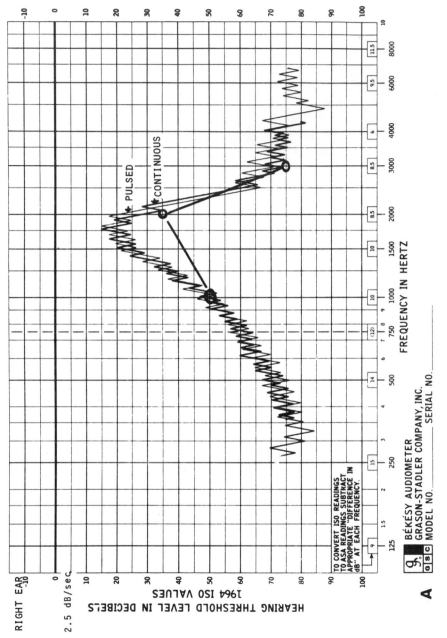

Fig. 5-2. Bekesy sweep frequency thresholds for pulsed and continuous stimuli, compared to discrete pure tone thresholds at 500, 1000, 2000, 3000, and 4000 Hz.

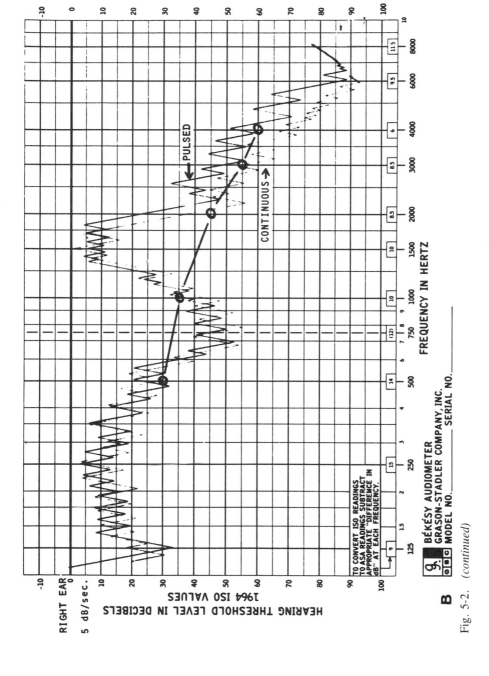

Fig. 5-2. (continued)

199

could be predicted from the corresponding unaided MCLs. Narrow bands of noise centered at 500, 1000, 2000, 3000, and 4000 Hz were employed. Sixteen normal right ears were used with the left ears plugged. Mild gain aids were used that had tapered volume controls and a maximum gain at any frequency of 18 dB. Custom made earmolds were employed. In the aided condition, MCL was measured directly in the subject's ear canal utilizing a probe-tube microphone with the tip of the mike 3−5 mm medial to the tip of the earmold canal portion. MCLs were obtained with written and verbal instructions, in a continuous ascending mode. Subjects were given practice. They adjusted the noise level in MCL 3−5 times, and a median value of the last three measures was recorded by the clinician.

MCL judgments at any given frequency were made at a constant SPL at the eardrum. By predicting the aided MCL from the unaided MCL at 1000 Hz the researchers showed that the predicted level would be within ± 5.5 dB of the true MCL in 68 % of individuals and within ± 8 dB of the true MCL in 68% of the individuals (Cox et al., 1978).

Shapiro (1977) also suggests using narrow bands of noise centered at 250, 500, 1000, 2000, 3000, and 4000 Hz to determine the use gain of hearing aids. He showed that hearing aid gain can be accurately and efficiently predicted on the basis of the MCLs for narrow bands of noise. The hearing-impaired subjects were found to be highly consistent in their MCL judgments for narrow bands of noise. *MCL for narrow bands of noise, therefore, appears to be a valid measure for specifying hearing aid gain and frequency response.*

Special Hearing Aid Considerations

BINAURAL HEARING AIDS

The decision to evaluate the patient with binaural hearing aids depends on his or her hearing loss, and on his or her vocational, social, and general communicative needs. Individuals with a hearing loss averaging from 50−80 dB to as high as 90−100 dB at 500, 1000, 2000, and 3000 Hz are excellent candidates. If the individual depends upon multidirectional sound input, then binaural hearing aids are critical. Binaural amplification should also be considered when monaural speech discrimination under earphones is poor. Predicting binaural speech discrimination from monaural information is risky. In any clinical practice, numerous examples exist of binaural amplification bringing significant improvement in speech discrimination compared to monaural under earphone speech discrimination. (Carhart, 1958; see Chapter 7).

The advantages of binaural amplification are difficult to demonstrate in a conventional sound room unless multidirectional sound sources are employed. Nevertheless, some specific alterations are easily possible. Olsen et al. (1967) recommend a procedure using two loudspeakers placed at a 45° azimuth to the right and left of a patient in a sound-treated room. The primary signal originates from the side of the best ear or the nontest ear. Compared to the unaided condition, the authors found improvement for the binaural aided conditions in the presence of noise.

Patients consistently affirm that binaural amplification allows better understanding of speech in the presence of competing speech and background noise. Consequently, any individual who communicates for a livelihood or depends on efficient communication socially, should be considered a candidate for binaural amplification. Binaural amplification can also be considered for ears that are asymmetrical where, for example, one instrument may provide a broad frequency response while the other instrument provides high frequency emphasis.

EYEGLASS MOUNTED HEARING AIDS

The decision to evaluate and recommend eyeglass type hearing aids demands that the patient wear eyeglasses consistently, or that he use two pairs of eyeglasses. The eyeglass aid affords easy manipulation of the volume control. For some patients, this is a sufficient reason to prefer this type of amplification. However, microphone location in the eyeglass aid may not be as favorable acoustically as in the ear-level aid. A patient who desires binaural eyeglass aids should be allowed a trial period to determine if the necessary adjustments can be made quickly, and if the glasses are removed frequently.

ASSESSING THE EFFECTS OF DIRECTIONAL
MICROPHONES

The purpose of directional microphones is to assist the user in the reception of sound from directly in front of him. This reduces the intensity of the sounds originating from behisnd him, and limits the negative influences of competing noise.

Lentz (1972) describes the equipment required for such evaluation. VArious speaker locations from around the patient's head are recommended. A variation from these recommendations is suggested by Frank et al. (1977) who vary the noise from either directly in front of the patient or in back, while speech is delivered from a loudspeaker at 45° azimuth from the midline of the subject's head (see Chapter 2).

CROS AMPLIFICATION

Persons who demonstrate a unilateral hearing loss will frequently complain of having increased difficulty in hearing when someone is speaking to them from their poorer hearing side. They also have difficulties hearing people in groups, in noisy surroundings, and have problems in localization (Harford et al., 1965). Harford et al.'s findings show that the intensity of the speech signal is attenuated approximately 60 dB across the head. Since higher frequencies are more distorted than low frequencies, poor speech intelligibility results. Intelligibility is also affected when a competing noise signal reaches the better ear as the speech signal reaches the poorer ear. These individuals are perfect candidates for moderate gain CROS amplification. Such amplification can also be utilized for the patient with a bilateral, high frequency sensorineural hearing loss. These individuals were previously considered unsuitable candidates for amplification because of their normal hearing sensitivity in the frequency regions of 1000 Hz and below. The problem of over-amplification by conventional broad frequency spectrum and high frequency emphasis aids is potentially solvable with a CROS aid. If spectrum shaping is not adequate electronically, then it can be modified acoustically by an open earmold (Jerger, 1971).

Benefits of high frequency emphasis CROS amplification are difficult to demonstrate. One approach that has been used with some success was previously referred to in the discussion of Bekesy Sound Field Audiometry. Schmitz et al. (1971) demonstrated that the increase in high frequency sound reception can be demonstrated with Bekesy tracking. Bekesy Sound Field, however, cannot differentiate between hearing aids of different frequency responses.

Even if differences between the aided and unaided condition can be demonstrated using Bekesy Sound Field Audiometry, the patient must experience an actual improvement in speech intelligibility.

Another approach to evaluating the effectiveness of CROS amplification is to obtain aided and unaided speech reception thresholds and discrimination scores with the patient's poorer ear facing 45° to a loudspeaker. Competing noise is used to assess the directionablity of the better ear. Speech and competing noise can be reversed. Speech and noise can also be presented binaurally through loudspeakers. Because of the placebo effect of CROS amplification (Reilly, 1971), it is imperative that a trial period be instituted. (See Chapter 7.)

CONSIDERATION OF SCALING TECHNIQUES FOR ASSESSING THE BENEFITS OF AMPLIFICATION

INTELLIGIBILITY RATINGS OF CONNECTED DISCOURSE

An additional tool for assessing the benefits of amplification is the use of connected discourse as a stimulus. In this technique, the listener scales intelligibility according to his or her own internal criteria of understanding. Rating scales from 1 to 9 are frequently employed for this purpose. The difficulties of such a scaling approach are the lack of sophistication of the patient and the time required for the task.

COMMUNICATIVE ABILITY SCALES

Self-assessment scales for hearing problems have been proposed by High et al. (1964), Noble et al. (1970), and Ward et al. (1977). Tannahill (1979) has applied High et al.'s (1964) Hearing Handicap Scale to measure hearing aid benefit for new hearing aid users with bilateral, sensorineural hearing losses. The scale was administered prior to and following 4 weeks of hearing aid use. As a result of the aided condition, significant changes in SRT, word identification, and Hearing Handicap Scale were recorded. Word identification ratings, obtained with the stimuli presented at conversational speech levels, were significantly related to the Hearing Handicap Scale score. The Hearing Handicap Scale utilizes a 20-item format with questions about daily listening. Answers are scaled from 1 to 5 from "practically always" to "almost never." Higher ratings reflect greater handicap. Reduced scores are associated with improvement in word identification at conversational levels. The author suggests that the Hearing Handicap Scale ratings "provide a more comprehensive profile of hearing aid benefit."

Scales have also been constructed by the Hearing Society for the Bay Area of San Francisco, and by Alpiner et al. (1975), known as the Denver Scale of Communication Function. The purpose of these scales is to enable the patient to record his communicative difficulties. The Denver Scale has enjoyed extensive use. The scale has been instrumental in furnishing insight into the individual's preamplification communicative problems, and into the problems that remain after amplification has been provided. The scale consists of 25 separate questions given in a time span of 10 min. The questions involve family, self-concept, and social-vocational and general communication. Results of the Denver scale are grouped in a profile that displays the area of needs. Pre- and post-assessment give insight into the benefits of amplification and the still remaining communicative problems. The scale may indicate those areas where other rehabilitative approaches are needed and where further attention should be directed. The patient is afforded the opportunity to review his communicative problems, which in turn helps him to examine the realities of his situation.

Giolas, et al. (1979) have constructed a Hearing Performance Inventory for adults which assesses the effects of hearing loss in a variety of typical listening situations. The six sections of the self-report questionaire consist of: understanding speech, intensity, response to auditory failure, social, personal, and occupational. This inventory can provide valuable information of the success of amplification in an auditory rehabilitation program.

Follow-up Procedures Involved in the Hearing Aid Selection

After the recommendation for a specific hearing aid has been made, the audiologist may wish to see the patient within the first week to assist him with any adjustment problems. The patient may have difficulties with the insertion of the earmold, adjusting the volume control, or acclamating himself to various acoustic situations and unexpected sounds.

The length of the trial period depends upon the patient's readiness to accept amplification, and his commitment to the experience. Hopefully, the patient's problems are solved within the 30-day period provided by law in which to claim a refund.

The trial period provides the patient an opportunity to utilize the hearing aid in a variety of demanding situations. Some suggestions that can be made for the patient are to use the hearing aid at home: (1) over various distances, (2) in the presence of other people speaking, such as the family conversation at the dinner table, (3) in a background of noise such as the television set, (4) while listening to radio and television, and (5) during public encounters such as the theatre, restaurants, church, lectures, and other meetings.

Follow-up procedures suggested by the American Speech and Hearing Association Conference on Hearing Evaluations (1967) are: (1) assessment of the electroacoustic properties of the hearing aid as worn by the patient; (2) assessment of speech reception and speech discrimination ability, as well as speech discrimination in noise at the use-gain setting of the hearing aid; (3) checking the patient's comfort with the earmold and his ability to insert the earmold easily and without discomfort and twisting of the tubing; and (4) reviewing with the patient the problem he is having with amplification, adjustment to the world of sound, frustrated expectations, inability to modify the aid's function in certain acoustical conditions, the problems with battery life, inability to manipulate the hearing aid's controls, and/or other expectations that have not been satisfied with the hearing aid.

Many clinical facilities incorporate a series of follow-up visits. The last follow-up usually takes place 6 months after the provision of the aid. The value of this appointment is questionable unless it is to check for progression of hearing loss. Adjustment problems will usually have resulted in the rejection of the aid prior to this period of time. If help is to be given to the patient, it should be instituted during the first weeks of hearing aid use.

If the patient is having an inordinate adjustment problem, then he should be seen more frequently. The sensitive clinician usually has a keen awareness of the patient who will be having adjustment problems to his own voice, to environmental noises, and to sudden unexpected sounds, or who will be having difficulty when inserting the earmold.

Follow-up evaluation procedures may result in:

1. A change from the skeletal mold to a half shell or canal hook mold that allows easier insertion.
2. Non-venting of the earmold if the patient would like to have more gain in the hearing aid but, due to feedback problems, cannot attain this. A change from a side branch vent to a parallel vent may allow more gain, as has been suggested by Cox's (1978b) research.
3. The use of external filters. The acoustic changes produced by sintered filters

may not be consistent from one filter to another. Electrical changes within the hearing aid are more consistent, but increase the cost of the aid and may produce additional distortion. However, filters do allow a more gradual adjustment to a world of sound.

4. The use of a power CROS if a high gain, ear-level type hearing aid causes feedback.
5. Changing the instrument for one that will allow volume setting at approximately the 50% rotation mark. If the volume control is being utilized beyond a 50% rotation, then the individual may encounter an unusually high increase in harmonic distortion (see Chapter 2).

Frequently, the audiologist will confront unrealistic expectations on the patient's part. The patient may be having difficulty acknowledging his problems, and may be defensive because of pressures from his family members and from others. If so, a training program is in order (see Chapter 10).

The Hearing Aid Evaluation Procedure in Summary

Figures 5-3 and 5-4 illustrate hearing aid evaluation forms useful in implementing all of the conditions previously discussed. The forms contain spaces for the following information:

A. The form indicates which ear is being aided.
B. The make of the hearing aid and the model are stated. The serial number can be stated if the same type of hearing aid is utilized with different specific modifications.
C. The volume control setting is indicated and is expressed in percentage of total available rotation.
D. MCL is established by rotating the volume control until a 73 dB SPL continuous-speech signal is found to be comfortable.
E. The pitch of the instrument is designated by marking the appropriate control location.
F. The battery type is indicated.
G. The type of earmold utilized in the evaluation process is indicated.
H. Speech reception thresholds or speech awareness thresholds are stated for comparison.
I. Word discrimination scores at 64 dB SPL, representative of normal conversational intensity level, can be expressed "for a noncompetitive situation" (quiet) and at various signal-to-noise ratios.
J. Word discrimination stimuli are specified so that the results are comparable. It is recommended that all stimuli, whether monosyllabic words, sentence tests, or nonsense syllables be presented in a recorded mode to allow test-retest with accuracy and reliability.
K. MCL and LDL should be established using a speech stimulus.

904 TOWN AND COUNTRY ROAD
ORANGE, CALIFORNIA 92668
(714) 558-2666

FASHION ISLAND MEDICAL CENTER
1441 AVOCADO · SUITE 208
NEWPORT BEACH, CALIF. 92660
(714) 640-5702

HEARING AID EVALUATION

Name: _____ D.O.B.: _____

CONDITION		UNAIDED	①	②	③	④
	Ear					
	Make					
	Model					
	Serial No.					
	Vol. Rot. % (73 dB SPL)					
	Pitch		↻	↻	↻	↻
	Power		↻	↻	↻	↻
	Gain		↻	↻	↻	↻
			↻	↻	↻	↻
	Battery					
	Earmold		Vented Standard Short	Vented Standard Short	Vented Standard Short	Vented Standard Short
	SRT/SAT	dB HL	dB HL	dB HL	dB HL	dB HL
WDS AT 64 dB SPL	Quiet	%	%	%	%	%
	S/N + 6 dB	%	%	%	%	%
		%	%	%	%	%
		%	%	%	%	%
	Stimulus					
	Rec.-Lv.					
	MCL	dB HL	dB HL	dB HL	dB HL	dB HL
	LDL	dB HL	dB HL	dB HL	dB HL	dB HL
WARBLE TONES	250	dB HL	dB HL	dB HL	dB HL	dB HL
	500	dB HL	dB HL	dB HL	dB HL	dB HL
	1000	dB HL	dB HL	dB HL	dB HL	dB HL
	2000	dB HL	dB HL	dB HL	dB HL	dB HL
	3000	dB HL	dB HL	dB HL	dB HL	dB HL
	4000	dB HL	dB HL	dB HL	dB HL	dB HL
	NOTES:					

Comments: _____

_____

_____

AUDIOLOGIST: _____

_____

DATE: _____

OUND FIELD CALIBRATED TO 13 dB SPL

Fig. 5-3.   Hearing aid evaluation worksheet

SOUND FIELD WARBLE TONE TESTING

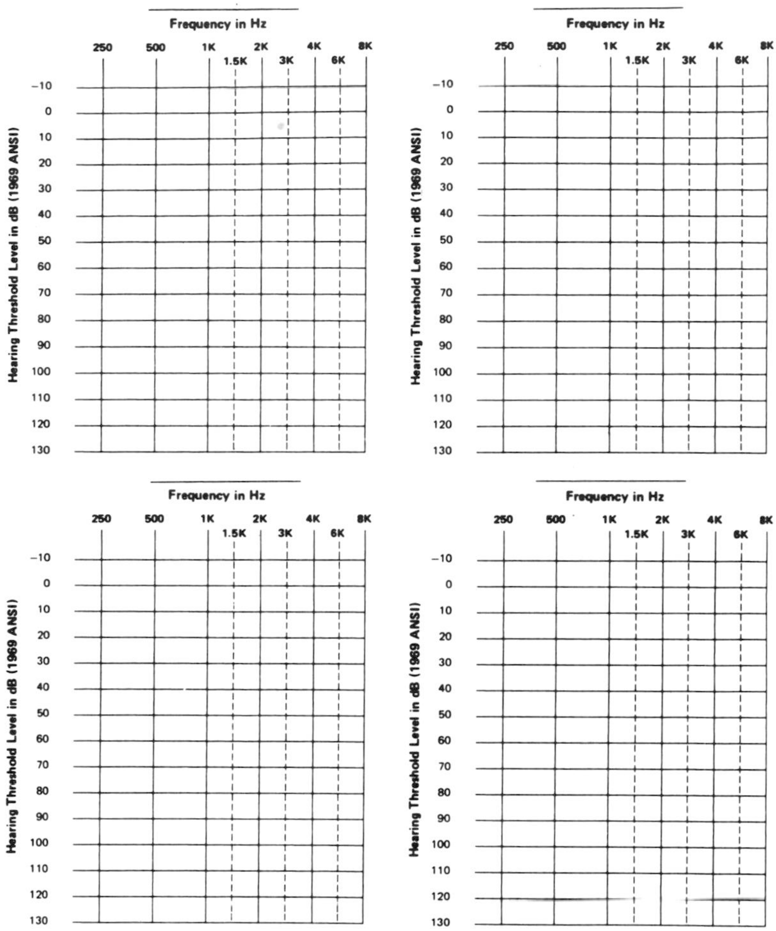

Comments: ______________________________

SYMBOLS

RIGHT EAR (Red)		LEFT EAR (Blue)
S	SOUND FIELD	S
A	SOUND FIELD (AIDED)	A
↓	NO RESPONSE	↓

Sound Field Calibrated To 13dB SPL

Fig. 5-4. Sound field audiograms

L. Warble tone thresholds are indicated for all frequencies, and represent
those levels expressed in dBHL. They can be translated into SPL
levels.

M. The "Notes" section is designed for recording the patient's comments
regarding a specific hearing aid.

N. The reverse side of the form (Fig. 5-4) allows thresholds to be graphi-
cally displayed for sound field warble tones or narrow bands of noise.
The four graphs are usually adequate to completely describe the performance of different instruments.

The hearing aid that is recommended for use is usually the instrument that
allows the greatest speech intelligibility in quiet and in a background of competing noises or speech babble. It is also the instrument that allows the greatest
reception of high frequency sounds, the greatest dynamic range, and the greatest
ease of manipulation of the hearing aid's controls.

Hopefully, the audiologist will not limit the use of evaluative procedures to
those indicated on the hearing aid evaluation form. When indicated, he will
utilize Bekesy Sound Field Audiometry, monosyllabic nonsense stimuli, connected discourse, and scaling techniques to arrive at a decision that has predictable benefits for the patient. The patient's adjustment and satisfaction with the
instrument will support the audiologist's commitment to exhaustive analysis.

BIBLIOGRAPHY

Alpiner JG: Client opinions of clinical hearing aid evaluations. J Acad Rehabil Audiol
6:58—60, 1973

Alpiner JG, Chevrette W, Glascoe G, et al: The Denver Scale of Communication Function,
in Pollack MC (ed): Amplification for the Hearing-Impaired. New York, Grune &
Stratton, 1973, 176—183

American Speech and Hearing Association: A conference on hearing aid evaluation procedures. ASHA Reports, 2:1—71, 1967

Beattie RC, Edgerton BJ: Reliability of monosyllabic discrimination tests in white noise
for differentiating among hearing aids. J Speech Hear Dis 41:464—476, 1976

Berger KW, Hagberg EN, Rane RL: A prescriptive method of hearing aid fitting. Audecibel 28:32—39, 1979

Berger JW, Millin JP: Hearing aids, in Rose DE (ed): Audiological Assessment. Englewood Cliffs, Prentice Hall, 1971

Burney P: A survey of hearing aid evaluation procedures. ASHA 14:439—444, 1972

Carhart R: Tests for selection of hearing aids. Laryngoscope 56:680—794, 1946

Carhart R: The usefulness of the binaural hearing aid. J Speech Hear Dis 23:42—51, 1958

Carhart R, Tillman T: Individual consistency of hearing for speech across diverse listening
conditions: J Speech Hear Res 15:105—113, 1972

Cox RM, Ward DJ: MCL at the eardrum in aided and unaided conditions. Paper presented
at the annual convention of the American Speech and Hearing Association, San
Francisco, 1978 a

Cox RM: Non-audible acoustic feedback: Effect on functional hearing aid performance. Paper presented at the annual convention of the American Speech and Hearing Association, San Francisco, 1978 b

Edgerton BJ, Klodd DA, Beattie RC: Half-list speech discrimination measures in hearing aid evaluations. Arch Otolaryngol 104:669−672, 1978

Elpern B: The relative stability of half-list and full-list discrimination tests. Laryngoscope, 71:30−35, 1961

Federal Trade Commission: Hearing Aid Industry Staff Report, November 1978

Fournier JE, Rainville MJ: Le controle des resultats d'appareillage par audiometrie automatique en champ libre. International Audiol 6:264, 1967

Frank T, Gooden R: The effect of hearing aid microphone types on speech discrimination scores in a background of multi-talker noise. Maico Audiological Library, 2:5, 1973

Garstecki DC, Bode DC: Aided and unaided narrow band noise thresholds in listeners with sensorineural hearing impairment. J Am Audiol Soc 1:258−262, 1976

Gengel R, Pascoe D, Shore I: A frequency response procedure for evaluating and selecting hearing aids for severely hearing-impaired children. J Speech Hear Dis 36:341−352, 1971

Gerstman HL: Development of a test instrument for speech discrimination, in Rubin M (ed): Hearing Aids. Baltimore, University Park Press, 1976, pp. 37−46

Giolas, TG et al. Hearing aid performance inventory. J Speech and Hearing Dis, 44: 169−195, 1979

Green D, Ross M: The effect of a conventional versus a non-occluding (CROS-type) earmold upon the frequency response of a hearing aid. J Speech Hear Res 11:638−647, 1968

Griffing T: Hearing correction is more than a hearing aid. Hear Aid J 6:62−65, 1978

Harford E, Barry J: A rehabilitative approach to the problem of unilateral hearing impairment: The contralateral routing of signals (CROS) J Speech Hear Dis 30:121−138, 1965

High WS, Fairbanks G, Glorig A: Scale for self-assessment of hearing handicap. J Speech Hear Dis 29:215−230, 1964

Hodgson, WR: Clinical measures of hearing aid performance, in Hodgson, WR and Skinner, RH (eds): Hearing Aid Assessment and use in Audiologic Habilitation. Baltimore, Williams and Wilkins, Co., 1977, pp. 127−144

Huizing HG, Kruisinga RJH, Taselaar M: Triplet audiometry: An analysis of band discrimination in speech reception. Acta Otolaryngol 51:256−259, 1960

Jerger J: Behavioral correlates of hearing aid performance. Bull Prosth Res 10:62−75, 1967

Jerger J: Synthetic sentence identification in the evaluation of CROS amplification. Paper presented at the Symposium on Amplification for Sensori-neural Hearing Loss, Audiology Center of Redlands Co., 1971

Jerger J, Speaks C, Trammell JL: An approach to speech audiometry. J Speech Hear Dis 33:318−328, 1968 a

Jerger J, Thelin J: Effects of electroacoustic characteristics of hearing aids on speech understanding. Bull Prosth Res 10:159−197, 1968 b

Jerger J, Speaks C, Malmquist C: Hearing aid performance and hearing aid selection. J Speech Hear Res 9:136−149, 1966

Jirsa RE, Hodgson W, Goetzinger C: Reliability of PB half-lists. J Acou Soc Am 2:47−49, 1975

Kalikow DN, Stevens, KN, Elliott LL: Development of a test of speech intelligibility in noise using sentence materials with controlled word predictability. J Acoust Soc Am 61:1337–1351, 1977

Kamm C, Dirks, DD, Mickey MR: Effect of sensorineural hearing loss on loudness discomfort level and most comfortable loudness judgments. J Speech Hear Res 21:668–681, 1978

Konkle DF, Beasley DS, Bess FH: Intelligibility of time altered speech in relation to chronological aging. J Speech Hear Res 20:108–115, 1977

Lamb SH: Speech Discrimination Assessment Scale (Experimental Form). Communicative Disorders Clinic, San Francisco State University, San Francisco, Cal. 94132, 1974

Lentz W: Assessment of performance using hearing aids with directional and non-directional microphones in a highly reverberant room. Paper presented to the annual convention of the American Speech and Hearing Association, San Francisco, 1972

Levitt H, White REC, Resnick, SB: Prescriptive fitting of wearable master hearing aids: A progress report, in Rubin M (ed): Hearing Aids. Baltimore, University Park Press, 1976, 149–159

Manning W, Shaw C, Mahi J, et al: Analysis of half-list scores on the PB-K 50 as a function of time compression and age. J Am Audiol Soc 1:109–111, 1975

McCandless QA: Loudness discomfort and hearing aids. Paper presented at 3rd Oticongress, 1973, 39–44

McCommons RB, Hodge DC: Comparison of continuous and pulsed tones for determining Bekesy threshold measurements. J Acou Soc Am 45:1499–1504, 1969

McConnell P, Silber E, McDonald D: Test-retest consistency of clinical hearing aid tests. J Speech Hear Dis 25:273–280, 1960

Niemeyer W: Speech audiometry and fitting of hearing aids in noise. Audiology 15:421–427, 1976

Noble WG, Atherly GRC: The hearing measure scale: A questionnaire for the assessment of auditory disability. J Aud Res 10:229–250, 1970

Olsen W, Carhart R: Development of test procedures for evaluation of binaural hearing aids. Bull Prosth Res 7:22–49, 1967

Pimonow L: The application of synthetic speech to aural rehabilitation. J Aud Res 3:73–82, 1963

Redell RC: Calvert DR: Selecting a hearing aid by interpreting audiologic data. J Auditory Res 6:445–452, 1966

Reilly MC: CROS and BICROSS follow-up evaluation of a V.A. population. Paper presented at the Symposium on Amplification of Sensorineural Hearing Loss, Audiology Center of Redlands, California 1971

Resnick D: Reliability of the 25 word phonetically balanced lists. J Audiol Res 2:5–12, 1962

Resnick DM, Becker M: Hearing aid evaluation—a new approach. ASHA 5:695–699, 1963

Ritter R, Johnson RM, Northern JC: The controversial relationship between loudness discomfort levels and acoustic reflex thresholds. J Am Auditory Soc 4:123–131, 1978

Ross M: Introduction and review of hearing aid evaluation procedures, in Rubin M (ed): Hearing Aids. Baltimore, University Park Press, 1976, 143–148

Ross M: Hearing aid evaluation. In: Katz J (ed) Handbook of Clinical Audiology, Baltimore, Williams and Wilkins, 1978, 532−534

Rubin M, Ventry I: The use of Bekesy audiometry in the measurement of the threshold of intelligibility for connected discourse. J Audit Res 12:255−260, 1972

Sanders JW: The successful hearing aid user, in symposium on sensorineural deafness. Otolaryngologic Clinics of North America, 11:187−193, 1978

Schmitz HD: Loudness discomfort level modification. J Speech Hear Res 12:807−817, 1969

Schmitz HD: Implications of high frequency, intraoctave sensitivity peaks in auditory pathology. Paper presented at the Tenth International Congress of Audiology, Dallas, 1970

Schmitz H, Egan J, Norland M: Bekesy sound field audiometry: Application to hearing aid performance. Paper presented at the Symposium on Amplification for Sensorineural Hearing Loss, Audiology Center of Redlands, Cal., 1971

Schumaier D, Rintelman W: Half-list vs. full-list speech discrimination testing in a clinical setting. J Audiol Res 16:16−17, 1974 (suppl)

Shapiro I: Hearing aid fitting by prescription. Audiology 15:163−173, 1976

Shore I, Bilger R, Hirsch I: Hearing aid evaluation: Reliability of repeated measurements. J Speech Hear Dis 25:152−170, 1960

Silverman SR, Pascoe DP: Counseling about hearing aids, in Hearing and Deafness. New York, Holt, Rinehart, and Winston, 1978, pp. 338−357

Tannahill JC: The hearing handicap scale as a measure of hearing aid benefit. J Speech Hear Dis 44:91−99, 1979

Thompson G, Lassman F: Relationship of auditory distortion test results to speech discrimination through flat vs. selective amplifying systems. J Speech Hear Res 12:594−606, 1969

Ward PR, Tucker AM, Tudor CA, et al: Self-assessment of hearing impairment: tests for the expanded hearing ability scale questionnaire on hearing impaired adults in England. Br J Audiol 11:33−39, 1977

Yantis PA, Millin JP, Shapiro I: Speech discrimination in sensorineural hearing loss: Two experiments on the role of intensity. J Speech Hear Res 9:178−193, 1966

Zerlin S: A new approach to hearing aid selection. J Speech Hear Res 5:370−376, 1962

Mark Ross and Carole Tomassetti

6

Hearing Aid Selection for Preverbal Hearing-Impaired Children

"For most hearing-impaired children, the early and appropriate selection and use of amplification is the single most important habilitative tool available to us." With these words, Mark Ross and Carole Tomassetti set the mood for this entire chapter—a realistic, holistic approach to the problem. One of the most frustrating aspects of selecting a hearing aid for a young child is not being able to quantify the accuracy of our decision. With this in mind, Mark and Carole present special considerations for dealing with these situations. Beyond this, they describe, in humanistic terms, suggestions for parent counseling as the key to the successful use of amplification by a child.

MCP

INTRODUCTION

The major problem of most hearing-impaired children is that they have trouble hearing!

Before you reject this remark as facetious or trite, let us look closely into its implications. Certainly, the congenitally hearing-impaired child's deviations in communication skills development and their resulting effect in all facets of his life are a direct consequence of the hearing impairment. Though there are differences of opinion regarding the specifics of the relationship between the degree, type, and configuration of the hearing loss and the consequent problems, no one could logically argue that a strong relationship does not exist. To what habilitative measures, however, do the professions involved with the hearing-

213

impaired child focus most of their time and energy? In what areas do the articles in professional journals and papers read at professional meetings show the greatest concentration?

Not, to answer the question negatively, on measures designed to reduce the problem at the source, namely, the hearing loss itself, but rather on efforts that are essentially remedial and focus on correcting abnormal developmental patterns.

The underlying premise of this chapter is that *for most hearing-impaired children, the early and appropriate selection and use of amplification is the single most important habilitative tool available to us.* Most of these children have a great deal of residual hearing (Goodman 1949, Huizing 1959, Elliot 1967, Montgomery 1967, Boothroyd 1972, Hine 1973), which, properly exploited with amplification, can give access via the auditory channel to the innate biologic mechanisms underlying speech and language development (Lenneberg 1967). By focusing on the auditory input in an enriched natural language environment, the child's own potential capacity for speech and language development is used as the most significant ally in the audiologist's educational and therapeutic endeavors. We have expanded on this point elsewhere in more detail (Ross 1967, 1972, 1978a). Once optimum amplification is accomplished, enriched language and speech experiences, special tutoring, and innovative media can be effectively applied to the remaining gaps and needs. The first step, however, must be focused on the quality and quantity of auditory input directed to the child so that the natural development of speech and language can be maximized.

It is not easy to ensure this first step when the selection of appropriate amplification is being considered. With adults, we see a diverse variety of preferred methods of selection, adjustment, and modification of hearing aids, all of which are subject to questins and ultimate validation. However, we can be informed and aware of the appropriateness of our selection procedures and the usefulness of the final product by the feedback we get from verbal adults who are able to express their preferences and concerns. In the infant and young child population, we have amassed a similar proliferation of selection procedures, but without the clear feedback regarding the status of our recommendations. Our preferred selection procedures may thus remain inappropriate or inadequate merely because we cannot get immediate constructive feedback from our client. We have not developed generally accepted procedures with them for judging the effectiveness of the final product, i.e., the appropriately fit hearing aid.

Our approach for systematically selecting and judging the effectiveness of the hearing aid is defined in five distinct yet interrelated steps. For the purposes of introduction, the steps will be briefly mentioned, although all will be explained in more detail in the ensuing pages.

The first and most basic step is quantifying the child's hearing loss. We need to know as much as possible about the child's hearing as quickly as possible, but what we don't know should not stop us from proceeding. We should always be aware that we will have to make modifications and perhaps even major changes as we learn more about the child and his auditory status.

We need to define the factors which optimize the auditory and language learning of our hearing-impaired child. We must incorporate information relative to the acoustic properties of the speech signal, the linguistic information in speech, and the psychoacoustic implications of the hearing loss. This second step requires that we are familiar with normal speech and language acquisition as well as with information relating to hearing-impaired adults from whom it is considerably easier to obtain repeatable results and subjective reports.

The third step is to define and provide the electroacoustic properties which would satisfy the demands we have outlined in step 2. It is at this step that we are judging the electroacoustic properties which a child requires and actually selecting an aid. We should not confuse this approach with the one by which the child is fitted with some standard amplification pattern.

Our fourth step is concerned with evaluating the adequacy and success of our selection criteria. In other words, in the interaction among the child, his residual hearing, and his electroacoustic system are we able to observe and measure the predicted growth in auditory skills and in speech and language development? Such substantiation will not come from sound field assessment alone. We should not expect that we will find all the answers in improved percentage or performance results, or in "once-in-a-while" assessment. We are looking for documentation from unsolicited and elicited reports from parents, teachers, and other managing adults; from documented growth in auditory skills and speech and language improvements; and from behavioral manifestations on the part of the child in the clinic, at home, in the classroom, and in other real-life situations.

Our fifth and final step is the process of modifying, adjusting, and monitoring the electroacoustic system as more data accumulates in any of the four steps previously mentioned. We may, for example, observe that the ambient noise in the child's home has an adverse effect on his behavior as well as on his auditory responsivity. These observations may provide sufficient information to indicate that the low-frequency gain, output, or both should be lowered for this child's particular instrument.

Implicit in this fifth step are two assumptions: first, *that the selection of hearing aids for preverbal children is an ongoing process that extends beyond one, two, or more clinic visits,* and beyond the typical confines of a "clinic," into the more important areas of a child's daily living. We are looking at a hearing aid evaluation as an integral part of a total habilitation program. Second, *all initial electroacoustic recommendations are tenative, subject to appropriate changes as information about the child's hearing and auditory development begins to accumulate,* and our knowledge in the areas of audition, linguistics, and electroacoustics increases and becomes more refined.

Throughout the process of hearing aid selection for the preverbal child, we are continually aware that it is only one phase, although an important one, in a total habilitative process. *Early emphasis on amplification cannot take place in a habilitative vacuum.* The successful use of amplification is apt to reflect the audiologist's ability to communicate the necessity for amplification to the parents, and their active participation in this phase of the child's program, which in turn depends on their understanding and their acceptance of their child and his problems. This is not a stage that can be taken for granted and it cannot be relegated to occasional casual contacts between parents and their therapists. "Parent counseling" does not occur magically because the audiologist sometimes talks to the parents or because this is what he labels his intentions. The services of a skilled, sensitive clinician who can assist the parents in working out the anxiety and guilt feelings that frequently accompany the discovery of their child's problems is a prerequisite for an optimally successful habilitative effort (see Luterman 1979, 1973, 1978; Ross, 1967, 1972; McConnell, 1968). A purely technical approach to habilitation, no matter how skilled, is apt to founder on the parent's misunderstandings and misapprehensions. Parents are the more important partners in a joint educational effort. They have more at stake and have the greatest impact upon their children, particularly the younger ones, and their informed participation can be crucial. The sooner a parent counseling guidance program is begun the better. Paradoxically, it is when the diagnosis of hearing loss is first confirmed, before the parents have been able to understand and deal with the fears, anxieties, and guilt ensuing from this confirmation, that they are most receptive to effective therapeutic intervention. In like manner, we know that we must extend our clinical appraoch to areas outside of the typical clinical situation. The practice of placing a hearing aid on a child and hoping for the best has not been paying dividends. The "perfect" electroacoustic system for a hearing-impaired child will be useless if it is not working or worn consistently once the child steps out of the clinic or if the use of audition is not encouraged and expected as reflected in therapeutic and educational strategies.

We reemphasize that although this chapter will be devoted to the procedures and technical aspects of selecting a hearing aid for young hearing-impaired children, it should nevertheless be understood that, *for the best results, these techniques must be embedded within a complete habilitative matrix.*

PRESELECTION CONSIDERATIONS

Accurate Diagnosis

The accurate diagnosis of a hearing-impaired child is an obvious preliminary to recommending a hearing aid. Does the child have a hearing loss at all? If so, what is the type, severity, and configuration? These are not easy questions to answer when infants are the subjects of the evaluations. Usually the audiologist is not sufficiently fortunate to obtain precise audiometric information on hearing-impaired infants before they are fitted with a hearing aid. Initial recommendations for a child, then, reflect, to some degree, uncertainty regarding the specifics of the hearing impairment. Although the advent and widespread use of physiological measures such as electrocochleography, evoked cortical and brain stem audiometry, stapedial reflex measures, and some autonomic response measures, as well as results from other approaches such as polytomes, are beginning to reduce the uncertainty of our observations, most of the information used in formulating a habilitation program for any individual child is based on the results of behavioral audiometry (Waldon 1973, Hodgson 1978).

We should not underestimate the value of information obtained through behavioral test techniques. In the hands of a skilled clinician who is experienced in observing and interpreting the child's response levels and response manner, such results can roughly define peripheral hearing acuity and suggest the child's ability to attend to, process, and respond to auditory signals in an age-appropriate manner. After one or two sessions, it is possible in the majority of children to formulate rough estimates on the degree of hearing loss, possible discrepancies in hearing acuity between ears, the configuration of the hearing loss, and whether it is conductive, sensorineural, or has elements of both. In detailing this information, it is necessary throughout to ask the question, "Is the child's manner of responding and his auditory behavior consistent with developmental age and peripheral hearing status?" If not, we must be continually alert to complicating factors other than hearing loss. The impedance battery, and the tympanogram at the very least, is an integral and routine part of the evaluation procedure. Not only does it provide unique information relative to the absence of presence of conductive dysfunction but it lends additional data on the degree of hearing loss.

Regardless of the evaluation technique employed, rarely is an accurate diagnostic picture complete before the ages of 2 or 3, or well into the maximum readiness period for speech and language development. Therefore, the audiologist is usually in a position in which he must either recommend a hearing aid on the basis of incomplete information or risk losing some very valuable time while he establishes precise diagnostic and threshold measurements.

We would hope that at the very least we do have minimal response levels established for speech and for the frequencies of 250 Hz through 4000 Hz. In the initial stages, a general approach is to assume the child's hearing acuity is approximately 10−15 dB better than demonstrated by his minimal response levels in conditioned orientating or play response procedures. *This approach, which may occasionally underestimate the degree of hearing loss, will minimize the danger of overamplification and subsequent rejection on the part of the child.*

Sometimes we may encounter the child who is not responding specifically to auditory signals and appears too deaf to benefit from amplification. Since it is only a minority of hearing-impaired children whose hearing is so poor that they respond only to low-frequency vibrotactile stimuli, and since even this limited information can provide some communication assistance (Ross et al. 1973), *it makes therapeutic sense to require hearing aids for all hearing-impaired children at the earliest age possible.*

A necessary qualification must be included here. Hearing aids should not be fitted to any child without prior otologic examination, clearance, and/or treatment. Not only will such practice ensure the good comprehensive medical care of the hearing-impaired child, but it may contribute to that child's initial successful adaptation to and use of amplification. In our own practice we have frequently seen prescribed medication relieve negative middle-ear pressure, which had previously contributed to annoyance with the earmold and an excessive amount of feedback.

Physical Characteristics

Although our primary focus is to define and provide an electroacoustic system which satisfies predetermined requirements, we must of necessity be concerned with the physical aspect of the hearing aid itself. These physical features are especially relevant to consider for children who are usually human tornadoes who spend much of their waking hours in sand, water, and highly active physical activities. Knowing this, we need to be concerned with the performance aspect of the instruments which we might recommend. For example, we should know whether the hearing aid has stable operating characteristics even when submitted to unusual use conditions, a decent maintenance record, and physical characteristics which are sufficiently sturdy. *The physical dimensions of the hearing aid should be appropriate to a child size user.* We still see many examples of ear-level hearing aids with the bottom microphones hidden in a coat or sweater collar, or a button receiver which is almost as large as a small child's pinna tending to pull the earmold out of his ear.

External controls should be clearly labeled so that parents and other managing adults may have reference points when monitoring their child's amplification. However, too many controls, screw adjustments, and labels may confuse and overwhelm a parent and should be avoided whenever possible. Other features which affect the performance or manageability of the hearing aid should also be considered. Such considerations as battery life, susceptibility of components to moisture, taper characteristics of the gain control, and degree of clothing noise generated will influence our final selection.

Some characteristics would be major reasons for excluding hearing aids from the selection process. The internal or circuit noise at "use" gain should permit at least a 30 dB S/N ratio at normal input speech levels. The questions of acceptable distortion levels require a number of rather arbitrary decisions. However, it is a desirable clinical practice to prefer instruments which have the lowest distortion value. A total distortion of 10 percent or more excludes a hearing aid from further consideration.

A primary preselection consideration is the type of hearing aid to be utilized, postauricle, in-the-ear, or body type. Although in-the-ear instruments are believed to offer some unique advantages on a theoretical level, we are hesitant to use them with little children because of their present restrictions in control flexibility, the inability to enlarge them easily as the child grows, and most important, the inability to switch instruments on a trial basis quickly once a commitment to that type of hearing aid is made.

In our own practice we prefer postauricle hearing aids. There are several models or combinations of models which now offer the flexibility, power, frequency response range, and practical features which were once only attributed to body instruments. Additionally, these instruments offer advantages of microphone placement in a more "normal" position, i.e., at or around the pinna area, and normal separation of the microphones for binaural listening.

We have found that modern postauricle hearing aids are appropriate for the majority of hearing-impaired children. However, for a very young child (under 3 or 4 years) who also has a very severe degree of hearing loss, we prefer the initial use of body instruments. Our clinical preference is primarily based on practical considerations. We have found that the use of ear-level instruments in this population requires persistent attention to the earmold fit. As the child grows, frequent remakes would be required to ensure control of feedback and appropriate use gain and output. This type of instrument would also be prone to more frequent repair and shorter battery life.

Our final consideration is whether a monaural or binaural fitting will be applied in the initial stages. At our facilities, binaural hearing aids are recommended initially almost in every case. In addition to the generally positive auditory effects (Ross 1977), this has been done primarily for two reasons: (1) Most of the children have eventually been found to have bilateral, fairly symmetrical losses with the ears rarely differing by more than 10 or 15 dB at specific frequencies. Therefore, with a moderate degree of assurance, both aids can be adjusted equally in terms of gain and output to the requirement of the better ear. (2) Parents are much more receptive to the concept of binaural amplification when the child is first being fitted with hearing aids. Two-ear amplification makes sense to them at this time and they very readily accept the recommendations. It is when binaural recommendations are made after a more or less successful adjustment to a monaural fitting that parental and, occasionally, a child's resistance to a second hearing aid is experienced. Our clinical procedure is acceptable from a financial point of view as well, since the family is never obligated to purchase two personal hearing aids before individual ear information is detailed. There is always a possibility that the aid selected is inappropriate for one ear, especially when we are relying on sound field results which may reflect the dimensions of the "better" hearing ear and underestimate the second or "poorer" ear. Until we can define levels and configuration bilaterally, clinic loaner instruments are utilized.

In summary, then, for the preverbal child with probable bilateral severe or profound hearing loss, we usually initiate our hearing aid trial with sturdy binaural aids with electroacoustic features that include minimal distortion, an adjustable power output that can be limited at various steps within a range of 120 to 135 dB, and an adjustable wide-band frequency response. In the present state of the art, limitations such as feedback, durability, and pinna size would make the use of body instruments advisable. In children with lesser degrees of hearing loss we may be concerned with power outputs adjustable to but not exceeding values such as 105, 115, or 125 dB, with the same low-distortion and desirable frequency responses features. Binaural ear-level instruments would be the preferred choice. The key word in the preselection of any hearing aid is *flexibility*. Since the initial information concerning the child's residual hearing may be limited and since the electroacoustics of the hearing aid must be varied frequently as more information is acquired, an aid whose electroacoustic characteristics can be modified to reflect the additional audiometric data is required. The aid we initially select may well not be the one ultimately recommended, and therefore trial hearing aid loaners are needed while we are in the process of defining the child's hearing and his hearing needs. This loaner option should be included in any program dealing with preverbal children.

Electroacoustic Rationale

The primary goal of amplification is to provide the child with the maximum auditory information consistent with his hearing loss. We are interested in providing maximum acoustic energy in the speech range in as many situations as possible without approaching or exceeding the level at which the reception of speech is uncomfortable. When possible, we are further interested in reducing the influence, or competition, of irrelevant acoustic energy which could potentially mask the speech signal.

To utilize such an approach, we would need to recognize and incorporate the acoustics of speech as a basis for our selection considerations (Levitt 1978, Boothroyd 1978, Ling 1978). What parameters of frequency, intensity, and duration of speech are the salient auditory cues for the perception of speech in the normal hearing child, and how can they be provided to a child with a hearing loss?

An electroacoustic approach toward the selection of a hearing aid can be applied to hearing-impaired individuals regardless of age, but it is particularly appropriate for young children with limited verbal skills. The procedures for "hearing aid evaluations" developed with adults cannot be employed with these children (see Chapter 5 and Ross 1978a for a discussion of adult hearing aid evaluations). We will, in this chapter, make frequent reference to findings obtained with adults, not specifically hearing aid evaluations per se but rather data relating to improved speech discrimination skills wrought by electroacoustic modifications. We are making the important assumption that any electroacoustic variation that has been shown to improve speech discrimination scores for adults will enable hearing-impaired children to maximally develop their speech discrimination skills. Furthermore, we are assuming that this optimization of the acoustic signal will be reflected in a more rapid and normal pattern of speech and language development. With preverbal children, the appropriate and carefully monitored choice of electroacoustic characteristics appears to have the greatest face validity in determining the selection of hearing aids (Gengel et al. 1971, Erber 1973).

In our own experience the practice of selecting a hearing aid on a comparative basis by observing the child's differential response to amplified sound presents too many confounding variables to be a sufficiently trustworthy technique in itself. In conjunction with electroacoustic hearing aid selection procedures, however, behavioral observations of the child can provide valuable information. Included in Chapter 12 is a trial amplification report for systematizing the behavioral observations of a child who is in the initial stages of amplification usage. To this list, we would add the observation of changes in the quality and quantity of speech output when using different aids and/or electroacoustic systems.

It is important to remember that, in our approach, the initial electro-acoustic recommendations depend upon available audiometric information and knowledge of the most salient perceptual cues present in the acoustic signal. The goal is to provide the child with maximum auditory information consistent with his hearing loss. We are not overly concerned with the brand name of a hearing aid, but with the electroacoustic response it embodies. This is an important distinction to make. The audiologist is not comparing brand X to brand Y but with electroacoustic system X compared with electroacoustic system Y. It is not the name monogramed on a hearing aid that interests us but whether its performance is likely to provide the most relevant acoustic information to a hearing-impaired child.

ELECTROACOUSTIC SELECTION PROCEDURES

SPL Reference Level

Our goal of packaging the most useful amplification pattern within the residual hearing range can be illustrated and observed by plotting all thresholds with the same reference level. In our judgment an SPL reference scale best lends itself to this purpose. The response characteristics of a hearing aid, the acoustics of speech signals, and ambient noise readings are all commonly plotted on an SPL reference scale. By utilizing the same scale for indicating hearing threshold level (HTL), comfort, and discomfort thresholds, the relevant dimensions for considering the performance of a hearing aid become almost directly comparable. The use of an SPL graph, moreover, can provide a visual representation of the more obvious electroacoustic dimensions which must be modified if the child is to receive more of the salient auditory cues in speech (Fig. 6-1).

Measurement Instrumentation

An electroacoustic selection procedure presupposes that we have some means of ensuring that we are actually delivering desired electroacoustic parameters. One requirement is electroacoustic measuring equipment, used with an understanding that there is a variation in the response generated in a 2-cm³ coupler as compared to that in a real ear. (Pascoe 1975, Skinner 1976, Dalsgaard and Jensen 1976). The difference may be significant and therefore functional evaluations should always be made if possible. For example, we know in general that 2cm³ coupler values will overestimate functional gain in the frequencies above 2000 Hz.

Despite this serious limitation, the consistent use of an electroacoustic measuring device provides us with verification that the particular model we are using is working as the manufacturer specified when it was first delivered and,

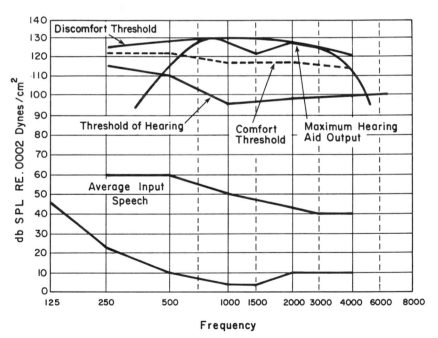

Fig. 6-1.   An example of the use of SPL reference level to plot the behavioral and electroacoustic measures on the same chart. The lower curve represents the minimal audible pressure (MAP) thresholds rounded out to the nearest 5 dB for ease in clinical computations.

more importantly, that the electroacoustic variables of that instrument remained stable over time and under various conditions of use. As practicing clinicians we have learned that we can never assume that the electroacoustic system we first put on the child is the same device 3, 6, or 12 months later. In fact, we are not surprised to find a completely different response in an instrument one day later when worn by a very active child after he has been involved in an hour of water play. Our experiences with this phenomenon has led us to routinely measure the hearing aids of little children on at least a monthly basis as a clinic-wide policy.

The electroacoustic measuring instrument is used to confirm preliminary estimates regarding the gain required by the hearing aid with further adjustments made as the child's reactions in behavioral assessment and observation would dictate. Such an approach is clearly preferred to the time honored methods of (1) setting the gain control by increasing the gain until acoustic feedback occurs, then reducing the gain just a bit until the feedback is eliminated. (2) Increasing the gain slowly, over a period of weeks or months until either feedback occurs or a discomfort reaction is elicited from the child. Unless we know the taper characteristics of the gain and volume control of that particular aid (assuming they are stable), either of these two latter methods involve too great a margin of error.

Finally, the use of a measuring device offers us one, but not the only, standard by which we might monitor the amplification characteristics of the hearing aid. The other standard is sound field aided and unaided assessment which will be discussed in a later section. Frequently, the discrepancies between what we have prescribed for a child and what the child consistently prefers to use has inspired us to investigate paramaters of the child's hearing aid via sound field testing which we otherwise might not have noticed or considered. In like manner, these discrepancies led us to investigate the interaction of the "prescribed" electroacoustic characteristics, measured both in a coupler and in a sound field, and the specific environmental acoustic situation confronting a child. This knowledge has enabled us to make desirable electroacoustic modifications, such as reducing the low-frequency response of an aid (Sweetow 1977).

Selecting Electroacoustic Parameters

Once we have determined that an electroacoustic approach will be used, we are then faced with establishing criteria for judging the particular response which will best provide for the child's needs. We must continually keep in mind the goal of providing the child with the maximum amount of auditory information consistent with his hearing loss without reaching intensity levels which would cause the child to reject the amplification.

Since we are concerned primarily with the perception of a speech signal, we must have some familiarity with its temporal, frequency, and intensity characteristics. The overall average intensity of a speech signal is about 65 dB SPL as measured 1 m from a speaker. The spectrum varies with frequency, with the energy at 4000 Hz approximately 20−25 dB less than the average intensity at 500 Hz. The variation in intensity is found within each frequency band as well; often one uses a single number to indicate the energy at a fixed point without realizing that this number also represents an average. Within each octave band the energy varies by approximately 30 dB. The total range between the highest energy in the low frequency band and the lowest energy in the high frequency band approaches 50 dB. However, for our purposes, realizing that we are using fixed intensity levels in our measurements, the average octave speech spectrum for normal conversation speech is approximately as follows (also see Fig. 2):

250	500	1000	2000	3000	4000
60	60	55	45	40	40

Our goal is to amplify this speech signal by the appropriate electroacoustic pattern and deliver to the child a 30 dB sensation level across the frequency range. With many severe and profound hearing losses, we may not be able to provide a 30 dB sensation level signal; our goal in these instances is to provide as

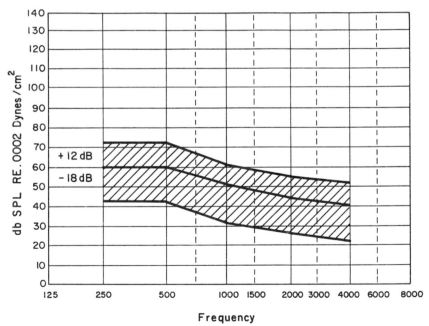

Fig. 6-2.   The approximate spectrum of average speech which is used for hearing aid selection purposes. Note the 30 dB range around the mean, 12 dB above and 18′ dB below, at each frequency point in the spectrum.

much as we can within the limits imposed by his auditory thresholds on the one hand and his loudness tolerance on the other. This general formulation will be qualified below.

As we begin to look at the variations in the spectrum of average speech, it becomes clear that a statement of gain or output which reflects one overall value is of little significance in the selection of an optimal electroacoustic system for a child. As an example, consider the child whose sound field thresholds are converted from HL to SPL values and displayed on the SPL graph of Figure 3. The relationship between the average speech and threshold of hearing varies as a function of frequency; thus it is apparent that this child requires different degrees of real-ear gain at each frequency if the speech spectrum is to be audible across the frequency range.

Maximum Output

In our clinical experience, *maximum output is the most important elec-troacoustic parameter to consider in fitting an aid on children.* It is, in our judgment, the major reason for their rejection of amplification. Constant or even

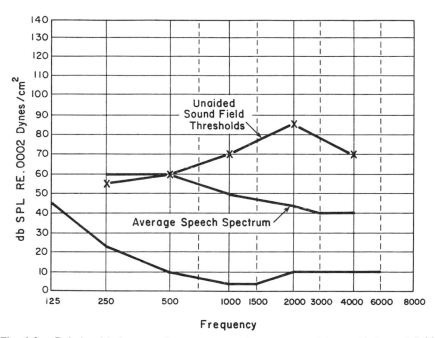

Fig. 6-3.   Relationship between the average speech spectrum and the unaided sound field thresholds of a hearing-impaired child. A first approximation of the amount of gain required at each measured frequency location in order to bring the speech signal above audibility can be determined from this plot.

occasional sounds which are uncomfortably loud or painful will elicit fear and rejection in the child not accustomed to amplified sound.

In defining this dimension for the amplification system of an adult, it is usually possible to obtain judgments of loudness discomfort level across frequency. However, these judgments are impossible to obtain from a preverbal child. In our own clinical approach, we are pleased when we are able to measure acoustic reflex levels with warbled tone or narrow-band stimuli presented in a sound field. Although reflex levels at each frequency do not precisely define the uncomfortable levels for differing acoustic stimuli (pure tones, warble tones, and narrow-band noise), the appearance of an acoustic reflex is the best objective information we have for inferring the threshold of discomfort and to establish the maximums of our amplification. When acoustic reflexes are measured, our first approach is to set the maximum output at the level which elicited the reflex. Our findings may be recorded on an SPL chart with reflex levels in SPL values representing the uncomfortable level. The area between our subject's sound field threshold and his reflex levels, therefore, define his dynamic range (Fig. 4).

It is necessary to reconcile the response differences between sound field stapedial reflex measures (used to estimate the real-ear required MPO) and coupler-defined output measures (how the information is actually reported). A

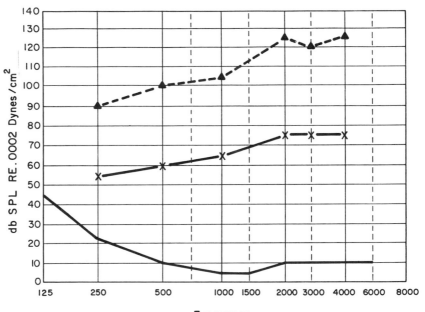

clinical method of making this reconciliation is to plot the functional gain as a frequency response and compare it to the coupler response of the same instrument (Pascoe 1978). Ordinarily there will be large differences, particularly at the higher frequencies. If we find that the coupler overestimates the frequency response at 2000 kHz by, e.g., 10 dB, and our reflex sound-field thresholds at this point is 125 dB, then we assume that the coupler MPO at this frequency should not exceed 135 dB. This procedure would be more accurate if aided reflex measures were made, since the variations produced by the receiver-mold combination would be included in the measurements. For a particular frequency, the functional gain plus the SPL of the tone which elicits the reflex provides a measure of the SPL in the ear canal. This figure is our MPO goal. The hearing aid output should not exceed the SPL which elicits an aided stapedial reflex. By applying the real-ear/coupler correction figure (the 10 dB in the above example) to the SPL in the ear canal when the reflex occurs, we can specify the coupler MPO which should not be exceeded for that frequency. The correction procedure can be applied at as many frequencies as desired, and precise instructions given to the hearing aid manufacturer, or adjustments made in available hearing aids, regarding the coupler-defined MPO curve across frequency. For the older child (or adult) this procedure would be more accurate if aided thresholds of discomfort (TD's), rather than aided stapedial reflex measures, could be measured, since this would give a direct estimate of loudness discomfort rather than an inferred one. This procedure would also be much more clinically useful if the clinician could adjust the frequency response at the saturation output; such a "fitting" option would permit a much closer congruence between the perceived TD's across the frequency and the output characteristics of a hearing aid. By precluding relatively narrow amplification peaks into the TD, the severely hearing-impaired person would achieve an actual increase in the aided dynamic range of hearing (his residual hearing).

In many of our cases, we are not able to elicit reflexes either because the child's hearing loss is too severe or because some degree of conductive loss or middle-ear dysfunction is involved. In these cases, we assume the reflex levels which have been found to occur with specified degrees of hearing loss. We are essentially making assumptions about reasonable maximum output levels which we desire at each frequency. For example, in normal hearers, reflexes will be established at 95−100 dB SPL. For mild losses up to 45 dB, reflex levels will not usually exceed 105 dB SPL; in moderate to severe losses to 80 dB, no greater than 115 dB SPL reflexes will be elicited whereas for severe losses of 90−100 dB HL reflex levels are not likely to exceed 125 dB SPL. Regardless of the degree of hearing loss, output levels beyond 130 dB SPL are recommended only occasionally.

This approach of establishing a maximum allowable output using acoustic reflex levels as a standard will lead us to establish lower maximum limits than have traditionally been suggested. However, with children it is always advisable to approach hearing aid selection conservatively and to increase the maximum output if and when we are able to document the necessity for such a change.

Gain and Frequency Response

Once we have established the maximum allowable output across frequency, we are able to consider gain as a somewhat independent parameter. In many newer hearing aids there are separate controls which are used to manipulate maximum output (usually a hidden screw adjustment) and gain (the volume control). This arrangement permits many gain-maximum output combinations.

As with output values, we are interested in specifying the required gain across frequency. We are aware of the dangers inherent in proposing a simplistic solution to a complex problem, particularly when the solution may almost be canonized by insecure practitioners. However, there is merit in proposing a procedure which can be used as a point of departure for further investigation, validation, and modification as new information accumulates. This approach, commonly recognized as the "prescription method," has been proposed by a number of others over the years. (Pascoe 1975, 1978, Skinner 1976, Victoreen 1960, Wallenfels 1967, Byrne and Tonnisson 1976, Powell and Tucker 1977, Martin 1973, Grainger 1977, Byrne and Fifield 1974, Byrne 1976, 1978, Berger 1976).

In determining the required gain across frequency, we use the so-called 50 percent law as our first approximation of functional gain required. Thus if the hearing threshold level (HTL) of an individual was 70 dB, then the first estimate of required functional gain would be 35 dB. We have found that using these values as a point of departure in determining functional gain gives us results very similar to that used by other clinicians employing slightly different procedures but with a similar electroacoustic rationale (Brooks 1973, Byrne and Tonnisson 1976, Byrne 1978, Berger 1976). In actual practice, we use somehwat less gain at the lower frequencies than 50 percent would predict. The amount of functional gain we can achieve in the high frequencies depends upon the dynamic range; we attempt to provide as many high frequencies as possible because of the significance of these higher frequencies in the perception and development of speech and language (the phoneme /s/, for example, which spreads acoustically from 3000 kHz upward, serves as a grammatical marker more often than any other phoneme in the English language). Unfortunately, and this is a sad commentary on the status of hearing aid developments, we are more often prevented from reaching this goal by the occurrence of acoustic feedback than the tolerance of the youngsters at these high frequencies (see Chapter 2).

Figure 6-5 illustrates the results obtained with this procedure. The HTL thresholds across frequency are given in the first row (this is the only time we depart from a strict SPL formulation for all computations). The estimated gain figure appears in row 2. It will be noticed that we estimate less gain at the low

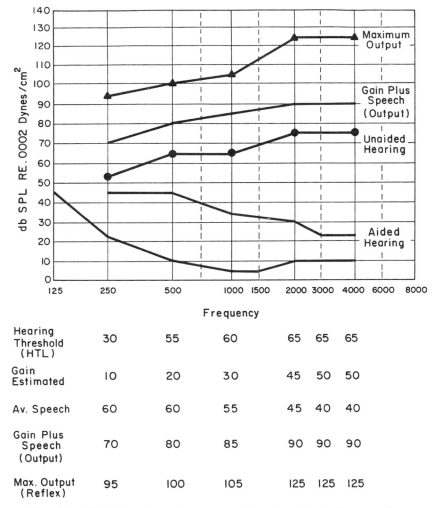

Fig. 6-5.   Worksheet for an electroacoustic hearing aid selection procedure.

frequencies and more gain at the higher frequencies than a strict 50 percent formulation would predict. The speech spectrum figures that we use is displayed in row 30. The acoustic output (gain plus input) appears in row 4. Row 5 gives the maximum SPL permitted in the ear, derived from stapedial reflex measures. As can be observed, the aided thresholds almost, but not quite, follow the uniform hearing level found by Pascoe (1975) to be most appropriate for individuals with gradually sloping losses. The aided output provides an acceptable audibility area across frequency (Skinner 1976) and appears quite close to an estimated MCL curve obtained through bisecting the thresholds of hearing and discomfort (Victoreen 1960, Wallenfels 1967).

Another example of how this procedure operates is given in Figure 6-6. This is a child whose hearing loss is greater in the high frequencies than that of the child in the previous example. He shows limited residual hearing between 2000 and 4000 Hz. If we assume that the output of the hearing aid is limited at the point where the stapedial reflexes occur, then it is not possible to place an amplified speech signal with a normal dynamic range (30 dB) between the thresholds and the output. Some parts of the speech signal will be inaudible although the peaks will be limited in some fashion (peak clipping or compression) by the hearing aid. This is the kind of child who can possibly benefit from

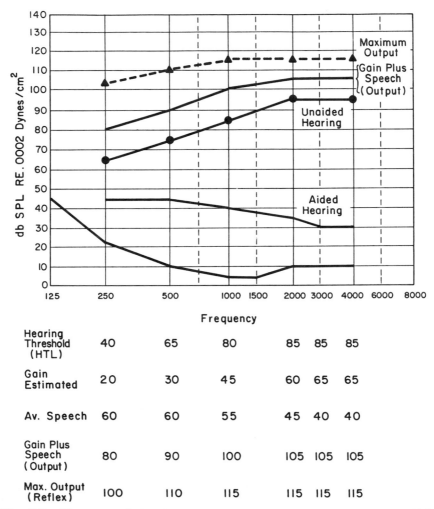

	125	250	500	1000 1500	2000 3000 4000
Hearing Threshold (HTL)	40	65	80		85 85 85
Gain Estimated	20	30	45		60 65 65
Av. Speech	60	60	55		45 40 40
Gain Plus Speech (Output)	80	90	100		105 105 105
Max. Output (Reflex)	100	110	115		115 115 115

Fig. 6-6. Electroacoustic hearing aid selection worksheet for a child with a high-frequency hearing loss.

the sophisticated signal processing techniques suggested by Villchur (1973). In this procedure, two separate bands of speech (an upper and lower band) are compressed and then filtered to follow an elevated, equal loudness contour, or placed at some point below the threshold of discomfort. The ratio and threshold of compression in the two bands can be adjusted, as can the filtered contour of the compressed speech.

EVALUATING THE APPROPRIATENESS OF ELECTROACOUSTIC SYSTEM

The basic premise throughout the whole of our approach to the selection of hearing aids for children is that all electroacoustic recommendations are tentative. When dealing with children we assume that we will not possess complete information relative to their hearing status and, furthermore, that this status may change over time. Unfortunate, but common, is the child with a progressive hearing loss. We have frequently encountered instances where progression is barely detectable except when viewed over a long period of time as well as where the progression occurs in dramatic threshold shifts. Modifications must be made in the electroacoustic parameters to reflect these changes in auditory status.

We can be assured that factors relative to the child, his acoustic environment, the present state of the art in electroacoustic knowledge and application will require that we modify our initial recommendations and selections. In fact, the same hearing aid worn by a child year after year without modification or replacement is strongly suspect. In all probability, it is no longer an "optimal" electroacoustic system for him.

The methods of evaluating the continued appropriateness of the system and identifying and providing the required modifications are not elaborate or theoretical. Simply stated, they involve long-term, consistent, and persistent monitoring, evaluation, and systematic application of remedial measures. In short, a very heavy "hands-on" approach.

In our program we develop and take advantage of four major evaluative situations. The first and most familiar to most audiology programs is the clinic evaluation. We see the little children in the clinic at least monthly and more frequently when a problem is reported or suspected. We rely on all the techniques discussed in this chapter, including electroacoustic measurement at "use" settings and sound field-aided assessment, to provide us with updated results.

Additional data have accumulated from other more formalized procedures (such as specific tests, scales, and performance measures) which are attempts to document changes and growth in speech; language; auditory, social-emotional, and cognitive development. With little preverbal children this technique may contribute the least amount of information relative to the other techniques employed but is valuable when it can be applied successfully.

We rely most heavily on directed observation of the child and useful reporting of his behavior in various situations by parents, teachers, speech pathologists, and other managing adults. A child's very active or overreactive behavior in free play segments of his preschool program may signal too much gain in the low frequencies an MPO set too high, or the need to consider noise control in that class segment. In any case, such behavior would signal that investigation and remedial measures are warranted.

Finally, the professionals responsible for electroacoustic selection, the audiologists, need to expand the skills of clinical observation to other situations. It is required that they leave the soundproof booth and be involved in the home and classroom situations—both of which are extensions of our traditional "clinic."

Aided Sound Field Audiogram

Measurement of functional gain is not new; it has been with us for as long as the profession of audiology has. In Mark Ross' 1958 M.A. thesis at Brooklyn College, evaluations with sound field audiometry dating back to World War II were referred to. Its use was reported by Liden and Kankkunen (1973), who used the technique to evaluate the capacity of 160 hearing-impaired children to benefit from amplification and as a tool for making educational prognoses.

In terms of evaluating the relative performance of hearing aids, it is most useful when young hearing-impaired children with little or no speech and language are the subjects. The child is only required to respond to the onset of sound; for younger children, who are unable to make a voluntary response to a sound, visual response audiometry (VRA) can be applied successfully. A precise correspondence between the unaided sound field thresholds and the better ear thresholds under phones is not necessary because it is the difference between aided and unaided thresholds under the same conditions in which we are primarily interested. Nonetheless, if we are interested in the correspondence, it has been shown that sound rooms can be calibrated to effect a close agreement between the thresholds (Green and Ross 1968; Morgan, Dirks, and Bower 1979).

The first step is to establish the unaided sound field thresholds. To preclude the possibility of standing wave effects, warble tones or narrow-band noises can be used as stimuli. The subject should be seated in a chair close to and facing the loudspeaker. The hearing aid is then placed on the child, set and marked in close approximation to the gain values we have determined by calculation and by electroacoustic measurement. An aided threshold is then obtained and the difference between the aided and unaided thresholds at each frequency represents the functional or real-ear gain. If this functional gain does not reflect the gain which we had initially selected, appropriate adjustments are warranted. Often the adjustments are minor variations in the tubing, earmold design, or volume or tone settings. Less frequently, the entire electroacoustic device must be changed. With each modification, aided sound field thresholds are repeated to measure the functional gain and monitor the approximation to our prescribed or optimal gain curve.

Sound field thresholds can also be used to compare the performance of hearing aids with different tonal adjustments and/or receivers. In Figure 6-7 the response of the same hearing aid is compared with a combination of different receivers and tonal adjustments. The gain control setting remained the same for all measurements. In this example, the high tone setting with receiver no. 1 provided the most acoustic information.

It should be noted at this point that those comparisons reflect the hearing aid's performance only at the aided threshold of hearing; the suprathreshold responses may possibly show a different picture of aided performance. This can be determined by electroacoustically evaluating a family of frequency response curves obtained with different and greater sound-pressure level inputs. If, for example, the input-output relationship of the best aid in Figure 6-7 proved to be nonlinear at normal SPL outputs, the aid would not be satisfactory in spite of the apparent advantages at the aided threshold. Additionally, by looking at aided output, one can judge the potential audibility of speech across frequency (Fig. 6-8).

The difference between the aided and unaided thresholds are a measure of the functional gain provided by the hearing aid. When we vary the intensity of

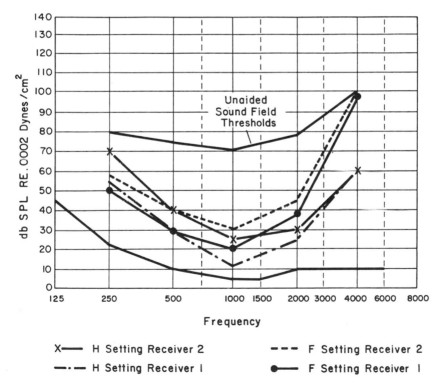

Fig. 6-7.   Changes in the sound field thresholds as a function of different receivers and tonal adjustments in a single hearing aid.

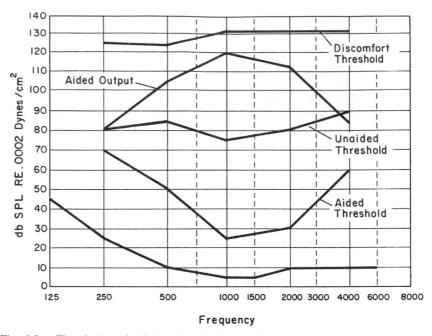

Fig. 6-8.   The plotting of aided and unaided sound field thresholds on an SPL reference scale. In this example, a hearing aid which appears to be the superior one of the three from Figure 6-7 is shown to provide inadequate amplification at 4000 kHz.

the inputs, however, we can directly measure whether or not the child's discomfort levels or reflex levels are likely to be approached or exceeded by the applied signal. For example, Figure 6-6 illustrates the SPL chart of a case whose amplification is set to deliver 45 dB of functional gain at 1000 Hz. Inputs up to 70 dB SPL would not be expected to elicit a reflex since the reflex threshold is 115 dB SPL, and in actual sound field-aided assessment, we find that this is the case. Additionally, we find that inputs of 80 and 90 dB do not elicit the reflex, indicating that functional output or output generated in the rear-ear canal under consideration does not exceed the maximum output levels which we predicted would be appropriate.

In our own clinical practice, we routinely rely on sound field-aided thresholds to provide us with information relative to the effects of different earmolds and earmold variations, and the stability of the child's amplification system over time and under the varying conditions under which the aid is used. For example, we will assess the child's aided sound field threshold with the aid set as he has been found to wear it in the classroom. If there are large discrepancies between thresholds obtained in a clinical setting (prescribed gain) and those with a preferred classroom setting (use gain), we would have strong indications that there is a problem in the classroom environment which must be remediated.

Finally, we have found that the graphic portrayal of aided versus unaided sound field thresholds enables us to communicate the function of the amplification system to the audiologically naive individual. The relative changes in the aided response of different hearing aids can assist us in explaining the need for a new one to the parents.

An additional advantage of sound field audiometry was reported by Liden and Kankkunen (1973). The recommend the cautious use of the technique for educational prognoses. They evaluated 160 hearing-impaired children and found three separate categories related to the child's capacity to use amplified sound. In the first category (example A, Fig. 6-9), there is a definite and clear-cut difference between the aided and unaided thresholds. Children in this category are excellent candidates for an auditory-oral program; their speech and language development begins relatively early (provided early management procedures are applied) and roughly follows a normal developmental course. The children in the second category (example B, Fig. 6-9, also demonstrate by the difference between their aided and unaided audiograms that they possess residual hearing capacity, although only at the low frequencies. They are also considered candidates for an auditory-oral approach, though their progress is lower than the children in the first category and their ultimate auditory status is more questionable. The children in the third category (example C, Fig. 6-9) represented approximately 10 percent of the 160 children that Liden and Kankkunen (1973) tested. These children showed no difference between their aided and unaided audiograms, indicating that measured thresholds represented vibrotactile responses (Nober 1968). On X-ray examination some of these children displayed missing or malformed inner ears. Similar medical findings were reported by Downs (1972), whose recommendations mirrored those of Liden and Kankkunen, namely, that some form of manual communication be taught to these children beginning at a very early age. However, the use of a hearing aid, which can deliver vibratory information to these children, should not be excluded.

In our work, we have not found the clear-cut categories reported by Liden and Kankkunen (1973). Instead it appears that every child for whom it was possible to measure unaided sound field vibrotactile thresholds showed better thresholds in the aided condition. It may be that we are simply increasing the sensitivity of the vibrotactile thresholds via sound amplification. A possible explanation is that we ensure that all children with residual hearing only in the low frequencies use hearing aids with an extended low frequency response. It was not possible to ascertain from the Liden and Kankkunen article whether this was also true of the children they evaluated.

For some older children it may be possible to measure their sound field thresholds with a Bekesy audiometer. This has the advantage of providing a continuous frequency plot across the entire frequency range of a hearing aid or the residual hearing. Octave step audiometry, or even half-octave steps, does not reflect what may be important information between the measured frequencies. A

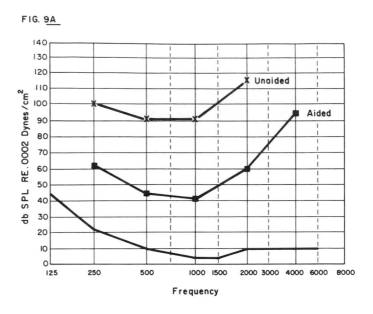

FIG. 9A

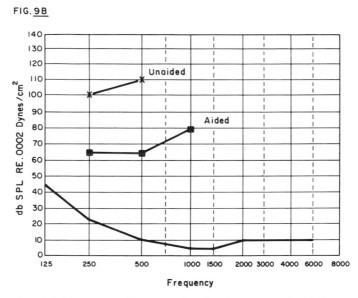

FIG. 9B

Fig. 6-9. Sound field assessment to make educational prognoses. In (a) the prognosis is excellent for an auditory-oral program; in (b), the prognosis is guarded for primary placement in an auditory-oral program; in (c), the prognosis is poor for maximum educational progress in an auditory-oral program.

FIG. <u>9C</u>

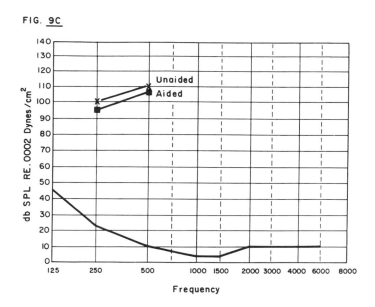

Frequency

Bekesy audiometer can be calibrated to approximate better-ear thresholds as measured under phones. Hearing aids and/or their adjustments can be compared as above by using this technique (Green and Ross 1968, Harford and Doods 1971).

Additional Electroacoustic Considerations

Although all details of the relationship may not be clear, we can safely assume that the pattern of amplified sound reaching a hearing-impaired listener bears some relationship to speech intelligibility. Furthermore, as indicated above, it seems reasonable to assume that the pattern, which has been shown to improve speech discrimination ability with hearing-impaired adults, would do the same with hearing-impaired children. The difference, of course, is that with adults modifications in signal processing increases their *recognition* ability, while with congenitally hearing-impaired children the same signal must be used for the *development* of speech and discrimination (and auditory language) skills. Since speech discrimination ability cannot be assessed directly in hearing-impaired infants, these assumptions are not only logical but necessary if we are to approach the selection of a hearing aid for children in an intelligent manner.

In an earlier section, we stated our procedure for estimating the low frequency gain. It is our practice to minimize but not eliminate the low-frequency gain and, particularly, output relative to the high frequencies when the child demonstrates significant residual hearing throughout the high frequencies. We base this preference on a series of studies completed at Gallaudet College (Danaher et al. 1978), where it was found that at high SPLs the presence of a low frequency first formant interfered with the perception of the higher frequency, second formant transitions. These transitions are known to be important cues to consonant perception. The elimination of the first formant, which normally is more intense than the second, resulted in improved discrimination of the second formant transitions for many subjects. Similar results were found (Sweetow 1977, Sung et al. 1971) when speech discrimination scores in noise were compared, with and without an extended low-frequency response pattern, for both normal and hearing-impaired adult subjects. Speech discrimination scores were superior when low-frequency amplification was reduced. The continuing practice of supplying broad-band high SPL signals for subjects with broad-band residual hearing is not supported by available evidence. We wish that the current engineering trend of providing hearing aids with lower and lower frequency ranges (fostered by the development of the electret microphone) would be matched by equal zeal in respect to improving the high-frequency capability of workable hearing aids. New earmold developments with a so-called "step" or "horn" bore are important steps to this goal (Villchur 1978).

In light of some convincing theoretical and clinical evidence, there has been a recent surge of emphasis in hearing aid design on extending the high frequency ranges of hearing aids. We know that much of the energy of voiceless phonemes, particularly /S/, /sh/, /f/, the unvoiced /th/, and /ch/, fall above 4000 Hz (Whetnall and Fry 1971). The child's reception of high-frequency sounds has both phonemic and morphemic implications. The /s/ and /t/ phonemes, for example, are also plural and past-tense markers, respectively. An electroacoustic system that filters potentially valuable acoustic information simply does not make sense. In this instance, one cannot generalize from adults to children. An adult who knows the language can function quite well with the elimination of a certain degree of the redundancy in the speech signal. Not so with a congenitally hearing-impaired child. He is attempting to learn speech and language through an impaired auditory system and a low-fidelity amplification device. Hence, the additional acoustic information provided by the high frequencies is likely not to be redundant at all, but the minimal cues necessary for developing certain speech and language skills.

A number of research studies have supported the extension of the upper frequency range of hearing aids (Watson 1960, Olson 1971, Pascoe et al. 1973 Triantos and McCandless 1974). Watson completed the only such study with hearing-impaired children as subjects. He tested speech discrimination skills for two groups of hearing-impaired children, one group with flat losses and the other with high-frequency losses, under types of conditions, one with an extended frequency range (to 8000 cps) and the other with the same equipment but with filters to reduce the frequency range to about 3000 Hz. He found improvement in discrimination ability for both groups of children when the higher frequencies were included, though more so for the flat than for the high-frequency loss group. All of these children presumably had had prior experiences with high-fidelity amplification while using group hearing aids, and for them the test was a simple speech discrimination task. One wonders how these children would have performed if they had never been exposed to the higher audible frequencies.

Olsen (1971) related various electroacoustic characteristics to the intelligibility of speech passed through different hearing aids. Of all the indices, he found that frequency band width was the one most predictive of speech intelligibility, with the wider band widths associated with improved intelligibility.

Pascoe et al. (1973) also demonstrated the importance of higher frequencies in their study. For one hearing-impaired subject who underwent extensive testing, they found an average improvement of 12 percent discrimination score as the higher frequency range was increased from 3150 to 6300 Hz. An additional finding in this same study has potentially great significance for the future design of the electroacoustic characteristics of hearing aids. They designed a master hearing aid, the frequency response curve of which inlcuded the head diffraction and ear canal resonance effects normally eliminated by the presence of an earmold (the so-called *insertion* loss that affects the normal field-to-eardrum transfer function.) This curve was flat to 1500 Hz, rose 19 dB at 3000 Hz, and continued at that level to 6300 Hz, at which point the termination of the frequency range began. They found that progressive reductions in the amplitude of the resonance from 0 to 10 dB lowered the discrimination scores by 15 percent. In an associated study, Miller (1973) speculated that the improvement in speech discrimination observed when hearing aids are coupled to open rather than closed earmolds is due to the restoration of the normal ear canal resonance that occurs with open earmolds.

Triantos and McCandless (1974) compared the speech discrimination ability in quiet and noise of both normal hearing and hearing-impaired adults under conditions of high-frequency cutoff, one at 3800 Hz and one at 5200 Hz. Both groups of subjects demonstrated an improvement in discrimination score of approximately 15 percent to the higher frequency cutoff when the tests were conducted in noise. No differences were found under quiet conditions. In terms of personal preference, the subjects selected the higher frequency cutoff over the lower frequency cutoff. The authors also observed that the response latency of the hearing-impaired subjects in noise was much less with the broader band than with the narrower band signal. Given the present technical capability of engineering hearing aids with upper frequency ranges to 5000 or 6000 Hz, there appears to be no good reason to deprive any hearing-impaired individual of this potentially valuable acoustic information. Children whose residual hearing is limited to the lower audible frequencies obviously require hearing aids with an extended low-frequency range (Leckie and Ling 1968). Some suppression of the higher frequencies, particularly at the points where the frequency response peaks, is advisable to reduce the production of acoustic feedback at these frequencies.

An electroacoustic modification mentioned but not covered in this chapter is the use of various kinds of sophisticated multiband compression amplification patterns. Theoretically at least, and with some experimental data beginning to accumulate (see Chapter 2 and Villchur 1978), this type of system shows possible significant advantages over traditional ways of limiting hearing aid output.

UTILIZATION OF FIRST HEARING AID

After the first hearing aid is selected, steps must be taken to ensure that the receiver mold or ear-level aid-mold combination stays in the child's ears. This is not a problem with adults: With young children it is a frequent problem and a nuisance. A child's ears are small, soft, and smooth and the earmolds may easily drop out of their ears, especially when weighted by either a heavy receiver or an ear-level hearing aid. To alleviate this problem in a receiver-mold combination, one can (1) tape the receiver to the pinna, (2) bend the cord up and around the back of the pinna and tape the cord to the mastoid process, or (3) use a shell mold, with tubing and an adapter to the receiver, which is then either taped behind the ear or hooked to the collar of the child's clothing. We prefer to minimize the length of tubing from the mold to the receiver because of the high frequency signal attenuation that will occur in this arrangement. In an ear-level/mold combination, hairdressing tape double-faced between the hearing aid and the mastoid process secures the aid enough under most circumstances so that it is not an additional weight on a well fitting earmold. A great deal of clinical ingenuity and frustration is involved in this process. However, the aid does the child no good if it does not stay in his ear, and attention to this detail is necessary.

We prefer a soft mold to minimize the effects of blows and other impacts upon the receiver and mold combinations, and to provide a secure but comfortable fit. However, we have seen many of the more popular earmold materials induce dermatological problems in tender skin, particularly during the humid summer months. A number of such cases has caused us to be very selective of earmold material, and watchful for minor irritations which might signal impending full scale eruptions.

If the child is to use a hearing aid with high gain and output capabilities, and since the distance between the microphone and the receiver cannot be very great in a small child, then the importance of an excellent earmold impression to reduce acoustic feedback is apparent (see Chapters 2 and 3). We assume that any cerumen has been removed by the otolaryngologist and there is no middle- or outer ear condition that precludes taking an earmold impression. We have made one observation in this respect regarding children. When a child has a middle-ear problem, e.g., a serous otitis media, feedback occurs at much lower gain levels than when the child does not have a middle-ear problem. Conversely, we have also noticed that the sudden presence of acoustic feedback at gain levels at which the child wore the aid previously with no problem can be an indication of a middle-ear problem. The reasoning is that increased impedance in the middle ear, due to negative middle-ear pressure or fluid, produces more sound reflections off the eardrum and thus more of the acoustic signal can be detected by the microphone. Clinically, this observation has been verified by middle ear impedance measures. Many of our hearing-impaired children have middle ear ventilating tubes. Additional precautions must be taken to minimize some adverse interaction of the earmold canal and the tube which would reduce the efficiency of sound conduction, the adequacy of the ventilating tube, or result in feedback. Obvious solutions include a short earmold shank, or conversely, use of a shorter version of aeration tube. Communication between the audiologist and otologist would be required to arrive at a workable resolution.

In the location we prefer to place body model aids—the shoulder socket on each side—feedback may well occur because of the close proximity of the receiver and the microphone. The hearing aids are located at this point to provide adequate spatial separation between the microphones of the two aids and to improve auditory self-monitoring. If, in spite of a well-fitting earmold, feedback is still a problem, then the aids are criss-crossed, with the microphone from one side led to the opposite ear and vice versa. With this arrangement the hearing aid gain can be increased with no apparent ill effects upon the child. Feedback cannot be alleviated as easily with ear-level placement; however, if adequate gain and output without feedback cannot be attained with expended effort over a reasonable period of time, we support the change over to body-type models. This is a decision that is not based only on convenience. Valuable auditory time can be lost—sometimes months—in an effort to fit the child to a type of instrument rather than selecting a type appropriate for him.

Child's Initial Adjustment to Amplification

In our experience, the initial adjustment to amplification is more of a problem to the parents and professionals than it is to a child. An insecure and fearful adult who approaches the child with a hearing aid in a tentative and uncertain manner can easily convey his trepidations to the child. Approached authoritatively, most children will accept amplification much the same way they accept being changed, fed, dressed, and so on. Involved recipes are not followed in preparing the young child to wear a hearing aid. The audiologist's goal is to put the aid on the child and keep it on him all day every day. Formulas that require 5 or 10 minutes of use daily, which is then slowly increased in time, bring too much attention to bear on the aid itself. The hearing aid, at least for some children, can then too easily become a point of dispute with parents. We prefer to view the hearing aid as an accepted and integral part of the child himself and transmit this attitude to the child and his parents. We do not put ourselves in the position where the child is given an option to wear or not wear the hearing aid; what if he says no?

The above should not be construed to mean that the fitting of a hearing aid on a child is a casual or thughtless affair. On the contrary, we assume that as few variables as possible are left to chance. All factors discussed previously have been considered and applied. The clinician has some workable estimate of the child's hearing threshold; he knows the characteristics of the aid, in particular that the maximum output does not exceed the child's discomfort level; that he is convinced of the potential benefits of amplification; that the earmold fits comfortably in the child's ear; and that the child and parents are enrolled in a follow-up program. Given these assumptions and the acceptance of the parents which has been developed with information, guidance, and support, the child is likely to make a good initial adjustment to amplification. The younger the child, the easier the acceptance of amplification seems to be. We have rarely had an instance in which a judicious combination of casualness (and cajolery, reward, and punishment when indicated) did not seem to give the desired results. The key factor, and it is worth restating, is a confident and competent clinician.

Parent Hearing Aid Orientation and Troubleshooting

The parents must be taught to take complete responsibility for the care and use of the hearing aid from the correct insertion of the earmold to the awareness of environmental conditions that detrimentally affect speech reception through the hearing aid. Some of the following comments and procedures will appear to be picayune considerations, unworthy of the attention of true "professional." In our judgment, however, more of our good intentions and theoretically sound advice have foundered on apparent trivia than perhaps any other factor. An excellent and detailed summary of the parent's role in maintaining a child's hearing aid was presented by Downs (1971).

The first step is to teach the parents how to insert and properly seat the earmold. The clinician should demonstrate how to manipulate the mold into the ear. This is accomplished by inserting the canal of the mold into the ear canal, with the superior tip of the mold facing forward, then while lifting the pinna up and out, the mold is screwed into the ear. When seated properly, the upper tip of the mold (the fossa portion) should rest securely in the antihelix fold of the pinna, with no air space visible between the mold and the concha. A very light coating of vaseline on the mold is occasionally necessary to reduce friction resistance.

The next step is to demonstrate the operation of the hearing aid. All of the adjustments on the aid should be fully explained and the specific ones used by the child noted. Volume controls should be marked for easy replication of gain settings. The battery compartment can be opened and the parents shown how to insert a battery. The cord prongs leading from the aid to the receiver should be disconnected and reconnected. The harness should be adjusted and fitted to the child by the parents. No detail should be assumed too simple for explanation and demonstration.

Troubleshooting procedures are both concurrent with and follow upon the explanation of the hearing aid's operation. The battery voltage is checked and the battery terminals examined for corrosion and poor contact with the battery. It is not good practice to use a battery in which voltage has dropped more than about 0.3 V. At and beyond this point, while the gain may still be adequate for a child, distortion products tend to increase dramatically. The aid, receiver, and cord are examined for physical damage, which may signify a malfunctioning hearing aid. The parents are asked to listen to the aid with their own earmold, or a commercially available hearing aid stethoscope. The cord should be rotated and bent where it inserts into the receiver and aid and any intermittancy or signal cessation noted. It is helpful if the parents develop a good subjective impression of the amplification pattern of the aid while it is operating optimally so that they can judge when differences are occurring. The extent of "clothing noise" and the effect of covering the microphone with several layers of clothing must be explained.

One of the first steps in any therapy session or visit is to remove the aid from the child and have it examined by the clinician-audiologist. Problems uncovered are discussed and demonstrated to the parents to ensure their comprehension. Without their active and informed cooperation, the full potential benefits of sound amplification cannot be realized. The results of a good orientation program can be observed when, after some period of time, the clinician finds the aid working satisfactorily at the commencement of all therapy or class sessions.

Signal-to-Noise Considerations

The primary purpose of sound amplification is to bring a desired signal within the child's residual hearing capacity. The entire rationale of an auditory approach to speech and language development rests on this factor. The speech signal must be perceived in order for it to activate the biologic mechanisms responsible for the normal course and sequence of this development. This cannot occur when the speech signal is constantly being buried in a noisy background.

It is an unfortunate fact that the hearing-impaired listener, particularly one with a sensorineural hearing loss, is more sensitive to noise-masking effects than the normal hearing individual listening to speech processed through a hearing aid (Finitzo-Hieber and Tillman 1978). As Tillman et al. (1970) state, "It is virtually impossible for a person with normal hearing to appreciate the handicaps to everyday listening that are experienced by the sensorineural patient because of such overmasking. . . . There are undoubtedly many times when hearing aid users cannot understand their companions even though all signals are sufficiently amplified and the background competition is so slight that a person with normal hearing would disregard it easily." These authors provide evidence to demonstrate that there is about a 30 dB spread between comparable conditions where listeners with normal hearing and those with sensorineural hearing loss could achieve a 40 percent intelligibility score. At a signal-to-noise (S/N) ratio of -12 dB, the listener with normal hearing obtained this score; the hearing-impaired subjects required a $+18$ dB S/N ratio before they could achieve this same 40-percent score. Related findings were reported by Gengel (1971), who showed that S/N ratios of $+15$ to $+20$ dB were necessary in order for a hearing-impaired subject to achieve his maximum intelligibility score for aided listening under noise conditions. At $+10$ dB and less, his subjects reported that listening required so much effort they would rather not use their hearing aids.

We should, at this moment, pause to consider the implications of these findings upon hearing-impaired children who are expected to develop speech and language via amplified sound. If hearing-impaired adults with existing language competencies are unable to recognize speech signals under only moderately adverse conditions, how then can children be expected to exploit these amplified speech signals for their language and speech development? The answer is, unfortunately, that they cannot. Rarely does it appear that there has been sufficient awareness where it counts, in our homes, clinics, and schools, of the deleterious effects of noise and reverberation upon speech perception. I (MR) have often visited schools and clinics and have had difficulty understanding the teacher's speech through my own hearing aid at the same time that the children were supposed to be listening and learning by means of this same speech signal!!

Although we live in an increasingly noisy world, it does not have to be noisy all of the time in the child's environment. It is possible to reduce noise levels at homes and schools, keeping in mind the admonition of Tillman et al. (1970) that acceptable noise levels for listeners with normal hearing may not be acceptable for hearing-impaired persons. One simple remedial measure to improve the S/N ratio is almost always possible, and that is to reduce the distance between the talker and the microphone of the hearing aid. Research on this effect, under various conditions, has been summarized elsewhere (Ross 1978b, Borrild 1978). By providing the child with the best possible S/N ratio, by clearly distinguishing foreground speech from background sounds, we can ensure, at the least, that the raw material of an auditory approach to speech and language development is available for neural processing and categorization. Without this provision, the child is supplied with the visible indication of his handicap—the hearing aid—but with no assurance that it can do the job it was designed for.

The relevance of the amplified sound reaching a child's ear is not only a product of the electroacoustics or the background sounds but also reflects the characteristics of the speech signal arriving at the hearing aid microphone. The concept of optimal amplification must of necessity encompass optimal input. The quality and quantity of conversation directed at a hearing-impaired child differs from that directed to his peers with normal hearing. This is not a volitional or conscious policy but, rather, seems to be a reaction to the child's inability to reinforce verbal communication with an appropriate response. As a consequence, the hearing-impaired child, while requiring enriched language experiences, actually receives a less satisfactory input than his peers whose hearing are normal (Goss 1970).

The speech directed at a hearing-impaired child must be clearly but not overly articulated. It certainly should not be mouthed or delivered in a whispered monosyllabic manner accompanied by natural gestures. Both of these tendencies are often found among parents and teachers who are often completely unaware of what they are doing. The emphasis on gestures will in the short run increase message reception, but at the expense of reducing exposure to the amplified speech input. It should be noted that the population of children we are referring to here are those who are candidates for an auditory-oral approach.

Ideally, the speech signal should be sufficiently intense at the hearing aid microphone to override ambient noise levels at the same location. A 65 to 70 dB SPL signal measured 3ft from the speaker would seem to be appropriate in most circumstances. This is approximately the average intensity for normal conversational speech. Within approximate limits, since the inverse square law does not hold in reverberant rooms, a doubling of halving of this distance would increase or decrease the sound intensity by about 6 dB. Shouting, to overcome distance effects, is not a good policy. The intensity range between the weakest (voiceless th) and the strongest (aw as in ball) phoneme is approximately 30 dB. We should aim whenever possible to provide a 30 dB SL signal within the dynamic range of the hearing-impaired child; this makes all the phonemes of the language potentially audible. Shouting increases the intensity of vowels relative to consonants and thus reduces the potential audibility of consonants, particularly voiceless consonants. Normal conversational speech close to the microphone of the hearing aid offers the best opportunity for clearly audible speech at the most favorable S/N ratio. Hearing aids that incorporate automatic gain control circuits can keep the output levels constant under various levels of input (or compress the input by some predetermined linear or nonlinear ratio); nevertheless, no matter what method is used to limit output, the S/N ratio at the microphone of the hearing aid must be highly favorable if the child is to receive the optimum signal (see Chapter 2 for a discussion of compression amplification and Chapter 8 for a detailed exposition on amplification for speech).

In this paragraph, only brief mention will be made of the vital area of the quality and quantity of language directed to the hearing-impaired child. This brief treatment reflects the nature of this volume rather than the significance of the area. A maturational, biologic view of how language is normally developed (Lenneberg 1967) presupposes that the child is exposed to an adequate sample of the language in order for the neural mechanisms to operate. van Uden (1970) forcefully expressed the need of hearing-impaired children for intensive and increased language exposure, which is tied to their maturation level and current experiences. Conversation is the key. As Brown and his colleagues (1969) point out:

> It seems likely that the many kinds of grammatical exchange occurring in discourse will prove to be the richest data available to the child in his search for a grammar. We suspect that the changes sentences undergo as they shuttle between persons in conversation are . . . the data that most clearly expose the underlying structure of language.

In other words, we must talk to children about what we and they are doing, always keeping in mind the child's interest and age level, and then listening for his responses and either expanding or expatiating accordingly.

ISSUES AND PROBLEMS

Effect of Hearing Aid Amplification on Residual Hearing

Even before the term "noise pollution" and its possible consequence on residual hearing capacity became fashionable, there had been reports and concerns published regarding the possible deleterious effect of hearing aid amplification. The logic appears inescapable. The output of hearing aids can easily reach $130-140$ dB and they are used by hearing-impaired individuals for all of their waking hours. The results of much of the early research has stressed the need for catuion, with some suggestion of thresholds shifts occurring for a significant number of hearing-impaired individuals (Ross and Lerman 1967). A comprehensive review and critique of the early literature has pinpointed some of the problems with this early research and suggested procedures for a more definitive analysis of the topic (Markides 1971). Since this review at least four research studies have investigated the topic again and have found no pattern of diminished hearing in an aided ear (Hine and Furness 1975, Darbyshire 1976, Markides 1976, Markides and Aryee 1978). Obviously, such events can occur in individual cases. I would recommend that clinicians be aware that further deterioration of residual hearing may occur in a few instances, but certainly amplification should not be permanently withheld from a child who, without it, cannot function auditorially at all. In questionable cases, a hearing aid can be used monaurally and rotated from ear to ear, the output can be reduced, otologic assistance solicited, and hearing acuity monitored frequently. These latter measurements can best be made both immediately after a hearing aid has been used and after the aid has not been used for a day or two.

Hearing Aid Malfunctions

None of our efforts to provide an appropriate electroacoustic system to hearing-impaired children will do any good if the hearing aids do not work or, when working, do not work properly. The record, insofar as children are concerned, is simply deplorable. Beginning with Gaeth and Lounsburys' article in 1966, in which they report that at the most only 50 percent of the hearing aids of 134 children could be considered adequate, the same dismal picture has been repeated in study after study (Zink 1972, Northern et al. 1972, Coleman 1972, Findlay and Winchester 1973, Skalka and Moore 1973, Porter 1973). It seems, if the reader will excuse this polemic cliche, easier to walk on the moon than to design "child-proof" hearing aids. Actually, the 50 percent estimate of operational hearing aids quoted above is somewhat optimistic when one considers that some portion of hearing-impaired children who should have hearing aids do not, that many of those who do, do not use them, that the acoustic situation in which they are worn precludes reception of an intelligible signal, and that the electroacoustic adjustments of hearing aids frequently leave much to be desired. The inescapable conclusion of this sad litany is that for most hearing-impaired children, the effective use of residual hearing is a myth shrouded with good intentions.

Binaural Hearing Aids for Children

Binaural hearing aids per se are discussed in Chapter 7. In this section, we would like to discuss briefly some unique aspects of this approach as they pertain to young hearing-impaired children. Earlier, we mentioned that our amplification goal with children was binaural, preferably ear-level hearing aids. In our judgment, supported by our interpretation of the evidence and our accumulated clinical experience, there is little doubt that most hearing-impaired children can benefit more from binaural than monaural hearing aids. It has taken years of research for this situation, as it pertains to adults, to become somewhat clear; it has been even more difficult to objectively demonstrate binaural advantages with hearing-impaired children (Ross 1977).

Our reasoning in recommending two hearing aids is similar to that we use to justify our preference for certain electroacoustic modifications. If binaural amplification is beneficial for most hearing-impaired adults, who can be objectively tested by many methods, then it should also be preferred for most hearing-impaired children for whom an objective estimate of superiority is much more difficult to obtain. In an attempt to circumvent the measurement problem, a study was accomplished (Ross et al. 1974) in which parents and teachers compared binaural-monaural amplification with several independent groups of children.

We found that parents and teachers rated their children similarly and that the parents of two separate groups of children scored binaural performance superior on the same four auditory dimensions. To us, this was a convincing demonstration of binaural superiority; unfortunately, this type of study is most convincing to those who are already "believers."

Yonovitz (1974) completed a study which appears to convincingly demonstrate binaural superiority for hearing-impaired children. He placed two speech spectrum noncorrelated noise sources 60° to the left and right of a listener. The signal source was placed directly in front. The signal was a recorded version of the WIPI test (Ross and Lerman 1971), which requires only a picture-pointing response from the child. The two channels of signal in noise were recorded at five S/N ratios via electret microphones placed in the ear canals of a young child. Twenty hearing-impaired children were tested with earphones under all S/N ratios for both the monaural and binaural mode. The results clearly demonstrate binaural superiority under all of the S/N (Fig. 6-10).

There are undoubtedly children for whom binaural hearing aids are not advisable. With the present state of our knowledge, however, we do not yet know for certain what types of losses and problems would be excluded from possible binaural candidacy (excepting those with a complete loss of hearing in one ear). Asymmetry per se may not be a contraindication. There is some evidence (Franklin 1972, Rand 1974) that asymmetrical signal bands applied to the two ears of hearing-impaired listeners may be more advantageous than broad-band amplification to both ears. In clinical practice, this situation can be duplicated by children who show different configurations of residual hearing in their two ears. Advantages, if any, under these circumstances, and for the gen-

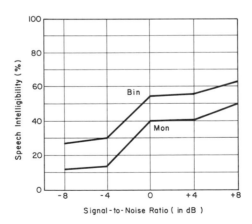

Fig. 6-10. Monaural and binaural WIPI scores for 20 hearing-impaired children under five different signal-to-noise conditions.

eral population of hearing-impaired children, may require long-term experience with the binaural signal and frequent observations to assess efficacy (Fisher 1964).

Recently, the entire topic of binaural hearing aids for children was examined in more detail (Ross and Giolas 1978, pp. 261–268). In addition to supporting our consistent view that for most hearing-impaired children binaural amplification is the recommendation of choice, the danger of not making early binaural recommendations is now becoming very clear. There is some very convincing evidence with auditory sensory deprivation studies with animals (and analagous visual deprivation studies with humans and animals) that clearly suggests permanent and irreversible binaural deprivation effects if early binaural amplification does not occur. Clinicians who "don't think there is enough evidence to support binaural hearing aids" should understand the consequences of their actions (in this case, omissions). The evidence is available and it is not ambiguous; clinicians must simply open their eyes to the literature and their minds to the implications of what they read.

CONCLUSION

In our judgment, the proper selection and use of amplification is the single most effective tool available to us in our remedial efforts with young, hearing-impaired children. We would not minimize the importance of parent counseling or any type of therapeutic endeavor; these will often set limits to the success of our efforts. Auditory amplification, however, is the only therapeutic tool specifically focused on the problem—the hearing loss itself. It is after all, the hearing loss that is the responsible agent for observed speech, language, and educational deviances. The effective exploitation of residual hearing will minimize these developmental deviancies and ensure the maximum effectiveness of other therapeutic endeavors.

We have presented the view that fitting a hearing aid to a young child requires the systematic application of time, information, sensitivity, and experience. To be most effective, the parents and the child should be enrolled in an educational program directly associated with the diagnostic audiology clinic. This association would facilitate the process of systematic, ongoing evaluation and modification that is generally required in the management of young children. Our amplification goal is to deliver the most, and most salient, speech and language signals within the residual hearing range. We can expect, once this is accomplished, that the child will himself prove to be a much superior "learner" of speech and language than we could ever possibly be as "teachers." The clinician will rarely make better use of his time or accomplish a more worthwhile objective than by making this possibility a reality.

BIBLIOGRAPHY

Berger KW: Prescription of hearing aids: a rationale. J Am Audiol Soc 2:71–78, 1976

Boothroyd A: Distribution of hearing levels in Clarke School for the Deaf students. SARP 3 Clarke School for the Deaf, Northampton, Mass., 1972

Boothroyd A: Speech perception and sensorineural hearing loss, in Ross and Giolas (eds): Auditory Management of Hearing-Impaired Children. Baltimore, Md., University Park Press, pp 117–144, 1978

Borrild K: Classroom acoustics, in Ross and Giolas (eds): Auditory Management of Hearing-Impaired Children. Baltimore, University Park Press, pp 145–180, 1978

Brooks D: Gain requirements of hearing aid users. Scand Audiol 2:199–208, 1973

Brown R, Cazden CB, Bellugi U: The child's grammar from I to III, in Hill JP (ed): 1967 Minnesota Symposia on Child Psychology. Minneapolis, University of Minnesota Press, 1969

Byrne D, Fifield D: Evaluation of hearing aid fittings for infants. Br J Audiol 8:47–54, 1974

Byrne D, Tonnisson S: Selecting the gain of hearing aids for persons with sensorineural hearing impairments. Scand Audiol 5:51–62, 1976

Byrne D: Gain and frequency response requirements of hearing aids for persons with sensorineural hearing impairments. National Acoustic Laboratories, Australian Department of Health, Report No 64, June 1976

Byrne D: Selection of hearing aids for severely deaf children. Brit J Audiol 12:9–22, 1978

Coleman RF: Hearing aid stability in an acoustic preschool nursery program. Nashville, Tenn., Bill Wilkerson Hearing and Speech Center, 1972

Dalsgaard SC, Jensen OD: Measurement of the insertion gain of hearing aids. J Audiol Tech 15:170–183, 1976

Danaher EM, Wilson MP, Pickett JM: Backward and forward masking in listeners with severe sensorineural hearing loss. Audiology 17:324–338, 1978

Darbyshire JO: A study of the use of high-power hearing aids by children with marked degrees of deafness and the possibility of deteriorations in auditory acuity. Brit J Audiol 10:74–78, 1976

Downs MP: Maintaining children's hearing aids: the role of the parents. Maico Audiological Library Series 10, Report 1, 1971

Downs MP: Relationship of pathology to function in congenital hearing loss. Audiology 11:330–336, 1972

Elliot LL: Descriptive analysis of audiometric and psychometric scores of students at a school for the deaf. J Speech Hear Res 10:21–40, 1967

Erber JP: Body-baffle and real-ear effects in the selection of hearing aids for deaf children. J Speech Hear Disor 38:224–231, 1973

Findlay RC, Winchester RA: Defects in hearing aids worn by preschool and school age children. American Speech and Hearing Association Convention, Detroit, 1973

Finitzo-Hieber T, Tillman TW: Room acoustics effect on monosyllabic word discrimination ability for normal and hearing-impaired children. J Speech Hear Res 21:440–458, 1978

Fisher B: An investigation of binaural hearing aids. J Laryngol Otol 78:658–668, 1964

Franklin B: The effect of a low-frequency bank (240−480 Hz) of speech on consonant discrimination in hearing-impaired subjects. Convention of the American Speech and Hearing Association, 1972

Gaeth JH, Lounsbury E: Hearing aids and children in elementary schools. J Speech Hear Disor 31:282−289, 1966

Gengel RW: Acceptable speech-to-noise ratios for aided speech discrimination by the hearing impaired. J Audiol Res 11:219−222, 1971

Gengel RW, Pascoe D, Shore I: A frequency-response procedure for evaluating and selecting hearing aids for severely hearing-impaired children. J Speech Hear Disor 36:341−353, 1971

Goodman AI: Residual capacity to hear of pupils in schools for the deaf. J Laryngol Otol 63:551−662, 1949

Goss, RN: Language used by mothers of deaf children and mothers of hearing children. Am Ann Deaf 115:93−96, 1970

Grainger JB: A non-verbal hearing aid selection procedure. Paper presented at 1977 American Speech and Hearing Association Convention

Green DS, Ross M: The effect of a conventional versus a nonoccluding (CROS-Type) earmold upon the frequency response of a hearing aid. J Speech Hear Res 11:638−647, 1968

Harford E, Dodds E: Bekesy audiometry in sound field. Sixth Annual Report of the Auditory Research Laboratories, Northwestern University, pp 27−29, 1971

Hine WD: How deaf are deaf children? Br J Audiol 7:41−44, 1973

Hine WD, Furness HJS: Does wearing a hearing aid damage residual hearing? Teach Deaf 73:261−271, 1975

Hodgson WR: Testing infants and young children, in Katz J (ed): Handbook of Clinical Audiology. Baltimore, Williams & Wilkins (ed 2), 1978

Huizing HC: Deaf mutism: modern trends in treatment and prevention. Ann Otol Rhinol Laryngol 5:74−106, 1959

Leckie D, Ling D: Audibility with hearing aids having low frequency characteristics. Volta Rev 70:83−85, 1968

Lenneberg EH· Biological Foundations of Language. New York, Wiley, 1967

Levitt H: The acoustics of speech production, in Ross and Giolas (eds): Auditory Management of Hearing-Impaired Children. Baltimore, University Park Press, 1978

Liden G, Kankkunen A: Hearing aid procedure in young deaf and hard of hearing children. Scand Audiol Suppl 3:47−54, 1973

Ling D: Auditory coding and recoding: an analysis of auditory training procedures for hearing-impaired children, in Ross and Giolas (eds): Auditory Management of Hearing-Impaired Children. Baltimore, University Park Press, pp 181−218, 1978

Luterman D: On parent education. Volta Rev 75:504−508, 1973

Luterman D: Counselling parents of hearing-impaired children. Boston, Little, Brown, 1979

Markides A: Do hearing aids damage the user's residual hearing? Sound 5:99−105, 1971

Markides A, Aryee DTK: The effect of hearing aid use on the user's residual hearing. Scand Audio 7:19−26, 1978

Markides A: The effect of hearing use on the user's residual hearing. Scand Audiol 5:205−210, 1976

Martin MC: Hearing aid gain requirements in sensori-neural loss. Brit J Audiol 7:21−24, 1973

McConnell F: Proceedings of the conference on current practices in the management of deaf infants (0-3 years). The Bill Wilkerson Center, Vanderbilt University, 1968

Miller JD: Possible importance of head diffraction and ear-canal resonance for speech perception and hearing-aid design. Eighty-sixth Meeting of the Acoustical Society of America, 1973

Montgomery GWG: Analysis of pure-tone audiometric responses in relation to speech development in the profoundly deaf. J Acoust Soc 41:53−59, 1967

Morgan DE, Dirks DD, Bower DR: Suggested threshold sound pressure levels for frequency modulated (warble) tones in the sound field. J Speech Hearing Disor 44:37−54, 1979

Nober EH: Air and bone conduction thresholds of deaf and hearing subjects before and during the elimination of cutaneous tactile interference with anesthesia. Final Report: Project 6-3073, Syracuse University, 1968

Northern JL, McChord W, Fischer E, et al.: Hearing services in residential schools for the deaf. Maico Audiol Libr Ser 11, Report 4, 1972

Olson, WO: The influence of harmonic and intermodulation distortion on speech intelligibility. Scand Audiol Suppl 1:109−125, 1971

Pascoe DP, Niemoeller AF, Miller JD: Hearing aid design and evaluation for a presbycusic patient. Eighty-sixth Meeting of the Acoustical Society of America, 1973

Pascoe DP: Frequency responses of hearing aids and their effects on the speech perception of hearing-impaired subjects. Ann Otol Rhinol Laryngol 84 (Suppl 23): xi−40, 1975

Pascoe DP: An approach to hearing aid selection. Hear Instrum 29:12−16, 36, 1978

Porter TA: Hearing aids in a residential school. Am Ann Deaf 118:31−33, 1973

Powell CA, Tucker IG: A method of determining the amplification needs of deaf children. Teacher Deaf 75:58−63, 1977

Rand TC: Dichotic release from masking for speech. J Acoust Soc Am 55:678−680, 1974

Ross M: A pilot project for hearing-impaired children, Part 1. Proceedings of the Forty-third Meeting of the Convention of American Instructors of the Deaf, 1967, pp 196−201

Ross M: Principles of Aural Rehabilitation. New York, Bobbs-Merrill, 1972

Ross M: Hearing aid evaluation, in Katz J (ed): Handbook of Clinical Audiology (ed 2). Baltimore, Williams & Wilkins, 1978a, pp 524−542

Ross M: Classroom acoustics and speech intelligibility, in Katz J (ed): Handbook of Clinical Audiology (ed 2). Baltimore, Williams & Wilkins, 1978b, pp 469−478

Ross M, Duffy RJ, Cooker HS, et al: Contribution of the lower audible frequencies to the recognition of emotions. Am Ann Deaf 118:37−42, 1973

Ross M, Hunt MF, Kessler M, et al: The use of a rating scale to compare binaural and monaural amplification with hearing impaird children. Volta Rev 76:93−99, 1974

Ross M, Lerman J: Hearing aid usage and its effect upon residual hearing. Arch Otolaryngol 86:639−644, 1967

Ross M, Lerman J: Work intelligibility by picture identification. Pittsburgh, Stanwix House, 1971

Ross M, Giolas TG: Auditory Management of Hearing-Impaired Children: Principles Prerequisites for Intervention. Baltimore, University Park Press, 1978

Ross M: Binaural versus monaural hearing aid amplification for hearing-impaired individuals, in Bess F (ed): Childhood Deafness: Causation, Assessment, and Management. New York, Grune & Stratton, 1977

Skalka EC, Moore JP: A program for daily "troubleshooting" of hearing aids in a day school for the deaf. Convention of the American Speech and Hearing Association, Detroit, 1973

Skinner MW: Speech intelligibility in noise-induced hearing loss: the effect of high frequency compensation. Ph.D. dissertation, St. Louis, Washington University, 1976

Stephens MM, Rintelmann WF: Influence of audiometric configuration on puretone, warble-tone, and narrow-bank noise thresholds for adults with sensorineural hearing losses. Convention of the American Speech and Hearing Association, Detroit, 1973

Sung GC, Sung RJ, Angelleli RM: Effect of frequency-response characteristics of hearing aids on speech intelligibility in noise. J Aud Res 11:318−321, 1971

Sweetow RW: Temporal and spread of masking effects from extended low frequency amplification. J Aud Res 17:161−170, 1977

Tillman TW: Carhart R, Olsen WO: Hearing aid efficiency in a competing speech situation. J Speech Hear Res 13:789−811, 1970

Triantos TJ, McCandless GA: High frequency distortion. Hear Aid J 27:9, 38, 1974

van Uden A: A world of language for deaf children, Part 1 (ed 2). Rotterdam University Press, 1970

Villchur E: Signal processing, in Ross M and Giolas T (eds): Auditory Management of Hearing-Impaired Children. Baltimore, University Park Press, pp 219−238, 1978

Villchur E: Signal processing to improve speech intelligibility in perceptive deafness. J Acoust Soc Am 53:1646−1657, 1973

Victoreen JA: Hearing Enhancement. Springfield, Ill., Charles C. Thomas, 1960

Waldon EF: Audio-reflexometry in testing hearing of very young children. Audiology 12:14−20, 1973

Wallefels HG: Hearing Aids on Prescription. Springfield, Ill., Charles C. Thomas, 1967

Watson TJ: Some factors affecting the successful use of hearing aids by deaf children, in The Modern Educational Treatment of Deafness. Manchester University Press, 1960

Whetnell E, Fry DB: The Deaf Child (ed 2). Springfield, Ill., C. C. Thomas, 1971

Yonovitz A: Binaural intelligibility: pilot study progress. Speech and Haring Institute, Texas Medical Center, Houston, 1974

Zink GC: Hearing aids children wear: a longitudinal study of performance. Volta Rev 74:41−51, 1972

Michael C. Pollack

7

Special Applications of Amplification

This is a conglomerate chapter, with four very distinct topics: binaural amplification; CROS hearing aids; tinnitus maskers; and in-the-ear hearing aids. Each of them could justifiably be a separate chapter, but various considerations dictated drawing them together. As throughout the rest of this book, the presentation here was aimed at being as practical as possible. Issues are presented and some conclusions are drawn, but the reader is left with many options in terms of how to use the information. More than anything else, I hope that this chapter will stimulate thought and discussion.

MCP

In recent years there have been numerous innovations as well as controversies in the use of amplification for the hearing-impaired. These include the CROS hearing aid and its many variations, in-the-ear hearing aids and tinnitus maskers. In addition to these more recent developments, there has been strong argument in the hearing health field concerning the utility of binaural versus monaural amplification. This chapter will consider each of these four "special applications" of amplification, attempting to present all sides of the issues and to draw some conclusions.

MONAURAL, BINAURAL, AND PSEUDOBINAURAL AMPLIFICATION

If the literature pertaining to the nonmedical management of individuals with bilateral hearing losses were to be reviewed, a major area of disagreement would be found among professionals concerned with hearing health care; whether the bilaterally hearing-impaired individual should use one hearing aid delivering sound to one ear (monaural), one hearing aid delivering sound to both ears (pseudobinaural or Y-cord), or two hearing aids (binaural). This disagreement has not been, and may never be, resolved to the satisfaction of all.

Historically, manufacturers and dispensers of hearing aids have strongly advocated binaural fittings, while audiologists have been more reluctant to do so. A great deal of formal and informal research has been performed in an attempt to demonstrate the advantage of binaural amplification. Positive case reports abound in the pages of professional publications. Yet, the disagreement continues.

Apparently, the problem is based on the fact that while users frequently report greater success with binaural than with monaural amplification, these improvements often cannot be demonstrated clinically. In fact, it has been infrequently demonstrated in the laboratory that binaural hearing is of significant advantage over monaural. Audiologists are often greatly concerned with the clinical, empirical exemplification of phenomena. It may be the lack of research evidence of the superiority of binaural hearing aids that often makes many audiologists very cautious about recommending such instrumentation. One could interpret this reluctance as suggesting a lack of confidence in binaural test procedures.

On the other hand, the dispenser often is at the other extreme, exhibiting the attitude that every individual with a bilateral loss should wear binaural hearing aids. He may base this philosophy solely on some user reports of success and satisfaction. He may also be influenced by manufacturer publicity claims of binaural superiority. The audiologist and the dispenser find it difficult to justify their positions to each other, especially when faced with the fact that some individuals find binaural amplification indispensable, while others are never able to properly adjust to two aids.

Rationales for Binaural Amplification

A wealth of clinical and experimental knowledge about binaural hearing has been accumulated, and many rationales behind recommendations for binaural amplification are based thereon. However, the vast majority of this information was obtained with subjects whose hearing was normal. Also, most studies have used adults as subjects, while we are most often concerned with children when considering binaural aids. The literature concerned with binaural hearing of the hearing-impaired and binaural amplification has produced varying results, leading to the realization that the advantages of two hearing aids over one must be viewed as equivocal.

Wright (1959) states that the purpose of binaural amplification is to create a sound environment for the listener that is a faithful reproduction of the original acoustic event so that he can take advantage of the intensity, time, and spectrum differences of the auditory signal at each ear. These differences, theoretically, provide the additional cues necessary for a more reasonable approximation of the hearing experiences of the normal-hearing population.

While binaural ear level aids provide these signal differences, a pair of body aids do not. Two microphones on the chest, especially with a child, are separated by no more than 2−3 inches, while the ears are separated by 7 or 8 in. Additionally, the head exerts a sound shadow between the ears. It is the presence of the head between the microphones that is primarily responsible for the intensity, time, and spectrum differences. Two body aids do not achieve the purpose of restoring a semblance of normal binaural auditory functioning; ear level aids do. With the advent of powerful ear level instrumentation, I have been recommending binaural amplification more often than in the past for both children and adults. In my experience, I have found that only in the most profound losses can I not find ear level aids that will provide suitable amplification.

It seems logical that hearing with two ears provides more information than hearing with one. Although speech can be intelligibly conveyed through a single neurological channel, there are circumstances when the understanding of speech should be improved considerably when it is heard through two ears. The higher level of redundancy with two-eared hearing theoretically should provide advantages in sound localization and discrimination in the presence of background noise.

Another implication of binaural amplification for congenitally hard-of-hearing children relates to the fact that a prerequisite to the appropriate processing of language information is the establishment of cerebral dominance. Referring to the work of Penfield and Roberts, Lankford and Faires (1973) raise the question of the validity of monaural amplification for these children "who must rely on the processing ability of both hemispheres in order to adequately analyze and synthesize previously unlearned language." Here is another important area in need of extensive research.

Although opinion differs on the degree of improvement of speech intelligibility, there is general agreement on the probable advantage of binaural hearing for localization of sounds (Hirsh, 1950; Bergman, 1957; Carhart, 1958; Wright, 1959). However, it is often difficult or impossible to demonstrate this clinically or experimentally. Speech discrimination scores have generally been accepted as one of the criteria in judging the superiority of binaural over monaural aids. As noted above, it is often difficult to demonstrate such discrimination improvement clinically. Here may rest the problem for the audiologist.

A careful examination of the studies that failed to demonstrate a binaural advantage suggests that many of them did not utilize speech intelligibility tasks rigorous enough to yield binaural results significantly better than monaural.

Clinical and Research Evidence of a Binaural Advantage

Langford (1970) summarizes many of the clinical and research observations, suggesting five potential advantages of binaural amplification—better sound localization, increased speech discrimination in noise, greater ease of listening, better spatial balance, and improved quality.

LOCALIZATION

It has long been an accepted fact that man needs two ears for satisfactory auditory localization (Bergman, 1957, Carhart, 1958, Wright, 1959). The rationale is that it takes analysis of input to two ears to determine effectively the distances and position in both azimuth and elevation of the sound sources. One exception is in highly reverberant rooms where differing times of arrival between direct and reflected sounds allows monaural localization with little effort.

SPEECH DISCRIMINATION

One of the most important advantages of binaural hearing seems to be an improvement in auditory figure-ground relationships. The listener is better able to interpret speech in a background noise. Koenig (1950) refers to this as a "squelch effect" in which ambient background noises seem to decrease in intensity and become less disruptive. He found such noises to be more disturbing with monaural amplification than with binaural aids. This phenomenon has also been studies by Dirks and Moncur (1967), who described it as an important advantage of binaural over monaural hearing for speech intelligibility in a reverberant environment.

Gelfand and Hochberg (1973) hypothesized that the "squelch effect" was responsible for their finding of better speech discrimination under reverberant conditions for binaural amplification. They state that this might be due to the ability of the binaural auditory system to squelch the effects of reverberation. This was the case for both normal and sensorineural hearing-impaired subjects.

Related to the "squelch effect" are data reported by Tillman *et al.* (1963) on the head shadow effect. They found sound field thresholds for speech to be almost 7 dB better at the ear nearer the sound source than at the far ear. In other words, the head exerts a block to the passage of sound from the near side to the far side. This is discussed in depth in the next section of this chapter, dealing with CROS hearing aids. Also presented in that section are the problems related to unilateral hearing loss. It is important to keep in mind that monaural amplification for a bilateral hearing loss creates, in essence, a unilateral hearing loss with its related difficulties.

There are many reports in the literature of subjective and clinical improvements in speech discrimination and intelligibility in noise with binaural systems (Harris 1965, Bergman 1957, Black and Hast 1962, Decroiz and Dehaussy 1964, Heffler and Schultz 1964, Zelnick 1970b). Markle and Aber (1958) and Belzile and Markle (1959) demonstrated significantly better speech discrimination scores with binaural than with monaural aids. However, their results must be carefully evaluated, as two body aids were used at ear-level to simulate a binaural situation. They overlooked differences in the responses of body and postauricular instruments due to such factors as body baffle and head shadow effects. Cherry and Bowles (1960) found that increased speech intelligibility is related to the binaural auditory system's ability to separate sounds spatially (figure-ground).

EASE OF LISTENING

Carhart (1958) indicated that "less effort is required for comfortable listening when this system (binaural) is used." Bergman (1957) and Hedgecock and Sheets (1958) related the greater ease of listening for speech to the binaural system's ability to minimize the effects of room reverberation on speech intelligibility (squelch). Langford (1970) reported that a binaural arrangement provides greater intensity to the auditory system than does a monaural aid. This allows the user to hear faint sounds with greater ease. He described situations in which binaural users turn up the gain of the reamining aid considerably if one aid is turned off. They appear to do this to maintain the signal intensity achieved with both aids on. Kodman (1961) summarized this aspect of the binaural use of hearing aids by suggesting that "another way of viewing the binaural effect is that the patient hears easier or with less effort, even though the intelligibility score is comparable, or even identical with, the monaural score. . . . It is suggested that binaural hearing prmotes an interaural effect which is reflected in better sound balance and ease of perception."

SPATIAL BALANCE

There appears to be an increased precision in auditory orientation when some binaural listeners are confronted with a complex acoustic environment. This may result from what Huizing and Taselaar (1961) report as an interaural integration of speech presented to both ears. They suggest that under certain circumstances, distorted signals are integrated more effectively binaurally than monaurally. Dirks and Wilson (1969) demonstrated a binaural advantage in subjects with sensorineural hearing loss when sound sources were spatially separated so that the individual could make use of the interaural time differences.

SOUND QUALITY

Numerous case studies have yielded subjective reports from users of binaural hearing aids that sound quality is considerably better than that obtained with monaural instrumentation (Heffler and Schultz 1964, Haskin and Hardy 1960, Kodman 1961). Binaural amplification appears to provide a greater "fullness" to sound. These subjective reports are most likely the result of a summation of the four characteristics described above—better localization, improved speech intelligibility, greater ease of listening, and improved spatial balance.

On the other hand, a number of research studies have attempted unsuccessfully to demonstrate a clinical advantage for binaural aids. Hedgecock and Sheets (1958) found no statistically significant differences between monaural and binaural performance in quiet. Others who have failed to show improved speech discrimination were Wright (1959), Wright and Carhart (1960), and Dicarlo and Brown (1960). Jerger and Dirks (1961) tried to replicate the Belzile and Markle (1959) results, but failed to confirm binaural superiority for speech intelligibility. Jerger, Carhart, and Dirks (1961) attempted to find objective verification for the numerous subjective reports of binaural advantage. Their results indicated that binaural systems produced little or no improvement in speech discrimination in quiet or noise.

Most reports showing an advantage for binaural amplification are based upon the reports of users rather than on empirical clinical data. At the present time, the clinical measures used do not adequately reflect subjective claims of improvement. This problem was pointedly demonstrated by Dirks and Carhart (1962), who examined the reactions of subjects who used a hearing aid. Those with binaural experience expressed a strong preference for two aids. The authors noted that users in whom binaural aids were successful could not perform differentially on clinical tests. They summarized the situation by stating that no clinical test battery has been able to demonstrate the superiority of binaural aids on the basis of measurements. In other words, those who used binaural aids reported a number of subjective advantages that cannot be measured at present by clinical techniques. The implication to be drawn from this is not that the advantages of binaural aids do not exist, but rather that our clinical evaluation tools are inadequate to measure them. Another area of future research is the need to develop tests sensitive enough to demonstrate the advantages of binaural aids.

A related drawback to a number of the studies that failed to show an advantage of binaural aids is they were not designed in a manner that would adequately measure true binaural performance. Testing is often performed in quiet where good intelligibility can be achieved with one ear. If it is going to be possible to demonstrate binaural superiority, speech and competing signals must be presented at a signal-to-noise ratio that will be difficult for a monaural listener. Additionally, there must be some angular (azimuth) displacement between the primary and competing signal sources. Only then will it be possible to see if the binaural mode causes a release from masking or "squelch" effect.

Pseudobinaural Amplification

Figure 7-1 depicts an amplification mode referred to as Y-cord or pseudobinaural, using one microphone, one amplifier, and two receivers. In essense, it is a monaural aid delivering sound to both ears. Available only in body hearing aids, the Y-cord arrangement is often used with severely or profoundly hearing-impaired children.

Lybarger (1973) described four advantages of a pseudobinaural system relative to a monaural arrangement:

1. Both ears are receiving auditory stimulation
2. Somewhat better speech discrimination—although not as good as with a true binaural system
3. Lower initial cost than binaural
4. Lower operating cost through less battery consumption than binaural aids

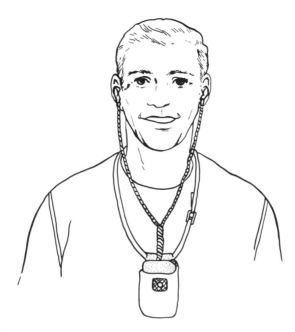

Fig. 7-1.   Pseudobinaural (Y-Cord) arrangement. (Adapted from Davis and Silverman, 1970.)

While such hearing aid arrangements may be required for economic reasons, the Y-cord system provides bilateral, not binaural, hearing. The signal from one aid is split between the two ears, losing the phase, time, intensity, and spectrum cues available from a true binaural hearing aid. Investigative data of Wright and Carhart (1960) and Black and Hast (1962) indicate that, although both ears are stimulated, pseudobinaural aided performance is not significantly better than monaural, and is not as good as true binaural in terms of discrimination and localization. The system is only duplicating the sounds the individual is hearing with one ear. The interaural differences in phase and intensity so necessary for localization, are absent.

Lybarger (1973) mentions the fact that not all body aids work well with Y-cord. When two receivers are used, an impedance mismatch is created that causes deterioration of the output signal. To overcome this, specially designed receivers must be used or the output impedance of the aid will be altered.

Another limitation of a Y-cord is a small loss in the output reaching each ear when the signal is split (3−6 dB). Related to this problem is the realization that the balance range in output that can be obtained is limited. Although a potentiometer can be placed in the circuit, more distortion is created at high output levels. The intensity reaching each ear must be approximately the same. Therefore, a Y-cord works optimally when the loss is symmetrical. If not, one ear may be underamplified or overamplified. Unfortunately, pseudobinaural aids are often recommended for young children before accurate threshold information is obtained.

Today, Y-cord arrangements are becoming less common. Generally, they are being used only when a true binaural system cannot be used due to cost, significant asymmetry between the ears, or other factors.

Guidelines for Considerations of Binaural Amplification

One consistent observation throughout the literature regarding binaural amplification is that while its advantages often cannot be demonstrated clinically, user reports after a period of experience with the two hearing aids often strongly point to the subjective benefits. The key is an adjustment period.

A program of auditory training is often necessary for a new binaural user so that he or she can take full advantage of increased sound cues for intelligibility and localization. The patient must learn to differentially adjust the gain of each aid so that the optimal summation effect occurs, resulting in potentially improved auditory perception. The implication to be drawn from this discussion is that there should be a trial period before one purchases the two hearing aids. However, I have seen numerous individuals who find binaural amplification untenable even after long trial and adjustment periods. My experience suggests that successful binaural use is a very individual phenomenon.

The idea of adjustment raises the argument of whether or not to fit both instruments immediately. Proponents of immediate fitting argue that since the user is going to eventually wear two aids, he should start with fittings that provide the most advantageous hearing response. From the start, he should learn to use and live with binaural amplification (Zelnick 1970a).

On the other hand, some of those in the hearing-health field suggest that adjustment to monaural amplification is often difficult enough. Therefore, the aids should be fitted one at a time, allowing the user to adjust to one before the second is fitted. I would tend to disagree with this philosophy, based on the experiences described above.

It has been observed that the user-adjusted gain setting of a monaural aid is generally lowered when a secnd instrument is introduced. With individual input to each ear, a binaural summation takes place, resulting in a lower gain setting for each instrument relative to that at which each would be adjusted monaurally. Although the binaural gain reduction is small $(3-6$ dB$)$, it is obvious and consistent and could produce a more favorable sound quality.

Who should use binaural amplification? This is a question that has plagued audiologists and hearing aid dispensers. There is no pat answer—each case must be viewed individually. The guidelines presented below are based upon clinical experience and common sense. They are intended only as generalized criteria.

The first consideration, naturally, must be the needs of the client. If he or she is frequently confronted with situations that demand functional binaural hearing, such as business conferences, academic settings (especially in the early school years) or social settings, binaural amplification should be given full consideration. Conversely, if the patient is not confronted with these types of conditions, careful thought must be given before binaural aids are recommended. For example, if the patient is retired or otherwise leads a relatively sedate life style, it may be difficult to justify the slight gain in auditory functioning provided by a binaural system against the expense. In some cases binaural aids cost twice as much as a single instrument. This does not imply that two hearing aids should not be considered, only that the needs of the patient be paramount.

Table 7—1 summarizes the possible benefits from binaural fittings for a number of categories of hearing losses. Again, it must be stressed that not every case exhibiting a particular loss will experience these advantages or lack of them. However, clinical experience suggests them as possibilities.

Binaural aids are not recommended or are of questionable value for most asymmetrical losses (more than a 15—dB difference between ears through the

Table 7-1

Potential Benefits of Binaural Amplification for Various Hearing Losses

Hearing Loss	Benefits			
	Improved localization	*Enhanced speech intelligibility in noise*	*Additional gain thru binaural summation*	*Questionable or little benefit*
Symmetrical bilaterally moderate	X	X	X	
Symmetrical bilaterally severe	X	X	X	
Symmetrical bilaterally mild				X
Symmetrical bilaterally profound			X	X
Asymmetrical better ear mild				X
Asymmetrical better ear moderate	X	X		
Asymmetrical better ear moderate, poor ear profound				X
Asymmetrical better ear severe-profound	X		X	X

speech range) for two reasons (a) either the better ear (if a mild loss) can compensate satisfactorily, or (b) the worse ear may cause the performance of the better ear to degenerate through the increased distortion presented to the auditory system. In these cases, a CROS instrument or one of the many CROS variations may be appropriate (see the next section of this chapter).

Again, the clinician should remember that the typical new binaural user will require thorough counseling and auditory training before he will achieve optimal benefit from the aids. Keep in mind also the advisability of a trial period before making a final decision. In no case should a patient be fitted with binaural instruments, given a pep talk, and bid a fond farewell.

Clinical Evaluation of Binaural Amplification

Zelnick (1970b) begins to delineate the problem of clinical evaluation of binaural hearing aids when he states, "if the benefits of binaural hearing aids are to be demonstrated, speech stimuli and competing noise would have to be presented at such relative intensities so that the relationship between the two results in a masking effect that prevents one ear from functioning as well as both ears." If such tests are to be constructed, what competition should be used? What signal-to-noise ratio should be employed?

Other questions that need further clarification:

1. What is the relationship between binaural amplification and such factors as recruitment and diplacusis?
2. How much benefit can be derived from binaural aids by a person with bilaterally profound hearing loss?
3. Is it possible or desirable to achieve a balance between ears through binaural amplification in a case with an asymmetrical sensorineural hearing loss?
4. How much should speech intelligibility be expected to improve in the presence of competing stimuli when binaural aids are utilized?
5. Since the better ear is generally left open in monaural fittings, and since the speech signal is frequently well above the threshold of the unaided ear, is it possible that the superior quality of the unamplified signal in one ear is of greater benefit than a second hearing aid? This may account, in part, for the success of CROS, i.e., the fact that a natural signal is being received in the frequency region where the loss is negligible.
6. What are the advantages, if any, of binaural over monaural amplification under natural reverberation conditions?

CROS AND ITS VARIATIONS

Historically there have been a variety of hearing loss types that have presented a confounding problem to the hearing health team. These include patients with one ear showing normal or near-normal responses and the other ear demonstrating a severe-to-profound hearing loss, and patients with bilateral or unilateral high frequency losses. In the past, a person with a high frequency or unilateral hearing loss was considered a poor candidate for a hearing aid. Since the early 1960s this problem has been greatly alleviated through the development and modification of the CROS (Contralateral Routing of Signals) hearing aid. In the basic CROS design, a microphone is placed on the side of the head with the bad ear, delivering amplified sound to the better ear. A nonoccluding or open earmold is necessary with CROS to allow natural sound to reach the good ear and to reduce amplified low frequencies. Since the introduction of the original CROS aid, many variations of this design have been developed. These have widely expanded its capabilities to a point where it is possible today to provide suitable amplification for almost any type of hearing loss.

Hearing Problems Associated with Unilateral Hearing Loss

Prior to the introduction of CROS instrumentation, there were two rehabilitative avenues generally used with unilateral hearing losses that were not medically correctable: no hearing aid or a monaural instrument on the bad ear. Often, neither was very satisfactory.

There was a time when audiologists and otologists underplayed the communicative problems associated with unilateral hearing loss. They often stressed to the patient that the hearing impairment was "minimal." Rehabilitation generally consisted of a pat on the shoulder, and a statement that in essence said, "You don't have any real problems—position yourself advantageously and learn to lipread—please pay the nurse on your way out."

As coarse as the above may sound, it is not without foundation. Two factors can be related to this attitude: a lack of appreciation for the many listening problems related to a unilateral hearing loss, and a lack of adequate remedial procedures. After all, the unilaterally hearing-impaired patient has no difficulty on the telephone if he uses his good ear, does not reflect any speech and language problems, does well on sound-field hearing tests in quiet, and is under no "real" handicap because he has only to "put his better ear forward." Also, because one ear is normal most people are totally unaware of the hearing loss.

In reality, this individual encounters numerous communication disorders, especially in less than ideal listening situations. These problems can be grouped into three categories.

SPEAKER ON THE SIDE OF THE IMPAIRED EAR

Tillman, et al. (1963) reported on a phenomenon known as the *head shadow effect*. If speech originates on one side of the head, the signal intensity will be lower at the ear farthest from the source (far ear) than at the ear closest to the source (near ear). When measured in sound field with the loudspeaker at a 90° or 270° azimuth, relative to the front of the head (facing one ear directly), the near ear SRT will be approximately 6.4 dB better than that of the far ear. In other words, the head exerts a shadow to sound traveling around it. This effect is even greater for high frequencies (15−30 dB above 2000 Hz) than for low frequencies.

If speech is coming from the side of the bad ear (or unaided impaired ear for a monaural user), the listener is at a decided disadvantage. He is hearing the speech at 6.4 dB less intensity. This relatively small intensity loss can result in a substantial discrimination loss. Of course, he can turn his head to correct this, but this is not always feasible.

The effect of the head shadow is not completely eliminated by increasing the signal intensity 6 or 7 dB. Such an increase does not compensate for the greater high frequency shadow. If the intensity is increased by 15−30 dB, excessive low frequency intensity results. Fletcher (1953) studied this phenomenon and concluded that the high frequency attenuation, although relatively small, can create sufficient distortion to impose a decrease in the quality of speech, particularly for sibilant phonemes, and a resultant decrease in speech intelligibility.

If the speech is coming from the poorer ear side and noise of equal intensity originates on the side of the good ear, the unilateral hearing loss patient experiences his great problem. In this case, the signal-to-noise ratio (S/N) at the bad ear is +6.4 dB and at the good ear is −6.4 dB, resulting from the head-shadow. In other words, this individual experiences almost a 13 dB deficit relative to a normal hearing person; the normal listener experiencing a +6.4 dB ratio at the near ear, while the unilateral listener experiences a −6.4 dB ratio at the near ear. If the conditions are reversed (speech on the good side, noise on the bad side) the unilateral listener is not at a major disadvantage relative to the normal hearer.

INCREASED DIFFICULTY HEARING IN GROUPS AND IN
NOISE

One of the most common complaints of individuals with unilateral hearing losses is difficulty understanding speech in the presence of competing sounds. The probable cause of this complaint is the absence of the squelch effect described in the preceding section of this chapter.

AUDITORY LOCALIZATION CONFUSION

The time and intensity differences between the ears, created by the head, are virtually eliminated by a unilateral hearing loss. Without these clues it is almost impossible to adequately locate the source of a sound.

Table 7−2 summarizes the various possible combinations of the primary speech (P) and secondary noise (S) signals and how the unilateral listener will function in each.

Two of the early rehabilitative approaches to unilateral hearing loss have been mentioned. The first, no hearing aid, has been described just above. The other remedial avenue involved a monaural hearing aid worn in the bad ear. This

Table 7-2
Matrix of Primary (P) and Secondary (S) Signal Locations and
Effects on Unilateral Listeners

Signal Conditions	Effects
P and S on side of good ear	No advantage or disadvantage over normal listener
P and S straight ahead	No advantage or disadvantage over normal listener
P ahead, S to either side	No advantage or disadvantage over normal listener
P and S on side of bad ear	Equal head shadow—discrimination decrease due to high frequency attenuation of speech by head shadow
P on good side, S on bad side	6.4 dB advantage due to head shadow
S on good side, P on bad side	Greatest problem—13 dB S/N difference relative to normal

was a common approach if the poorer ear had usable residual hearing. Unfortunately, a monaural instrument for unilateral hearing loss is limited in terms of success factors.

There are a number of serious limitations to the successful use of a monaural hearing aid by an individual with unilateral hearing loss. First, there are many unilateral conductive hearing losses that can be remediated medically. If this is done after a hearing aid has been fitted, the instrument is then only temporary. Although not common today, in the past most otolaryngologists were quite reluctant to operate on a conductive ear if the opposite ear was normal. Their advice to these patients was often to position themselves advantageously and to supplement their hearing with speech reading. Second, there are people who have good speech discrimination ability in the impaired ear but who find it impossible to adjust to the combination of normal sound in the good ear and the "hollow" amplified sounds in the impaired ear. Third, if discrimination in the poorer ear is relatively good but the sensitivity loss is in the severe range, a body aid would probably be required. If so, the user loses the advantages of localization ability and the cosmetic appeal of ear-level instrumentation. Fourth, there are many unilaterally hearing-impaired individuals with such poor speech discrimination ability in the bad ear that useful amplification is precluded on that side. As Harford and Musket (1964) indicated, "where the impaired ear does not offer usable residual hearing for speech, a different approach is necessary to alleviate the communicative problems of one-eared hearing."

History of CROS

Working independently of each other, Wallstein and Wigand (1962) and Harford and Barry (1965) developed similar amplification devices for unilateral hearing losses. The former researchers did not receive favorable reactions from their subjects, and apparently did not pursue the matter. Harford and Barry called their instrument CROS—Contralateral Routing of Signals. The original objective was to eliminate the head shadow as a deficit. Figure 7−2 depicts the original CROS arrangement in eyeglasses. A microphone is located on the eyeglass temple on the side of the bad ear. The sounds picked up are routed through a wire to an amplifier and receiver in the opposite temple, from where the amplified sound is delivered to the good ear. This arrangement can be, and today most often is, incorporated into ear-level instruments, with the signal routed either through a wire or length of tubing. With this configuration, sounds from the side of the bad ear are directed to the good ear. Since this is done electronically, the effect of the head shadow is essentially eliminated. Thus, one of the major complaints of the unilaterally hearing-impaired, difficulty hearing and understanding speech from the side of the bad ear, is compensated for by delivering sound from that side to the better ear.

It is important that you keep in mind that the original CROS hearing aid was intended to provide amplification for persons with no aidable hearing in one ear, and normal or near-normal hearing in the opposite ear. Because of this intent, only minimal gain was required to overcome the 6−7 dB head shadow. After all, since the sound is going to a normal or near-normal ear, one would need only a minimum of amplification. However, there are a great number of hard-of-hearing individuals with one unaidable ear whose better ear is not normal. With these persons in mind, many variations on the original CROS have appeared. They will be described below.

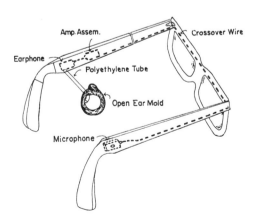

Fig. 7-2.   CROS (from Harford and Barry, 1965)

What is meant by the term "unaidable"? Harford (1966) describes four conditions under which an ear would be considered "unaidable.": (a) an ear with a sensitivity impairment beyond a point where amplified sounds can be perceived with any appreciable degree of usefulness in terms of intelligibility; (b) an ear that manifests a severe discrimination deficit, regardless of the degree of sensitivity loss; (c) an ear in which the use of an earmold is noticeably contraindicated; and (d) an ear that exhibits a markedly reduced tolerance limit and is therefore unable to utilize amplified sound.

An historic sidelight: Schaudinischky (1965) reported the development of the "audiomon" for unilateral hearing loss. This device consisted of a small microphone for sound collection in the external meatus of the bad ear which transferred the sound to a bond-conduction vibrator on the mastoid bone of the better ear. No further reports or additional data on this device have appeared.

Benefits of CROS

Experiences of clinicians, hearing aid dispensers, and CROS users have demonstrated a number of practical advantages of CROS, both anticipated and unexpected. Successful use of this hearing aid configuration has dispelled the once classic axiom that individuals with unilateral hearing loss cannot utilize amplification. Also, since the good ear receives the sound, high gain instrumentation is not required.

The greatest and most consistent advantage reported by users is increased ease in hearing speakers from the side of the poor ear. The reason for this appears to be the elimination of the head shadow. While this benefit holds true in a relatively quiet environment, CROS appears least helpful in conditions of high ambient noise—cafeteria, social gatherings, and so on. That is, in these situations CROS may not provide any advantage over normal hearing. An exception to this is when the origin of the noise is on the side of the good ear and the speech is on the other side. If the S/N ratio is negative, the noise greater in intensity than the speech, CROS is of little help even under the above conditions.

Harford (1969) reported an unexpected dividend of CROS; an improvement in auditory localization ability by some individuals. Apparently some people can utilize the difference in quality, between sounds entering the better ear naturally and CROS-amplified sounds, to localize. If the sound is natural, the source is on the side of the good ear. If the sound is "metallic," "hollow"," or "echoic," the source is on the side of the bad ear. Another factor that may account, in part, for improved localization is the time-of-arrival difference between natural and amplified sounds.

Shortly after CROS instrumentation gained popularity, the status of the better ear was found to have a direct bearing on the success that the user will have. A person with some degree of high frequency loss in the good ear will generally experience greater success than a person with normal hearing (Harford and Dodds 1966, Harford 1967a). This phenomenon is explained on the basis of the CROS arrangement providing greater high frequency than low frequency amplified sound to the good ear. The presence of even a mild high frequency loss reduces the chances of over-amplification or poor subjective quality in this range. As will be explained in the next section, the tubing delivering sound from the receiver nozzle to the ear either rests alone in the canal, with no mold, or is held in place by a plastic ring. This allows the sound from this side to enter the ear naturally. Lybarger (1967) measured the response of CROS aids with their special earmolds and demonstrated a marked decrease of response below 1500 Hz, with little or no gain below 800 Hz. Lybarger (1968) followed-up on these results by writing that the "really great importance of CROS lies in its ability to give good hearing to the bilateral case where the hearing (better ear) is nearly normal in the low frequencies and drops down or off rapidly above . . . 1000 Hz." He is pointing out that as a result of the shunting of low frequency gain, CROS can be applied to these individuals without fear of overamplifying. Low frequency sounds reach the ear naturally. This application of CROS was not originally anticipated.

In a recent follow-up study of CROS users, Aufricht (1972) sent questionnaires to 60 veterans. Of the 54 replies, 85 percent reported satisfaction with the instrument. These results support the findings of Harford and Dodds (1966) in which great user satisfaction was reported. On the other hand, my own experiences and those of a number of other audiologists, lead me to question these results. Apparently, even with extensive counseling and hearing aid orientation, a considerable number of CROS users eventually abandon their aids. This was demonstrated by Smedley et al. (1974) in another study of veterans. Approximately 80 percent of their CROS subjects reported using their aids less than one-half of the time. On the basis of the criteria they employed, the authors concluded that one-half of the CROS users were not obtaining sufficient benefit to warrant continued use on any consistent basis.

Special Earmolds for CROS

The primary rationale behind CROS hearing aids is to deliver sound from the side of the bad ear to the side of the good ear while, at the same time, the good ear receives sound normally from that side. If a conventional earmold was used in the good ear, sound would be prevented from entering normally. An unoccluded meatus in the better ear is an essential element of the CROS principle.

Generally, two approaches can be employed: open or free-field mold, or no mold. The open mold is essentially a plastic ring that holds the tubing from the receiver nozzle in place (see Chapter 3), for ear-level CROS instrumentation, it also provides support for the aid. Since the anchor is not essential for eyeglass aids, the open mold is often dispensed with, leaving the tubing suspended in the canal. Both of these approaches allow natural sound into the ear in addition to the amplified sound. Ron Morgan and I describe these couplers in more depth in Chapter 3.

Another important reason for leaving the canal open is the resulting damping action on the low frequency components of speech and other sounds. Since most of the intensity of speech and ambient noise is in the low frequencies, and since the typical CROS user has normal hearing below 1000 Hz, without this shunting effect overamplification of the good ear would be a major problem. A typical CROS aid with an open mold gives little or no gain below 800 Hz and relatively uniform gain above about 1500 Hz. Figure 7-3 shows the response of the same aid with a closed and an open mold. The dramatic reduction of low frequencies with the open mold is obvious.

Various other investigations into the clinical importance of the open mold have confirmed the resulting marked decrease in low frequency amplification and a concommitant increase in speech discrimination scores and subjective user evaluation (Lybarger 1967, Lybarger 1968, Dodds and Harford 1968, Green and Ross 1968, Green 1969, Harford 1969, Dunlavy 1970). Lybarger (1968) summed it up by stating: "with the open canal arrangement, both the gain and saturation output are cut by the acoustical systems of the ear and even very loud sounds in the low frequencies would not produce an uncomfortable level through the hearing aid, as would be the case with the closed mold."

Criteria for CROS Recommendations

When considering the advisability of a CROS hearing aid, the clinician must take into account a number of factors. First, as with any fitting for a hearing aid, medical clearance should be obtained prior to a final decision. This is especially true in the case of a unilateral loss, because it may be indicative of a serious and

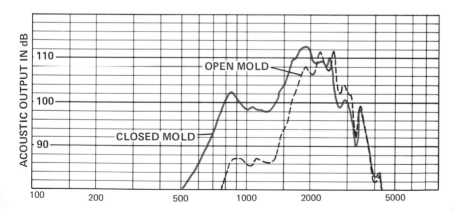

Fig. 7-3. Hearing aid response with a closed and open mold. (Courtesy of Zenith)

possibly medically treatable disorder, such as chronic middle ear pathology, Meniere's Disease, or acoustic neurinoma. Second, no final decision regarding a CROS aid should be made until after a trial period of at least 3 or 4 weeks. It is often difficult to clinically demonstrate advantages for a CROS. A trial period is essential for proper evaluation. Third, it is imperative to consider nonaudiometric factors in the selection of an appropriate hearing aid. For CROS, there are at least four areas of special consideration.

1. What are the communication demands placed on the patient's hearing? What are his communication needs? A safe rule of thumb is the greater the demand, the greater the potential benefits. Does the patient's job require frequent group conferences in which people speak to him from all directions? Is he commonly in social group situations?
2. What is the status of hearing in the better ear? As noted above, the better the hearing in this ear, the less are the chances for successful CROS use. If the good ear has a hearing loss, even if not enough to warrant an aid, the chances are greater for favorable reaction to CROS. However, the presence of normal hearing should *not* preclude a trial with CROS if it would otherwise be considered. Perhaps one of the CROS variations would be more appropriate.
3. What is the patient's motivational level? If he is highly motivated to improve his communication ability, the more likely he will be to benefit from CROS. It takes a considerable adjustment period to successfully use CROS. Without proper motivation, as with any hearing aid, it is likely to end up in a dresser drawer. It is incumbent upon the clinician and dispenser to determine the motivational level and, if necessary, attempt to improve it.
4. Age and age at onset. Although the age of the patient at onset of the hearing loss should not influence the decision about CROS, his present age is a factor. This is related to communication needs. A young child or a retired person may not have communication demands that would justify CROS. Ordinarily, a preschool child would not find a unilateral hearing loss enough of a handicap to justify a hearing aid. An exception, of course, would be the presence of a high-frequency loss in the better ear. However, when the child enters school, CROS should be considered.

For any one individual the clinician may find there are other factors to be considered. The above four areas are felt to be generally the most important. They have been derived from my clinial experiences as well as the experiences of others (Harford and Barry 1965, Harford and Dodds 1966, Harford 1969, Harford and Dodds 1974).

Dunlavy (1968) and Harford (1969) discuss the use of CROS with individuals having bilateral high frequency sensorineural hearing loss, with a precipitous drop in sensitivity above 1000 Hz. Two related problems often reduce the probabilities of successful conventional monaural hearing aid use with these cases.

First, it is difficult to adequately attenuate the low frequencies (normal hearing in this range cannot tolerate much amplification) and maintain adequate high frequency response. Second, since venting is commonly employed in earmolds for high frequency losses, output is limited by feedback. If CROS is utilized for this type of hearing loss the low frequencies are dampened considerably by the open mold, and feedback problems are reduced because the head offers the necessary attenuation between microphone and receiver.

CROS Variations

As CROS instrumentation gained popularity in the mid 1960s it became apparent that there were many hearing-impaired individuals for whom this arrangement was not satisfactory. Using great imagination and creativity, members of the hearing health team have developed a number of variations on the original "Classic CROS." These variations involve modifications of the design and applications for particular types of hearing losses. Using or eliminating the head shadow and relying on earmold modifications for frequency response alteration, these variations are allowing individuals to benefit from amplification who otherwise might not. It is now possible to meet the amplification needs of the vast majority of the hard-of-hearing population.

The first group of variations are those retaining the original CROS principle, but modifying the hearing aid/earmold coupling, the sound pick-up system or the frequency response of the amplifier.

CLASSIC CROS

For review, the Classic CROS, housed in either eyeglass or ear-level casings, consists of a microphone on the poorer ear side and a receiver on the better ear side. Sound picked-up on the impaired side is delivered to the good ear via an open earmold. The objective of this mode is to provide the person with better hearing for speech that originates on the off (poorer) side. Classic CROS is optimally used in cases of unilateral hearing loss with a mild high frequency hearing loss in the better ear. Figure 7-2 presents a diagrammatic view of Classic CROS.

HIGH CROS

Identical to Classic CROS in configuration, High CROS utilizes high frequency emphasis (HFE) instruments to further reduce low frequency response. It is intended for bilateral high frequency hearing losses for which Classic CROS would not provide sufficient gain. High CROS utilizes the head shadow by using the natural attenuation of the head to provide more amplification of the high frequencies without feedback. An open mold is used with this modification.

MINI-CROS

When it was discovered that the original CROS arrangement was not adequate for a better ear exhibiting normal responses, the Mini-CROS was developed. It is the same as Classic CROS except that there is no tubing from the
receiver nozzle. Sound escapes directly from the nozzle, which is simply directed
toward the concha. Moderate to high gain instruments are frequently utilized
because much of the amplified sound dissipates before reaching the ear. Since the
microphone and receiver are separated by the head, higher output can be used
without feedback problems. In other words, Mini-CROS both uses and eliminates the head shadow.

FOCAL CROS

Some individuals with precipitous high frequency hearing losses cannot
successfully use High-CROS. Apparently they do not receive sufficient high
frequency amplification. Focal-CROS instruments are designed with a nozzle at
the microphone port. A length of tubing is attached to the nozzle and extends into
the meatus of the off-side ear. Thus, sound is picked-up in the canal, taking
advantage of the resonant characteristics of the external meatus to enhance high
frequencies. Some Focal-CROS instruments have the microphone at the canal
end of the tubing. Others retain the microphone within the aid case. With either
arrangement, Focal-CROS reduces the need for high gain since the meatus en-
hances the frequencies between 2500 and 5000 Hz by $8-12$ dB, resulting in less
low frequency amplification and lower distortion.

Harford and Dodds (1974) suggest two additional possible uses for Focal-
CROS. One would be for persons working outdoors. The sound pick-up may
reduce annoyance from wind noise. The other is in noisy environments. The aid
may reduce background noise amplification by increasing the S/N ratio through
capitalizing on the acoustic attenuation offered by the pinna.

POWER CROS

Conventionally, a person with a severe-to-profound hearing loss in both ears
receives a recommendation for a body aid in order to utilize maximum gain and
output. Frequently the patient refuses this recommendation for cosmetic reasons.
Even with a tight fitting earmold, an ipsilateral ear-level aid cannot provide the
needed output without feedback problems. Power-CROS utilizes the head
shadow attenuation by employing a powerful postauricular aid in a CROS mode
and using an occluding earmold in the onside (aided) ear.

The next two variations utilize two microphones delivering sound to one
ear. Coincidentally, one of the first references in the literature to a special
hearing aid for unilateral hearing loss employed this principle (Fowler 1960).

BICROS

Figure 7-4 illustrates this principle, in which there is one microphone on each side sending signals to one receiver. BICROS is used in cases with one ear unaidable and the other aidable, i.e., a profound loss in one ear and a moderate loss in the other. With this arrangement, sound is picked-up from both sides and delivered to the better ear, in essence, giving the user two-sided hearing with one hearing aid. The off-side microphone pick-up eliminates head shadow effects. A standard occluding earmold is employed to allow the use of maximum gain when needed.

OPEN BICROS

This configuration is the same as BICROS except that it utilizes an open earmold or tubing alone rather than an occluding mold. It is most appropriate in cases exhibiting one unaidable ear and one ear with a high frequency hearing loss. In this situation an open mold is necessary to the comfort and effective amplification use derived from the resulting low frequency damping.

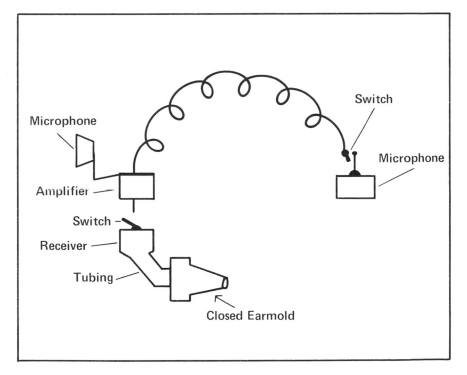

Fig. 7-4.   BICROS

UNICROS

Dunlavy (1968) reported on the development of a CROS variation for use with individuals exhibiting asymmetrical hearing loss, both ears aidable, i.e., a loss in one ear that might be aidable by Classic CROS or High-CROS and a loss in the other ear that would benefit from a conventional monaural instrument. This configuration is called UNICROS. It consists of two receivers, two volume controls, and one microphone located on the side of the poorer ear. In other words, UNICROS is a combination of a monaural instrument for the poor ear and a Classic or High-CROS for the better ear. It contains all the components of a true binaural system except that there is only one microphone. The bad ear is fit with a standard earmold while the better ear utilizes an open mold or tubing alone to shunt low frequencies. Because UNICROS is employed with asymmetrical hearing losses, the two volume controls allow differential gain to each ear. Additionally, two receivers and/or amplifiers with different frequency response characteristics can be used.

MULTI-CROS

If an individual exhibits one unaidable and one aidable ear and has a wide variety of listening needs, one may consider Multi-CROS. Harford and Dodds (1974) call this configuration the "epitome of flexibility." This instrument can be used as a Classic CROS, BICROS, Open-BICROS, or conventional monaural aid. It is essentially a BICROS instrument with a separate on/off switch for each microphone. Examples of the uses that can be made of Multi-CROS are:

1. In social settings or meetings where speech is originating on both sides, both microphones are on in a BICROS mode.
2. For conversation with only one person or in a noisy location, only the off-side microphone is on in a classic CROS mode.
3. If excessive ambient noise arises from the poorer side, only the on-side microphone is activated in a monaural mode.
4. Multi-CROS can also be constructed as Focal-CROS, Mini-CROS, High-CROS, or IROS (see below), depending on the needs of the individual.

Although Multi-CROS is potentially very flexible, one must consider the warning of Dunlavy (1970) that ". . . anytime you add another switch, another wire, another microphone, another receiver, or divide the instrument in any way, you are creating a potential source of trouble (breakdowns and repairs)."

The next two variations are considered by some as not true CROS modifications. However, they do employ certain CROS principles.

IROS

Ipsilateral Routing of Signal instruments are monaural hearing aids using an open earmold. This term was coined by Green (1969) to differentiate it from monaural aids in which a closed mold is used. Since the aided ear is open and low frequencies are therefore damped, IROS can only be used in instances requiring relatively low gain; most often with high frequency hearing losses. If the user has two aidable ears, binaural IROS can be employed. Of course, it can be used monaurally.

The rationale for IROS is that if adequate gain can be achieved ipsilaterally without feedback, there is no reason to locate the microphone on a contralateral ear. If one carefully examines the configurations previously described, it is apparent that one of the primary reasons for placing the microphones on the off-side is to take advantage of the head shadow to obtain greater gain without feedback.

CRIS-CROS

Ross (1969) points out that when two body aids are worn by an individual with severe bilateral hearing losses, these instruments do not provide true binaural hearing. The primary drawback is that the microphones are not separated by the 6−7 inches between the ears and do not have the head between them for attenuation. He suggests using two complete ear-level instruments in a double CROS or CRIS-CROS arrangement. In this way the user can take advantage of the head shadow to obtain maximum gain in each ear and still retain the two-eared differences.

One of the major innovators in CROS-type variants has been Alfred Dunlavy, a long-time hearing aid dispenser in New York. He has been credited with the development of IROS, Uni-CROS, and Power-CROS. In addition he has been granted patent rights to four other configurations (Dunlavy 1974b), FROS, BiFROS, Double FROS, and BiFROS 270. All of these variations can be used only in eyeglass hearing aids. They are illustrated in Figures 7−5 to 7−8.

FROS

Front Routing of Signals is a refinement of the IROS principle in which the microphone is located in the frame rather than the temple piece of the glasses. This increases the separation between the microphone and receiver, allowing greater gain than IROS. Dunlavy (1974b) has reported that all of the FROS variations are very directional in that there appears to be a decrease in background noises resulting from the back-to-front head shadow. It also allows the user to look at and have the microphone facing the speaker.

BiFROS

Binaural front routing of signals utilizes two microphones, one on each side of the frame, each of which sends signals to a receiver in the temple on the same side. In essence, BiFROS is a true binaural system, but has the advantages of greater gain capability, directional characteristics, and open molds if necessary.

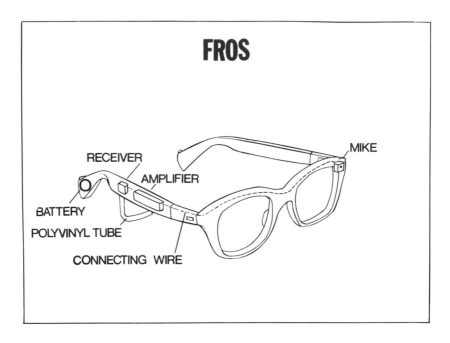

Fig. 7-5.   FROS (Courtesy of A. Dunlavy)

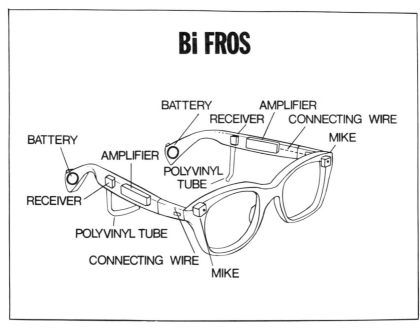

Fig. 7-6.   BIFROS (Courtesy of A. Dunlavy)

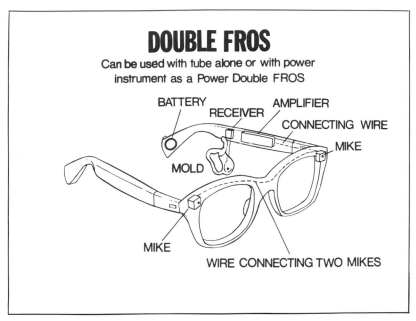

Fig. 7-7.   Double FROS (Courtesy of A. Dunlavy)

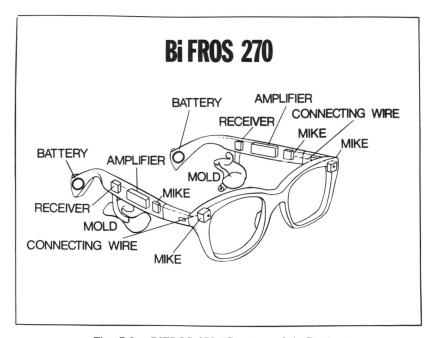

Fig. 7-8.   BIFROS 270 (Courtesy of A. Dunlavy)

DOUBLE FROS

Two microphones, but only one receiver, are employed. It can take the place of BiCROS fittings in some cases.

BiFROS 270

BiFROS 270 is the newest FROS variation. As of this writing it is still experimental. BiFROS 270 uses four microphones and two receivers. Two microphones are located in the frame and one in each temple. In other words, the two microphones on each side deliver signals to the receiver on the same side. According to Dunlavy (1974b) this 270° sound stimulation provides "a more full-rounded sound" and potentially allows front-back localization, which is not often demonstrable with most hearing aid configurations.

Comments

It is my opinion that the "naming game" of CROS variations is getting out of hand. The potential number of variations on the original arrangement are probably infinite—modifying tubing or earmold, changing microphone location, altering amplification characteristics of the aid, and so on. These devices are designed to overcome some of the off-side, feedback, and response shaping problems. I believe it is much more efficient to think in terms of two arrangements, modified as needed—CROS and BiCROS.

The classic CROS can be modified in many ways: a high frequency emphasis aid (High-CROS) can be used; receiver tubing (Mini-CROS) eliminated; sound pickup altered (Focal-CROS); a closed mold and a high gain unit(Power-CROS) used; or two CROS aids can be used simultaneously(CRIS-CROS).

BICROS can also be modified in many ways: use an open mold (Open BICROS); employ two volume controls and two receivers (Uni-CROS); place the microphones in the frame rather than the temples of the eyeglasses (Double-FROS); or put in a switch to control either or both microphones (Multi-CROS).

IROS, FROS, BiFROS, and BiFROS 270 do not really belong in a consideration of CROS hearing aids; none of them employ the CROS principle. IROS, for example, is nothing more than a mild-gain monaural fitting with an open mold. They have been included in this discussion because they make use of a development arising out of CROS—an open mold.

Conclusions

When one becomes familiar with the countless CROS-type hearing aids now commercially available, one realizes that great strides have been made in our ability to meet the communication needs of the hearing-impaired. The clinician can now choose amplification devices that begin to maximize communicative abilities. Although there are now CROS modifications for almost any unilateral and most bilateral hearing losses, it is inevitable that the future holds even more variations. The clinician must always be careful not to be lulled into thinking that any hearing aid solves the patients communication problems. It is a major step, but must be supplemented with other appropriate habilitative and rehabilitative measures.

IN-THE-EAR HEARING AIDS

In the past five years, there has been a tremendous increase in sales of in-the-ear hearing aids (2.6 percent of the market in 1974 versus 29.5 percent in 1978). One reason for this phenomenon was the introduction of the so-called custom unit contained within the earmold. It was touted as having a response custom designed for the user's loss and being less visible than ear-level aids. These traits, naturally, appeal to both the user and dispenser. It is a great sales tool for the dispenser, appealing to the vanity issues often presented by first-time users.

One other appealing factor has not been widely discussed. Since all the dispenser has to do is take an impression of the ear and send it to the manufacturer along with an audiogram, he has to do almost nothing in terms of selecting the appropriate aid for the user. All he has to do is fit the aid when it comes from the manufacturer. The effect of such a system is to take responsibility for failure of the fitting off the shoulders of the dispenser. After all, if the user is dissatisfied, the dispenser can say "It's not my fault, they designed the aid for your loss. You must be wrong." As ridiculous as this may sound, I have been told by users in my vicinity that they have been confronted by such statements by traditional dealers in our area.

Conversely, if the fitting is successful, the dispenser takes all the accolades.

As you can tell from this description, I am not enamoured with the in-the-ear (ITE) hearing aid. In my practice, generally speaking, we have had nothing but trouble with them. Of the ITEs we have ordered for our patients, all but two had to be returned to the factory because either we believed the response was inappropriate for the user or the fit was bad. Of those that eventually were fit, only four remain in use. The remainder resulted in dissatisfied users or, when we allowed the patient an opportunity to compare the performance of the ITE with an appropriate ear-level aid, they invariably preferred the ear-level.

I do not mean to imply that all ITE fittings are poor. We do fit some, but generally only under two circumstances: (1) if the patient absolutely refuses to consider anything else, or (2) if we believe that the size of his pinna and the space behind it will not be suitable for an ear-level aid.

There are three primary reasons for our attitude. First, as shown in Figure 7—9, as soon as a closed mold, such as an ITE, is placed in the ear, there is an immediate insertion loss (a hearing loss caused by the mold), which must be

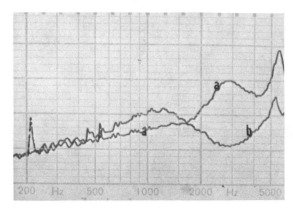

Fig. 7-9.   Insertion loss caused by a closed mold as measured on KEMAR

overcome by the amplification characteristics of the aid before any gain to compensate for the loss becomes effective. Since the ITE is limited in gain by feedback because of the proximity of the microphone and receiver, this situation seriously limits the effective gain of the ITE.

Second, many of the losses fit with an ITE are relatively mild or high frequency in configuration. As was demonstrated in Chapter 3, such losses can more optimally be fit with a free-field earmold. It is physically impossible to put a very large vent, such as would be seen in an IROS mold, acoustic modifier mold, CROS mold, or free-field mold, in an ITE. I believe that many people fit with an ITE could be more optimally fit with an ear-level aid using an open or free-field mold.

Third, a dispenser cannot rely on the response of an ITE he receives from a manufacturer. To investigate this problem, the audiogram shown in Figure 7−10 was sent to five manufacturers, with proper ear impressions and an order for an ITE with a large vent. Figure 7−11 is a composite of the five frequency responses we received. As you can see, there is great variability. Who is to say which of these five responses is most appropriate for this hearing loss?!

Thinking that there may have been a human error in the design of some of the instruments, the same audiogram was again sent to the five manufacturers with an order for ITEs. Figure 7−12 is a composite of the five responses received the second time. Again, you can see the large variability. Figure 7−13 is the audiogram with the ranges of the two sets of responses superimposed.

The main questions that arose from this data were: (1) how much would there be overamplification below 1000 Hz? (2) Considering the data from Chapter 2 on differences between 2 cc coupler and KEMAR measurements, are any of these responses appropriate? (3) Since each manufacturer apparently uses its own formula for determining necessary gain by frequency, and since each results in different responses, who is right?

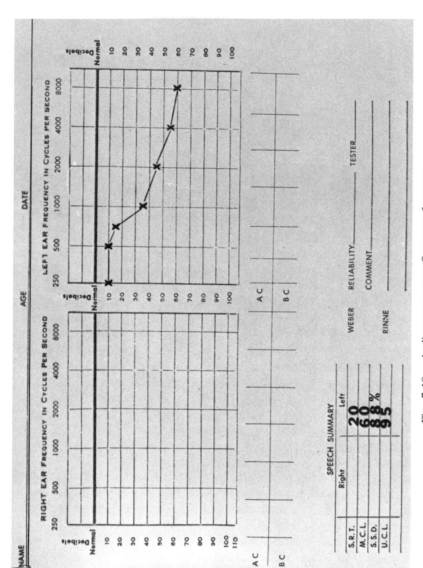

Fig. 7-10. Audiogram sent to five manufacturers

283

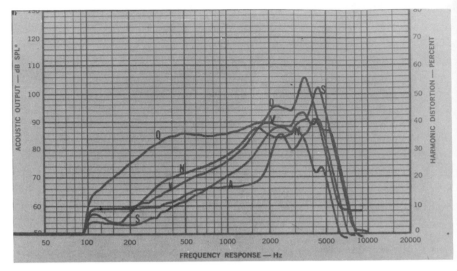

Fig. 7-11.   Responses of five ITE aids

As an aside: of the ten aids received, four did not fit properly. The impressions from which they were designed were carefully made and were considered by us to be highly acceptable.

As an audiologist and a hearing aid dispenser, I believe that my primary responsibility is to do the best I can for my patients. I do not believe that, in most cases, I can do this with in-the-ear aids. Until the myriad problems with ITEs are resolved and they become more reliable, I will continue to recommend ear-level rather than ITE instruments.

TINNITUS MASKERS

The Problem of Tinnitus

Perhaps the most common symptom associated with hearing loss is head noise, or tinnitus. Although most often reported in the presence of a hearing loss, tinnitus is also often present when there is no demonstrable hearing loss. It is a very subjective phenomenon for which there are no concrete objective indicators. As Vernon (1977) has indicated, tinnitus is a symptom of some disease or damage state of the ear, and is not a disease in and of itself. Various studies (Jones and Knudsen, 1928; Ventri 1953; Reed 1960) have shown that tinnitus is generally associated with some form of hearing loss and that only 7−8 percent of tinnitus patients demonstrated no hearing loss in the measurable range.

Tinnitus is reported in various ways by those suffering from it. It is often episodic or intermittent, and it is also often reported as fluctuating. Most people

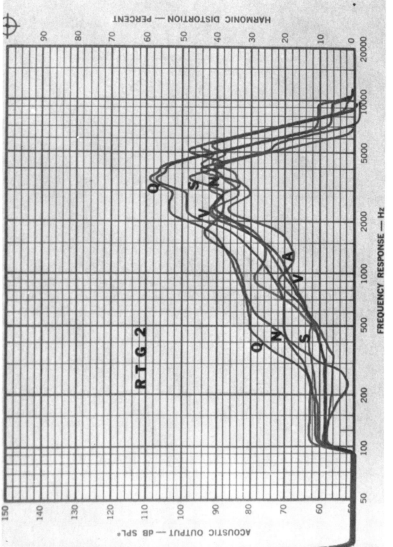

Fig. 7-12. Responses of five ITE aids after second order

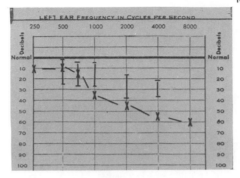

Fig. 7-13.   Audiogram with ranges of responses

indicate that their tinnitus seems worse when they are tense, nervous, or tired, and about 6 percent of tinnitus patients generally report that the head noises keep them awake at night or awaken them from sleep (Vernon 1978a). When questioned carefully, the reported fluctuations seem to be in the loudness of the tinnitus, not its subjective pitch or sound spectrum. As Vernon (1978b) has indicated, patient reports of fluctuation in the tinnitus are encouraging in that more individuals with fluctuating tinnitus demonstrate a spontaneous remission over a period of months or years than do individuals reporting a steady state of tinnitus.

According to Reed (1960) and Vernon (1975) most tinnitus clinically seen in patients is reported as a high frequency tone, rather than a low frequency tone or a band of noise. Reed's study in 1960 found that 76 percent of his cases reported such high frequency tinnitus.

Most of us have experienced some tinnitus at one time or another, although it is generally very short-lived and mild. However, even a brief experience with head noises can give us some greater appreciation of the problem faced by those individuals who experience this on a consistent basis. A high-pitched ringing tinnitus can be an extremely distracting and nerve wracking phenomenon, inhibiting the individual from concentrating on other stimuli, both auditory and otherwise, in his life.

Tinnitus Types

Reported cases of tinnitus generally take on one of several forms. Tinnitus can be reported as either a high- or low-pitched tone, a band of noise, or a combination of the two. Because of the lack of objective indicators for this subjective phenomenon, tinnitus can be described by many different terms. Some of the more common terms used by patients to describe their tinnitus include: ringing, bells, hissing, buzzing, crickets, steam from a radiator, whistling, clanging, whistles, and ocean roar.

As will be described later in this chapter, methods have been developed to give us a better objective measurement of tinnitus as well as a very promising treatment for this problem.

Theories of Cause and Cure Attempts

Over the years a wide range of theories have been put forth as to the cause of tinnitus. Stevens and Davis (1938) felt that it was due to increased spontaneous activity of the VIIIth nerve. As described by Vernon (1977), tinnitus can arise from many insults to the auditory system, including concussion, whiplash, noise exposure and diseases such as otosclerosis, diabetes, hypertension, and hydrops. Some causes of tinnitus are correctable, such as wax against the tympanic membrane, otitis media, otosclerosis. However, less than 5 percent of tinnitus cases seen clinically demonstrate tinnitus due to these causes.

Over the years, tinnitus has been most often treated with various drugs, such as nicotinic acid, vitamin A, and morphine. Myers (1975) described the use of placebos as probably the best known treatment for tinnitus. None of these pharmaceutical approaches have shown much success. In severe cases, a rather drastic treatment approach is to section the VIIIth nerve. This is generally only done when the sufferer of tinnitus is becoming very desperate. Unfortunately, such an approach relieves the tinnitus in only about 37% of the cases, while it destroys the hearing on the operated side (Vernon 1978b).

In recent years, Dr. Jack Vernon and his associates at the Kresge Hearing Research Laboratory in Portland have been developing an alternate treatment approach to tinnitus, involving the use of external masking noises. Their research (Vernon and Schleuning 1978; Vernon 1977; Vernon et al. 1977) have demonstrated complete relief in up to 70 percent of cases when the tinnitus masker is used. It is important to realize that the masker only provides relief from the tinnitus and is not a cure of the problem. It has been found that the degree of relief from the tinnitus depends to great extent on the spectrum of the head noise relative to the pitch of the tinnitus. In other words, if the tinnitus falls within the band width of the external noise masker, the chances are increased of some degree of relief while using the masker. Vernon (1978a) reports that they found that a noise-type tinnitus can be masked either by a tone or a narrow band of noise centered at the frequency of the tinnitus.

Severity and Loudness of Tinnitus

Before describing the tinnitus maskers in more depth, a discussion of subjective severity and subjective loudness of tinnitus is in order.

As part of his study of 200 tinnitus patients, Reed (1960) developed a three point severity scale. He described *mild* tinnitus as "not always present," "noticed only in quiet places or at bedtime," and "as a head noise from which the patient can be easily distracted by other stimuli." He described *moderate* tinnitus as being "constantly present, but more intense in quiet surroundings." He describes it as being "bothersome when the individual attempts to concentrate or get to sleep." *Severe* tinnitus is described as being "very debilitating, a condition in which the patients complain bitterly and cannot concentrate on anything else for very long." These patients report that they can often think of little other than their tinnitus.

Various studies have been done to determine the loudness of tinnitus. Patients variously describe tinnitus as being faint to extremely loud. Reed (1960) and Fowler (1943) have done perhaps the two most extensive studies on the loudness of tinnitus and both found that when matched against a similar type of external noise, most tinnitus matches at a maximum of $10-15$ dB sensation level. In Reed's study, 69 percent of his cases matched their tinnitus at less than 10 dB sensation level, while 87 percent matched it at less than 20 dB sensation level. A point to consider here is that while objectively tinnitus most often is not very loud, subjectively it can be very debilitating to the individual.

TREATMENT OF TINNITUS

Hearing Aids

All the approaches to relieving tinnitus that will be described in this chapter are based on masking of some sort—*an attempt to present an external sound stimulus to the patient in such a way that it will mask his tinnitus.* There are four basic approaches that will be described: *Hearing aids, FM radios, tinnitus maskers* and *tinnitus instruments.*

An important point to keep in mind when thinking about tinnitus masking is that *there does not appear to be a good relationship between the subjective pitch of the tinnitus and the frequency range of the hearing loss.* The tinnitus is often located in the region of the loss. Vernon and Schleuning (1979) report that tinnitus is usually not found in the region of maximum loss, but in a region about one third the way down the sloping audiometric function. This is an important observation when considering masking as a treatment approach.

Hearing aids were first suggested for the relief of tinnitus in 1949 by Saltzman. *The basic premise underlying this approach is that amplification of ambient environmental noises may mask the tinnitus.* Hearing aid dispensers have known this for years from client reports. I encourage you to keep in mind that *if it appears that a hearing aid would suffice as a tinnitus masking device, it should be used before any tinnitus maskers.* In other words, if a hearing aid is indicated for an individual's hearing loss, fit it and see if the tinnitus is also masked to some degree. My experience has been that as soon as the hearing aid is put on and the patient questioned, if the masking works, it will be apparent to him or her immediately.

Hearing aids are especially good for masking tinnitus associated with high frequency losses, the type of loss described in Figure 7-14. This type of hearing loss was previously thought to be unaidable due to the then available hearing aids and earmold technology. As I described in Chapter 3, with the advent of the free-field mold and tube fitting, such hearing losses can now be easily and successfully fit. Vernon (1977, 1978a) has reported, and my personal observations confirm, that *hearing aids work best at masking tinnitus in the range of 2000–4000 Hz*. In other words, if an individual's tonal tinnitus or noise band tinnitus is located in this range, the chances are increased that a hearing aid will prove effective as a masking device. Generally, hearing aids have proven ineffective for tinnitus that is greater than 4500–5000 Hz, as most hearing aids do not amplify much above this range.

If a hearing aid works as a masking device, it provides the individual with a double benefit in that it not only improves his hearing but also subjectively reduces his tinnitus. It has been noted that unlike the benefits obtained in many cases with tinnitus maskers, a hearing aid as a masking device does not result in any residual inhibition. This is the phenomenon of a continued reduction or absence of the tinnitus for a period of time after the removal of the masker. This will be described in great depth later in this chapter.

In summary, three points are important to consider regarding the use of hearing aids in treatment of tinnitus. First, this approach cannot be used when the individual's hearing is normal. Second, a hearing aid will work best as a tinnitus masker if the tinnitus is in the range 2000–4000 Hz. The hearing aid will be ineffective if the tinnitus is higher in frequency than the upper limit of the frequency range of the hearing aid. Third, while hearing aids do prove to be effective maskers for some tinnitus patients, no residual inhibition is generally seen.

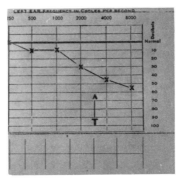

Fig. 7-14.   High frequency hearing loss with matched frequency of Tinnitus indicated.

FM Radio

For those tinnitus patients who report that their sleep is disrupted by the head noises, an FM radio has often proven to be an effective device. If the FM radio is tuned to the hissing static between stations and adjusted in volume to a point where it just masks the tinnitus, it often results in an alleviation of the sleep problem. This approach is most often used for individuals who report not being bothered by their tinnitus during their daily routine; who describe their tinnitus as mild, according to Reed's scale. FM masking does not work well for patients with extensive high frequency hearing losses and high frequency tinnitus. FM radio static is essentially a white noise, so that in the above cases the person hears too much sound in the region in which she or he hears well and does not need masking, and too little where he does need masking. If she or he raises the noise level to mask the tinnitus, the overall loudness can interfere with sleep. Work is presently under way to develop an all-in-the-ear masker for use while sleeping.

The FM radio seems to mask the tinnitus enough to allow patients to sleep comfortably. This approach is even used by some individuals with more severe tinnitus who do not like to wear a hearing aid or a masking unit while they sleep because of the physical discomfort of the earmold and the behind-the-ear-unit.

Tinnitus Maskers

As mentioned above, a series of units has been developed in ear-level hearing aid cases that produce various types of noise bands for use in masking tinnitus. The premise involved is that *this masking is an external noise and as such can more readily be ignored than the internal tinnitus*. All of us in our everyday lives have unconsciously learned to tune out environmental noises of which we do not need to maintain a general awareness. It appears that tinnitus has an inertia that makes it extremely difficult to ignore or tune out. In other words, the tinnitus masker produces a sound that not only masks the tinnitus but is generally more acceptible to the individual than his own head noise. A band of noise is less unpleasant than the high-pitched screech of a tone being constantly present. The masker effectively covers the individual's tinnitus, and the person, for perhaps the first time, has control over the presence and absence of his head noise. The output of the masker is controlled by the patient.

Maskers are especially good when the individual has no hearing loss and a hearing aid cannot be used, or if the tinnitus is too high or low in pitch for effective masking by a hearing aid.

Vernon (1977) reports that in the development of the tinnitus maskers, attempts were made to shape the response of the noise bands to avoid the speech frequencies. In other words, attempts were made to present as little energy as possible in the range from 300−3000 Hz. This would permit the use of the masker without appreciable interference with speech perception.

At the present time there are three types of tinnitus maskers available: *high frequency emphasis noise; low frequency emphasis noise;* and *broad-band noise*. In all cases, the response of the masker can be modified by the earmold configuration, especially by tube fitting. Figure 7-15 shows the responses of four commercially available tinnitus maskers. The curves in Figures 7-15A and 7-15B are of two different high frequency emphasis maskers; the graph Figure 7-15C is the low frequency emphasis masker; and the curve in Figure 7-15D represents the broad-band masker. The curves represent measurements made on KEMAR with a tube fitting.

The type of masker selected will depend upon the results of the tinnitus evaluation, the procedures for which are described below. To some extent, the benefits of the masker can be attributed to psychological factors, but the presence of residual inhibition points to some physiologic basis for the masking phenomenon. This will be discussed in more depth in the section on residual inhibition.

In some cases in which the tinnitus is bilateral, it can be masked in both ears by a masker in only one ear. This is a rare situation, but one that needs to be attempted in such cases of bilateral tinnitus. The effective masking of tinnitus in two ears by one masker (contralateral masking of the one ear) suggests a central rather than a peripheral locus for the tinnitus.

In some cases of severe-to-profound hearing loss with severe tinnitus, if a

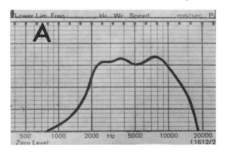
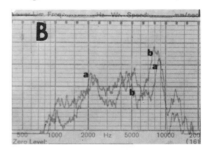
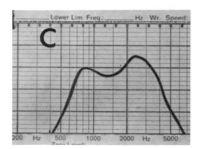
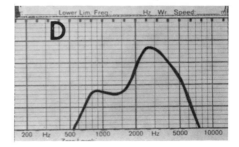

Fig. 7-15.   Frequency response of four tinnitus maskers measured on KEMAR: *A*, Vicon 564 high frequency masker; *B*, Audiotone T-500 high frequency masker; *C*, Vicon 574 low frequency emphasis masker; *D*, Vicon 344 broad-band masker.

masker on the affected ear (even with a closed mold) does not prove successful, attempts can be made for direct contralateral masking. If it is successful, it again points to a central mechanism for the tinnitus. When it works, a relatively low intensity of masking noise to the opposite ear can achieve the masking. However, if the tinnitus is due to a peripheral phenomenon, the contralateral masking will not be effective.

Tinnitus Instruments

In some cases where a hearing loss is present along with the tinnitus, a hearing aid may not be a sufficient treatment. In such cases the use of a tinnitus masker alone may alleviate the problem of the tinnitus but does not help, and may even exacerbate the communication problems resulting from the hearing loss. Therefore, the *tinnitus instrument* has been developed, a combination unit of *a high frequency emphasis hearing aid and a high frequency emphasis masking noise*. The frequency response of the hearing aid and the response of the masking noise are shown in Figure 7-16. Both the masker and the hearing aid circuits are combined in a single ear-level hearing aid case with separate volume controls for each of the circuits. Such a unit provides the advantages of both the hearing aid and the masker.

I have fit this unit and have had both success and failure. Unfortunately, the masking circuit in this unit does not provide as high a frequency emphasis as does the high frequency emphasis masker. Because of this, the masking circuit has

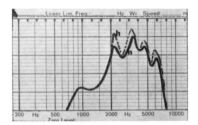

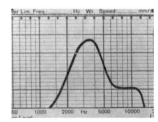

Fig. 7-16.   Vicon 244 tinnitus instrument responses as measured on KEMAR: *top*, hearing aid response; *bottom*, masker response.

proven to be not as effective for some individuals as the masking in the high frequency emphasis masker. For example, Figure 7-17 shows a case in which we fit the tinnitus instrument binaurally because of the hearing loss and the tinnitus. In this case the tinnitus was measured at about 8000 Hz. The masker had no effect at all on the tinnitus, but the hearing aid was very effective for the hearing loss. As a result of this we eventually replaced the two tinnitus instruments with high frequency emphasis hearing aids. This patient felt that the hearing loss was his major problem and wanted relief from that more than the relief from the tinnitus that could have been provided by the high frequency emphasis masker. I am hopeful that a tinnitus instrument can be developed that will give a spectrum of noise similar to the high frequency emphasis maskers as well as the hearing aid response presently available.

SPECIAL CASES

The following are two special applications of the tinnitus masker we have seen in our facility. The first, presented in Figure 7-18, is the case of an individual with a severe unilateral loss and tinnitus. Amplification in the bad ear was not useful and a CROS-type hearing aid was considered appropriate. A special unit was designed that would give us a mild CROS hearing aid as well as a power masker for the bad side. In other words, the bad ear unit had both a microphone for the CROS hearing aid and the power masker. At this writing, this individual is doing quite well with the two units, having the benefits of the CROS amplification as well as the masking.

The other case, which in a sense is related to the first, is that of masking tinnitus in a severe-to-profoundly deaf ear. In this case, we cannot use a hearing aid but we can mask. We would not use an open mold or a tube fitting but must use a closed mold. The individual may be aware of hearing some of the masking noise but the tinnitus may be markedly reduced, subjectively. The important point to remember here is that unlike most cases in which the tinnitus masker is fit with a free-field mold, *the severe-to-profound ear must be fit with a closed mold,* so as to provide the higher levels of masking required. With a tube fitting, too much of the noise would be shunted off.

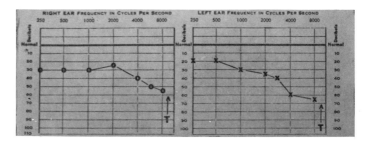

Fig. 7-17.   Audiogram of case unsuccessfully fit with binaural tinnitus instruments.

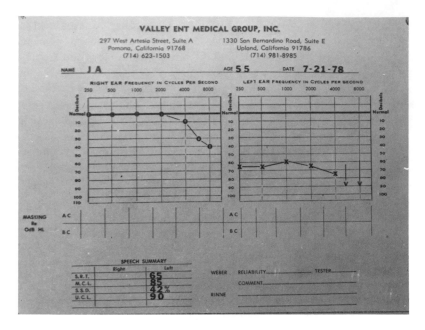

Fig. 7-18.   Case of unilateral loss and tinnitus.

Residual Inhibition

The phenomenon of *residual inhibition* was first formally commented upon by Feldman (1969a,b 1971) when he described a phenomenon where the masking effect is prolonged beyond the duration of the masking noise or tone. With the use of tinnitus maskers, after the masking noise is removed, the tinnitus does not immediately return to its premasking subjective loudness. This persistence of the masking effect on tinnitus following cessation of the masking sound is not displayed by all users. For some it is not present at all and for others it is only partial. Vernon *et al.* (1977) report that 70 percent of their tinnitus masker users display residual inhibition.

Although there is no, as yet, established correlation between the duration of the masking and the duration of the residual inhibition, Vernon and Schluning (1978) have reported that in many of their cases, if the residual inhibition is complete, daily use of the masker often leads to a production of extended periods of residual inhibition. They also report that residual inhibition is most commonly seen and is of longer duration in individuals exhibiting a tonal type tinnitus. It has also been noted that the higher of the subjective pitch of the tonal tinnitus, the greater is the duration of any residual inhibition effect. It has been observed that the duration of residual inhibition is related to how well the masking sound matches the frequency composition of the tinnitus. This relates to how well the noise masks the tinnitus. In other words, if the frequency of the tinnitus is not correctly identified, we may get some satisfactory masking, but little if any residual inhibition. We must again stress the importance of the clinical measurement of tinnitus, which will be described later in this chapter.

Vernon *et al.* (1977) have also reported that if no residual inhibition is experienced, this may indicate faulty masking and/or improper identification of tinnitus. They also indicate that some tinnitus is not amenable to residual inhibition. In other words, the absence of residual inhibition may mean that the masker does not include all the appropriate frequencies of the tinnitus. Therefore, the masking noise does not easily mask the tinnitus or produce complete masking, much less residual inhibition.

I have observed that residual inhibition is not found with hearing aids as tinnitus maskers. Apparently, the amplification of ambient environmental noise is enough to distract the tinnitus sufferer from his head noises, but does not produce the residual inhibition effect.

It has also been noted that residual inhibition is not seen with contralateral masking. Residual inhibition is restricted to ipsilateral masking. This leads me to suspect a peripheral mechanism for residual inhibition, since contralateral masking is accomplished through a central mechanism. Since we often achieve masking but no residual inhibition and since a hearing aid often masks the head noise but also does not provide the residual inhibition, it would seem that the mechanism producing relief from the tinnitus with masking is not the same as the mechanism that produces residual inhibition.

However, the presence of the residual inhibition does suggest that the masker may be interfering in some way with whatever process it is that produces the tinnitus.

Vernon *et al.* (1977) suggest that if ipsilateral masking does not produce residual inhibition, it may be an indication that the tinnitus is due to a central rather than peripheral process. If so, the presence or absence of residual inhibition may be a test to separate central and peripheral locations of tinnitus.

Another possibility for the use of the phenomenon of residual inhibition is that during the evaluation process the presence of residual inhibition may indicate how well the patient will respond to masking, since patients who display residual inhibition usually do gain a significant amount of relief from the masker, often more so than those who display the residual inhibition.

Clinical Measurement of Residual Inhibition

As part of the clinical evaluation and measurement of tinnitus, it is beneficial to administer a test to measure the presence or absence of residual inhibition.

After the tinnitus is matched as to frequency and intensity, according to the procedure outlined below, present a noise that will completely mask the tinnitus. This could be either a narrow-band or a broad-band of noise. The noises used are those most often found on clinical audiometers. Present the sound about 10−15 dB above the measured intensity of the tinnitus, or at a level that will completely mask out the tinnitus. Present the sound continuously for 1 min. After this time, turn off the noise and immediately ask the patient to describe his or her tinnitus. Specifically ask if there has been any change in the tinnitus.

The tinnitus may be gone completely or partially for as long as 30−40 sec. It will gradually return to its prestimulation level in 30−40 sec. This process is depicted in Figure 7-19. This graphic schematization of residual inhibition shows that after the masking is maintained for 60 sec, upon its termination the masking is at the 100-percent level (tinnitus completely absent) and gradually returns to the 100-percent level (prestimulation subjective level) after 30 sec to 1 min.

Figure 7-20 shows the audiogram and tinnitus identification information for a patient seen in my office. During the evaluation, after 1-minute stimulation with the masking noise, she displayed complete residual inhibition for 1 min.

After wearing a tinnitus instrument (hearing aid/masker combination) for as short a time as 3 hr, she reported complete residual inhibition lasting for as long as 3−4 hr. After wearing the masker for a full day, she reported that the tinnitus was absent at night when she went to sleep and was not present for almost an hour after she woke up in the morning.

Admittedly, this case is an ideal example, and not all patients will exhibit the same results. However, it does serve to demonstrate the potential effects of tinnitus maskers for a great many of our patients.

TINNITUS EVALUATION

The clinical evaluation of tinnitus consists of three very important sections: Otologic evaluation and tinnitus questionnaire; audiological evaluation; and tinnitus evaluation.

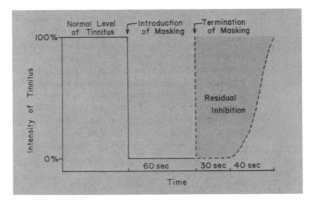

Fig. 7-19.   Graphic representation of residual inhibitation

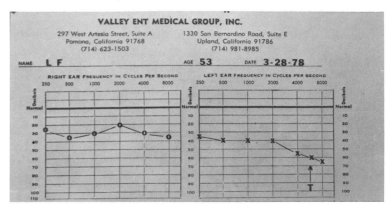

Fig. 7-20. Sample case demonstrating complete residual inhibition

Otologic Evaluation and Tinnitus Questionnaire

Medical clearance is essential prior to the fitting of any tinnitus masker in order to determine if there is any pathologic condition causing the tinnitus that is medically treatable. It is also important in order to determine if there are any medical contraindications to the use of the instrument. Another aspect of this part of the evaluation is the tinnitus questionnaire we have been using in our clinic. It is adapted from the questionnaire used by Vernon and his associates at the Kresge Lab in Portland. The questionnaire is presented at the end of this chapter.

We have the patient complete the questionnaire privately and then we go over each of the questions during the interview. It has been found that duration and rate of onset of the tinnitus are relatively unimportant in terms of the sucess of the masker. Any measures of the severity of the tinnitus are very subjective, and to a great extent indicate how the individual is coping with the problem. The main difficulty is that the patient has no language to describe the tinnitus and to identify and describe its subjective pitch and loudness.

Although the individual may indicate that the tinnitus is present only in one ear or the other, this may not, in fact, be accurate. It is possible that the tinnitus can be asymmetrical in terms of its loudness, and would therefore appear to be located only in the ear demonstrating the louder tinnitus. Methods for determining this will be described below.

Note that on the questionnaire there are two semantic differential questions (questions 4 and 7). These scales are most useful when carefully explained to the patient so that she or he has a more accurate basis upon which to make his selection on the scale. This is especially true for the pitch scale. It is very helpful to describe the scale as a piano keyboard.

Audiological Evaluation

A standard audiological evaluation can be performed. It is often helpful to use a pulsed rather than a continuous tone, thereby making it easier for the individual to differentiate between the clinically presented tone and a steady state tinnitus, especially one of tonal nature.

Tinnitus Evaluation

During this evaluation, we attempt to duplicate the frequency and the intensity of the tinnitus by matching it to various stimuli presented to the patient. The pitch match is the most important measure because it is the measure that will determine the type of tinnitus masking that will be employed. The evaluation can be done either in sound field or under phones. However, if the tinnitus is reported as bilateral or symmetrical, and there is a suspicion that it is neither, more accurate information could be obtained under phones.

The evaluation begins by demonstrating to the patient various narrow band noises and pure tones simply as a demonstration of the meaning of pitch and sound spectrum. A useful analogy is to describe the pure tone as the sound of a single piano key and a noise as the sound of a group of piano keys or some other equally descriptive term. The first question that should be asked is, "Is your tinnitus a tone or a noise?" This gives you a starting point in your matching procedure.

The first match will be to the pitch of the tinnitus, then to its loudness. If the patient has indicated that his tinnitus is of a tonal nature, present a 1000 Hz tone at $10-15$ dB above his pure tone threshold in the ear under test and then present a higher frequency tone as a comparison. Ask the patient which one sounds more like the tone of his tinnitus. Follow this procedure moving up and down in frequency and bracket the tinnitus carefully. If it is found that the tinnitus is reported to be at a frequency higher than the highest frequency on a clinical audiometer, a Bekesey audiometer can be used to present higher frequency tones. An alternative is an inexpensive audio oscillator that can be incorporated into the diagnostic equipment for this purpose.

It is important to remember that when matching the tinnitus to external sound, especially pure tones, harmonic confusions are often made by the patient. He therefore may match to his tinnitus a tone that is in reality a harmonic of the frequency of the tinnitus. It is important that the clinician be careful of this and use successive approximations to check the match against its harmonics. This becomes especially important for the test of residual inhibition as a choice of sound spectrum in the masker to be used.

If the patient has indicated that his tinnitus is more of a noise than a tone, follow the same procedure using narrow bands of noise. It is important to also make comparisons between narrow bands and white noise during the evaluation. At times it may also be necessary to make a comparison between narrow bands and complex or saw-tooth noise.

As I mentioned above, it is important to remember that even if the patient indicates that his tinnitus is unilateral, check under earphones to see if it is asymmetrically bilateral, especially if a hearing loss is present. This can be done by presenting a masking noise to one ear, once the pitch and loudness of the tinnitus have been identified, and then asking the individual if the tinnitus is present in the other ear.

Once the pitch is identified, it is then necessary to identify its loudness. In our procedure, we present a signal (tone or noise, whichever is appropriate) at the identified frequency at 20 dB above the pure tone threshold in the ear under test. The patient is then asked to indicate whether the external sound is subjectively louder or fainter then the tinnitus. In this way the loudness is bracketed until it is clearly identified. My experience has been consistent with that of the authors cited previously in that most patients exhibit tinnitus at a sensation level of only 10–15 dB.

Vernon (1978b) indicates that he first matches for loudness, then pitch, since the loudness of a sound influences its perceived pitch. I have found it more effective to first identify pitch, then loudness. I then rematch the pitch to verify.

Once you are sure of the match for intensity and frequency, the test for residual inhibition can be undertaken. This should always be done first under earphones, especially if there is an asymmetry or bilateral nature to the tinnitus. Present an appropriate masking tone, as determined during the previous part of the evaluation, at 10–15 dB above the matched loudness of the tinnitus. If the individual reports that the tinnitus is completely masked, you can begin the procedure. If not, vary the intensity of the masking noise until the tinnitus is maximally masked. When this is accomplished, turn on the stimulus for 1 min, and follow the procedure outlined in the previous section for the measurement of the residual inhibition.

In cases of bilateral tinnitus it may be necessary to use bilateral instruments to completely achieve optimal masking. In some cases both ipsilateral and contralateral masking can be achieved with one unit. This needs to be measured also.

Once the evaluation is completed you will have enough information to determine which of the available tinnitus units will be best for your patient. As I mentioned previously, if the individual has a hearing loss as well as the tinnitus, and if the tinnitus is in the range below 4000–5000 Hz and also within the range of amplification of what you would consider an appropriate hearing aid, the hearing aid should be your first step. If the hearing aid also functions to mask the tinnitus you may not need to proceed further. If the hearing aid does not sufficiently mask the tinnitus to your and the user's satisfaction, a tinnitus masker or tinnitus instrument may be used.

AMERICAN TINNITUS ASSOCIATION

In 1975, the American Tinnitus association (ATA) was formed for the purpose of raising funds and accumulating support for research into problems associated with tinnitus. One of the Association's functions was the collection of information about tinnitus from those who suffer from it and the dissemination of this information to its members.

At the present time, all tinnitus units (high frequency masker, low frequency masker, broad-band masker, tinnitus instrument, and a prototype design power masker) are available only through the American Tinnitus Association headquarters in Portland, Oregon. According to Vernon and Schluning (1978) the Association has established the following guidelines to control distribution.

1. No patient may be fitted with any tinnitus masker without the medical clearance for *that fitting* by either an otologist or an otolaryngologist.
2. Those eligible to dispense the various masking units must be certified by ATA. Certification is obtained by successfully completing an ATA-sponsored course on the testing of tinnitus.
3. It is strongly encouraged that new tinnitus clinics involve the team approach, combining the talents of an otologist or otolaryngologist, an audiologist, and a hearing aid dispenser.
4. Those participating in the program will be asked to make data available to a central collection agency.
5. It is requested that patients fitted with any of the masking devices be re-checked at the end of 1 month and at the end of 1 year.
6. Patients being fitted with a tinnitus masker should be tested with that unit in the clinic to ascertain the degree of masking the patient can expect.
7. In no way, implied or otherwise, should any patient be lead to expect an increasing amount of residual inhibition that might ultimately free them of tinnitus.
8. Those desiring more information should contact the American Tinnitus Association, P.O. Box 5, Portland, Oregon, 97297.

Additionally, the Association guidelines prohibit any advertising of tinnitus units without the express written consent of the Association, and generally will only allow the use of Association-prepared advertising material.

TINNITUS SYNTHESIZER

At the time of this writing, efforts are under way to develop a *tinnitus synthesizer,* an instrument that will be made available for the clinical evaluation of tinnitus. The prototype units now under test contain frequencies from 100 to 20,000 Hz in a continuously variable sweep frequency configuration. Also present is a continuously variable noise window from 100 to 20,000 Hz with variable bandwidths of 3, 6, 12, or 25 percent of the center frequency. The noise bands will have steep skirts of 30 dB with minimal roll-off. The synthesizer will also have a maximum output to the masking of 120 dB SPL in 1 dB steps. The controls will allow various masking signals to be presented to one or two ears and the unit will be calibratable.

Although the tinnitus synthesizer will allow a more accurate determination of the tinnitus and the optimal masking noise for its masking, with the present technology available in the masking units, it is my opinion that synthesizer is not a vitally necessary clinical tool. My experience has been that the information obtainable from clinical audiometers provides sufficient information to make a determination of the type of masking unit to use. The masking units are limited at the present time in terms of their characteristics. At some time in the future, if tunable maskers become available, the synthesizer would then be a useful tool. Work in these areas is presently underway by at least three hearing aid manufacturers.

CONCLUSION

At the time of this writing, tinnitus units are available through the ATA from two different manufacturers. The Vicon Instrument Company produces four units: high frequency masker, low frequency masker, broad-band masker, and tinnitus instrument. Additionally, they are developing a power masking unit. Audiotone is also developing and beginning production of a high frequency masker with an indeterminate high frequency limit.

I have found the possibilities of tinnitus masking to be very exciting in my clinical practice. For the first time we are able to offer many individuals who suffer from tinnitus a practical and an effective treatment protocol. It is my expectation that with continued research and development, tinnitus masking units will be made available that can do even a better job than those presently available.

BIBLIOGRAPHY

Monaural/Binaural/Pseudobinaural Hearing Aids

Belzile M, Markle DM: A clinical comparison of monaural and binaural hearing aids worn by patients with conductive or perceptive deafness. Laryngoscope 69:1317−1323, 1959

Bergman M: Binaural hearing. Arch Otolaryngol 66:572−578, 1957

Black JW, Hast MH: Speech reception with altering signal. J Speech & Hear Res 5:70−75, 1962

Bocca E: Binaural hearing: another approach. Laryngoscope 65:1164−1171, 1955

Breaky M, Davis H: Comparison of thresholds for speech: words and sentence tests; receiver vs field; and monaural vs binaural listening. Laryngoscope 59:236−250, 1949

Briskey RJ: Binaural hearing aids and new innovations, in Katz J (ed): Handbook of Clinical Audiology. Baltimore, Williams & Wilkins, 1972, 590−601

Carhart R: The usefulness of the binaural hearing aid. J Speech & Hear Disor 23:41−51, 1958

Chappel RG, Kavanaugh JF, Zerlin S: Monaural versus binaural discrimination for normal listeners. J Speech & Hear Res 6:263−269, 1963

Cherry EC, Bowles J: Contributions to a study of the cocktail party problem. J Acoust Soc Am 32:884, 1960

Decroix G, Dehaussey J: Binaural hearing and intelligibility. J Audit Res 4:115−134, 1964

DiCarlo LM, Brown WJ: The effectiveness of binaural hearing aids for adults with hearing impairments. J Audit Res 1:35−76, 1960

Dirks D, Carhart R: A survey of reactions from users of binaural and monaural hearing aids. J Speech & Hear Disor 27:311−322, 1962

Dirks D, Moncur JP: Interaural intensity and time differences in anechoic and reverberant rooms. J Speech & Hear Res 10:177−185, 1967

Dirks D, Wilson R: The effect of spatially separated sound sources on speech intelligibility. J Speech & Hear Res 12:5−38, 1969a

Dirks D, Wilson R: Binaural hearing of speech for aided and unaided conditions. J Speech & Hear Res 12:650−664, 1969b

Gelfand SA, Hochberg I: Binaural and monaural speech discrimination under reverberation. Annual Meeting of the Acoustical Society of America, 1973

Harris JD: Monaural and binaural speech intelligibility and the stereophonic effect based upon temporal cues. Laryngoscope 75:428−446, 1965

Haskins H, Hardy W: Clinical studies in stereophonic hearing. Laryngoscope 70:1427−1432, 1960

Hedgecook LD, Sheets BV: A comparison of monaural and binaural hearing aids for listening to speech. Arch Otolaryngol 68:624−629, 1958

Heffler AJ, Schultz MD: Some implications of binaural signal selection for hearing aid evaluation. J Speech & Hear Res 7:279−289, 1964

Hirsch IJ: Binaural hearing aids—a review of some experiments. J. Speech & Hear Disor 15:114−123, 1950

Huizing HC, Taselaar, M: Experiments on binaural hearing. Acta Otolaringol 53:151−154, 1961

Jeffress LA, McFadden D: Differences of interaural phase and level in detection and lateralization. J Acoust Soc Am 49:1169−1179, 1971

Jerger J, Carhart R, Dirks D: Binaural hearing aids and speech intelligibility. J Speech & Hear Res 4:137−148, 1961

Jerger J, Dirks D: Binaural hearing aids, an enigma. J Acoust Soc Am 33:537−538, 1961

Keys JW: Binaural versus monaural hearing. J Acoust Soc Am 19:629−631, 1947

Kodman F: Successful binaural hearing aid users. Arch Otolaryngol 73:302−304, 1961

Koenig W: Subjective effects in binaural hearing. J Acoust Soc Am 22:61−62, 1950

Langford BG: Why Binaural? Audecibel 1970, 151−158

Lankford S, Faires W: Objective evaluation of monaural versus binaural amplification for congenitally hard of hearing children, Meeting of the American Speech and Hearing Association, Detroit, 1973

Levitt H, Rabiner L: Binaural release from masking for speech and gain in intelligibility. J Acoust Soc Am 42:601−608, 1967

Lewis D, Green R: Value of binaural hearing aids for hearing impaired children in elementary schools. Volta Rev 64:537−542, 1962

Liden G, Norlund B: Stereophonic or monaural hearing aids. Acta Otolaringol 53:361−365, 1960

Lybarger SF: Advantages and limitations of the 'Y' cord. Hear Aid J 26:6,34, 1973

Malles I: Hearing aid effect in unilateral conductive deafness. Arch Otolaryngol 77:405−408, 1963

Markle DM, Aber WA: Clinical evaluation of monaural and binaural hearing aids. Arch Otolaryngol 67:606−608, 1958

Melnick W, Bilger R: Hearing loss and auditory lateralization. J Speech & Hear Res 8:3−12, 1965

Ross M, Hunt WF, Kessler M, et al: The use of a rating scale to compare binaural and monaural amplification with hearing impaired children. Volta Rev 76:92−99, 1974

Schubert E, Schultz M: Some aspects of binaural signal selection. J Acoust Soc Am 34:844−849, 1962

Shaw A, Newman EB, Hirsh IJ: The difference between monaural and binaural threshold. J Exp Psychol 37:229, 1947

Tillman T, Kasten R, Horner J: The effect of the head shadow on the reception of speech. Convention of the American Speech and Hearing Association, 1963

Whetnall E: Binaural hearing. J Laryngol Otol 78:1079−1089, 1964

Wright HN: Binaural hearing and the hearing impaired. Arch Otolaryngol 70:485−494, 1959

Wright HN, Carhart R: The efficiency of binaural listening among the hearing impaired. Arch Otolaryngol 72:789−797, 1960

Zelnick E: Effectiveness of binaural hearing aids for speech intelligibility. Natl Hear Aid J Part I August 1969; Part II September 1969; Part III October 1969

Zelnick E: Options in the fitting of binaural hearing aids. Natl Hear Aid J 23:8−37, 1970a

Zelnick E: Comparison of speech perception utilizing monotic and dichotic modes of listening. J Audit Res 10:87−97, 1970b

Zelnick E: Effectiveness of binaural hearing aids, Second Annual Oticongress, Copenhagen, 1971

Zelnick E: Binaural hearing aids for infants. Hear Aid J 26:7, 1973

CROS and its Variations

Aufricht H: A follow-up study of the CROS hearing aid. J Speech & Hear Disor 37:113−117, 1972

Bergman M: Binaural hearing. Arch Otolaryngol 66:572−578, 1957

Dodds E, Harford E: Modified earpieces and CROS for high frequency hearing losses. J Speech & Hear Res 11:204−218, 1968

Dodds E, Harford E: Follow-up report on modified earpieces and CROS for high frequency hearing losses. J Speech & Hear Res 13:41−43, 1970

Dunlavy AR: CROS: A review of application of fittings utilizing contralateral routing of signals. Natl Hear Aid J:1−5, 1968

Dunlavy AR: CROS: The new miracle worker. Audecibel 29:141−148, 1970

Dunlavy AR: Tips on making and repairing the CROS aid. Hear Aid J 1973

Dunlavy AR: Patent 3,789,163, Hearing aid construction, granted January 29, 1974a

Dunlavy AR: Personal communication, March 15, 1974b

Fletcher H: Speech and Hearing in Communication. Princeton, Van Nostrand, 1953

Fowler EP: Bilateral hearing aids for monaural total deafness: a suggestion for better hearing. Arch Otolaryngol 72:57−58, 1960

Green DS: Nonoccluding earmolds with CROS and IROS hearing aids. Arch Otolaryngol 89:512−522, 1969

Green DS, Ross M: The effect of a conventional versus a nonoccluding (CROS-type) earmold upon the frequency response of a hearing aid. J Speech & Hear Res 11:638−647, 1968

Green DS, Yanagisawa E, Smith HW: CROS hearing aids: a breakthrough for the unilaterally deaf patient and for others with special hearing problems. Connecticut Med 31:855−858, 1967

Harford E: Bilateral CROS. Arch Otolaryngol 84:426−432, 1966.

Harford E: Recent developments in the use of ear-level hearing aids. Maico Audiol Libr Ser 5:3, 1967a

Harford E: Innovations in the use of the modern hearing aid. Int Audiol 6:311−321, 1976b

Harford E: Is a hearing aid ever justified in a unilateral hearing loss? Otol Clin North Am 153−173, 1969

Harford E, Barry J: A rehabilitative approach to the problem of unilateral hearing impairment: the contralateral routing of signals (CROS). J Speech & Hear Disor 30:121−138, 1965

Harford E, Dodds E: The clinical application of CROS. Arch Otolaryngol 83:455−464, 1966

Harford E, Dodds E: Versions of the CROS hearing aid. Arch Otolaryngol 100:50−58, 1974

Harford E, Musket C: Binaural hearing with one hearing aid. J Speech & Hear Disor 29:133−146, 1964

Hodgson W, Murdock C: Effects of the earmold on speech intelligibility in hearing aid use, J Speech & Hear Res 13:29−297, 1970

Jetty AJ, Rintelmann WF: Acoustic coupler effects on speech audiometric scores using a CROS hearing aid. J Speech & Hear Disor 13:101−114, 1970

Johnson EW: The physician and CROS types of amplification. Audiotone Publications series, 1972

Lotterman SH, Kasten RN: Examination of the CROS type hearing aid. J Spech & Hear Res 14:416−420, 1971

Lybarger SF: Earmold acoustics. Audecibel 16:9−20, 1967

Lybarger SF: Some comments on CROS. Natl Hear Aid J 21:8, 1968

Miller AL: A case of severe unilateral hearing loss helped by a hearing aid. J Speech & Hear Disor 30:186−187, 1965

Ross M: Changing concepts in hearing-aid candidacy. Maico Audiol Libr Ser 7:10, 1969

Schaudinischky LH: New hearing aid for the monaurally deaf restoring binaural hearing. Arch Otolaryngol 60:461−466, 1965

Smedley TC, v Khaelssberg J, Clement JR: Success and failure paterns among CROS and BICROS users. Meeting of the American Speech and Hearing Association, Las Vegas, 1974

Tillman T, Kasten R, Horner J: The effect of the head shadow on the reception of speech. Convention of the American Speech and Hearing Association, 1963

Wullstein HL, Wigand ME: A hearing aid for single ear deafness and its requirements. Acta Otolaringol 54:136−142, 1962

Tinnitus Maskers

Feldman H: Untersuchumgen zur Verdeckung Subjektiver Ohrgeräusche. Ein Beitrag zur
    Pathophysiologie des Ohrensausens. Z Laryngol Rhinol Otol 48:528−545, 1969a
Feldman H: Homolaterale und Kontralaterale Verdeckung von Subjektiven Ohrgeräschen
    durch Breitbandgeräusch, Schmalbanderäusche und Reine Töne. Arch Ohr Nas
    Kehlkheilk 194:460−466, 1969b
Feldman H: Homolateral and contralateral masking of tinnitus by noise bands and by pure
    tones. Audiology 10:138−144, 1971
Fowler EP: Head noises in normal and diseased ears. Arch Otolaryngol 39:498−503,
    1943
Jones HH, Knudsen VO: Certain aspects of tinnitus, particularly treatment. Laryngology
    38:597−611, 1928
Myers D: Tinnitus. Hos Med 55−64, 1975
Reed GF: An audiometric study of two hundred cases of subjective tinnitus. Arch
    Otolaryngol 71:94−104, 1960
Saltzman M: Tinnitus aurium in otosclerosis. Arch Otolaryngol 50:440−442, 1949
Stevens SS, Davis H: Hearing. New York, Wiley & Sons, 1938
Ventrus RS: Discussion of tinnitus aurium. Proc R Soc Med 46:826−829, 1953
Vernon J: Tinnitus. Hearing Aid J. 13:85−86, 1975
Vernon J: Attempts to relieve tinnitus. J Am Aud Soc 2:124−131, 1977
Vernon J: Tinnitus and its treatment. Course at 12th Otology-Audiology Workshop, Vail,
    Colorado, March 1978a
Vernon J: Personal communication, 1978
Vernon J, Schleuming A: Relief of tinnitus by masking. Audiology & Hearing Educ, 1979
Vernon J, Schleuming A, Odell L et al: A tinnitus clinic. Ear. Nose & Throat J
    56:181−189, 1977

Appendix

TINNITUS QUESTIONNAIRE

Name _____   Age _____
Address _____   Phone _____
_____

1. I have had tinnitus in its present form for: (circle one)
   a. Less than a year   d. Three to five years
   b. One to two years   e. Longer than five years
   c. Two to three years

2. Prior to my present form of tinnitus I had a mild tinnitus for _____ years.
   (number)

3. My tinnitus seems to be primarily located in: (circle one)
   a. The left ear   d. Both ears but unequal
   b. The right ear   e. My head
   c. Both ears equally

4. The severity of my tinnitus in its worse form, according to the scale below, is
   represented by the number:

1	2	3	4	5	6	7	8	9	10

mild   moderate   extremely
tinnitus   severity   severe

5. The loudness of my tinnitus is: (circle one)
   a. Fairly constant from day to day.
   b. Fluctuates widely, being very loud on some days and very mild on other days.
   c. Usually constant but on rare occasions will decrease markedly.
   d. Usually constant but will increase markedly.

6. If my tinnitus changes from time to time, these changes are caused by _____
   _____

7. On the scale below indicate the pitch of your tinnitus. It might help to imagine the scale
   as if it were a piano keyboard.

1	2	3	4	5	6	7	8	9	10

low   middle   high
pitch   pitch   pitch

8. Circle any items below that describe how your tinnitus sounds: (Circle all appropriate)
   a. Hissing   f. Ringing
   b. Cricket-like   g. Steam whistle
   c. Pounding   h. Bells
   d. Pulsating   i. Clanging
   e. Whistle   j. Ocean roaring

9. My tinnitus appears worse: (circle appropriate letters)
   a. When I am tired   c. When I am relaxed
   b. When I am tense and nervous   d. After use of alcohol

10. Do you smoke?   Yes   No
    If so, for how long have you been a smoker? _____ years
    If so, how many cigarettes per day? _____

11. Do you drink coffee?   Yes   No
    If so, how many cups per day? _____

12. Circle any of the following items that give you any relief from your tinnitus.
    a. Listening to radio or T.V.   d. Medication (_____)
    b. Traffic sounds   e. Changes in altitude
    c. Sounds of running water (e.g., shower)   f. Other

13. Have you ever received a head injury?   Yes   No
    If so, were you knocked unconscious?   Yes   No
    How long ago was the accident? _____ years

14. Have you been exposed to loud sounds?   Yes   No
    Explain briefly   _____

16. Do you wear ear protection in the presence of loud sounds?   Yes   No

17. Have you ever worn a hearing aid?   Yes   No
    If yes, do you currently wear it?   Yes   No

18. Do you have any of the following? (circle the appropriate letters)
    a. High blood pressure   c. Allergies
    b. Diabetes   d. Other _____

19. Does tinnitus cause you problems getting to sleep?   Yes   No

20. If you are a hearing aid user, how does the aid effect your tinnitus?

   _____

21. Are you taking any medications?   Yes   No

22. What medications? _____ _____

23. Have you any history of ear disease? Explain _____

   _____

24. Have you a hearing loss?   Yes   No   Right ear   Left ear

Additional Comments:

Daniel L. Bode

8
Speech Signals and Hearing Aids

One of the most common misconceptions held by the general public is that hearing aids can restore hearing to normal. If a person with this belief begins to wear an aid, he is suddenly made aware that this is not the case. I believe that this is the number one reason why so many hearing aids end up in a dresser drawer. In another chapter of this book, Derek Sanders points out the importance of providing the hearing aid user with realistic expectations. Understanding why hearing aids do not generally restore normal auditory functioning and being able to explain this to your clients is a major step in realizing these expectations.

In this chapter, Dan Bode undertakes the task of explaining many of the questions often asked by lay persons and members of the hearing-health team. Relating basic principles of speech acoustics and noise interactions to hearing aid hardware and physiological dysfunction in the ear, Dan describes some of the complex relationships between speech signals and hearing aids.

MCP

This chapter will be an overview of the major interactions among speech signals, noise, hearing aids, and impaired listeners. The topic is complicated because of the many variables associated with (A) speech acoustics, (B) noise spectra, (C) electroacoustics of hearing aids, (D) complex speech-noise interactions, (E) ear mold acoustics, and (F) variability among sensorineural listeners in the degree and configuration of their hearing impairment, together with any consequent processing problems.

Any one of the above topics could be the sole focus of this chapter; in fact enough has been published in each area to constitute, from a literature review perspective alone, an entire book. Of necessity, then, discussion in this chapter will be descriptive rather than technical. The other chapters in this book and the present references will aid the interested reader who wishes to pursue further the specifics of a particular topic or issue that is briefly introduced here.

I am basically addressing two questions regarding persons with sensorineural hearing impairment: (1) Why do hearing aids typically *not* restore hearing to normal? (2) Why are we not able at present to prescribe hearing aids? The review will proceed from speech acoustics to speech-noise interactions, then to sources and types of distortion along the path from talker to listener, and finally, to a discussion of these topics and the two questions posed earlier. Throughout the review I will emphasize the research needs and the practical limitations of current clinical knowledge.

CHARACTERISTICS OF SPEECH SIGNALS

Complexities of Speech

Speech acoustics are quite complicated, due to the instant-to-instant interactions of sound pressure, frequency, phase, and duration. Sound pressure levels (SPL) for soft, conversational, and loud speech at a distance of 1m are approximately 50, 65, and 80 dB, respectively. These average values typically describe overall measures of low frequency vowel components. Consonants, which are generally more important for speech perception, may have average levels considerably less than these values (House *et al.* 1965). However, the acoustic cues used by listeners for consonant perception cannot be easily considered independent of the vowel environment. Many important cues are contained within vowel-consonant and consonant-vowel transitions as a consequence of coarticulation during production (Liberman *et al.* 1967).

In the frequency domain, speech contains components that are important for speech perception covering a range from about 100 Hz to at least 5000−6000 Hz. However, it is nearly impossible to say which frequency components are most important to a listener because this judgment requires at least three considerations: the type of listener, the type of listening task, and the specific objectives of a given audiologist in a given situation, e.g., diagnostic testing, hearing aid evaluation, auditory training, or prediction of an individual's performance and needs in a specific work, academic, or social environment. With hearing aids one must consider the whole frequency range from 100 to 6000 Hz as potentially important, depending upon many considerations. For example, in working with a child who is learning speech and language we may wish to emphasize low frequencies (100−1000 Hz) during some listening conditions so that the child might benefit from prosodic cues (pitch, duration, loudness), whereas under other listening conditions (e.g., noise backgrounds, consonant perception training) emphasis of high frequencies may be the practical goal.

Durational characteristics of speech further complicate our topic. Vowels and some consonants may have durations at average talking rates of approximately 100−200 msec while many consonants (plosives in particular) may be as short as 40−50 msec (Liberman *et al.* 1967). Normal listeners can easily make use of these cues, despite the fact that their hearing sensitivity decreases substantially as the duration of a signal is reduced. Temporal integration and other time-oriented characteristics of auditory perception *may* be dramatically worsened for some sensorineural listeners (Hirsh 1967; Gengel 1972).

Some hearing aid transducers during high-level output at the receiver stage probably are not able to follow short duration signals without considerably distorting the speech. That is, the aid may add transient distortion by altering the speech signal and by continued response after the original signal ceases, possibly masking the next phoneme. (See Chapter 2 for a description and discussion of transient distortion).

Many of the acoustic components in speech occur simultaneously (in parallel) as a result of coarticulation of phonemes. The acoustic results of primary interest here are the transient features of plosives (p, b, t, d, k, g, ch, dz). These phonemes represent about 25 percent of the consonants in spoken English and thus are considered to be very important for speech perception. Not only do some impaired listeners have difficulty hearing these cues through high-fidelity earphones, but there is a question of whether output transducers of hearing aids are able to reproduce faithfully these transients at high output levels without distortion.

Since transient speech sounds by definition have rapidly changing sound pressures, frequencies, and durations, it is amazing how well normal listeners handle these cues. It is even more surprising when hearing aids and impaired listeners interact to process and use these complex and subtle features of speech. This is particularly striking when these cues are competing with environmental noises and with cues from other talkers during everyday listening. Contextual restraints and redundancy cues in connected speech account for these abilities (Sanders 1971).

Speech Perception

A fairly recent development in hearing aid research and evaluation has been the increasing awareness that criterion speech discrimination scores can be subjected to analytic study. That is, rather than only assessing performance on the basis of the percentage of correct perception of monosyllables, some efforts have been made to determine the types of errors and confusions that impaired listeners make under aided and unaided conditions (Picard 1974). Given that we could know the types of errors a listener makes and the acoustical characteristics of the phonemes involved in the errors, we then might be in a better position to prescribe amplification.

A great deal of research is needed since the topic is more complex than often believed. The relevant acoustic cues for speech perception by normal listeners still are being studied. A variety of speech materials and analysis systems are available for research and clinical use. Nevertheless, normative data regarding perception of specific material have not been established, possibly because few audiologists are trained in and/or use available analysis systems.

Knowledge regarding the interactions among speech acoustics, electroacoustics of hearing aids, and characteristics of impaired performance at suprathreshold levels is inadequate for prescription of hearing aids. Until more is known of these complexities, and until we have demonstrated reliable and valid assessment procedures, educated and insightful clinical evaluations remain the most pragmatic approach.

One of the major obstacles again is that we do not understand fully the normal speech perception processes, let alone those of hearing-impaired listeners with or without hearing aids. Many times for analysis and/or instructional purposes we break down the total communication system into components for convenience and ease of study. However, it then becomes very easy for us to concentrate only on the components. To consider the total communication process seems essential if we are to understand the relevant effects of specific components. The need exists for operational theories of speech perception processes, based on data integration and considerable effort. We seem especially to be lacking data regarding speech perception by listeners with hearing impairment. Major attempts though have been made in terms of normal processing (Stevens and House 1970; Liberman et al. 1967) and a few preliminary hypotheses have been offered regarding impaired reception and discrimination (Carhart 1967a; Boothroyd 1968). A constructive interchange among audiologists, psychologists, speech scientists, and other disciplines interested in speech perception continues to be needed. This broad-based perspective would contribute toward development of theories of speech perception.

Intelligibility versus Prosodic Cues

Efforts are often directed toward making speech more intelligible for hearing-impaired listeners. Of considerable value to human communication are the prosodic cues present in conversational speech (Lieberman 1972). Pitch, duration, loudness, and juncture are important cues for language perception since the subtle meanings of sentences in English are often conveyed through the prosody factors. The two following sentences emphasize the importance of juncture cues:

1. The sons raise meat.
2. The sun's rays meet.

Given that contextual cues are not present, these types of sentences can be easily confused by all of us, but potentially more so for the impaired listener who cannot detect these subtle cues in speech. A striking example is the severely or profoundly hearing-impaired child whose hearing loss occurred prior to the development of language. In the absence of amplification and auditory stimulation, the question arises as to whether or not the child will develop appropriate language skills and intelligible speech. If the child does not hear prosodic cues, how can he be expected to utilize these cues either in his understanding of other's speech or in his own expressions of language? Appropriate prosodic features are often missing in the speech of these children.

This topic has been of concern for some time, and becomes complicated by other associated questions. One such question in recent years has been the masking effect of low frequency vowel sounds on higher frequency components of speech (Danaher *et al.* 1973; Danaher and Pickett 1975). It is suggested that amplified vowels can reduce impaired listeners' ability to discriminate and identify second-formant transitions. The paradox then becomes: Do we provide such individuals with hearing aids that emphasize low frequencies (for prosodic cues), high frequencies (for intelligibility cues), or some combination thereof?

At least two approaches are possible in the absence of definitive research. One is to select an aid that has a suitable tone control capability so that highs and lows can be independently controlled depending on the educational objective and the person's needs. Another approach is to select two aids, one delivering low frequency cues to one ear and one delivering high frequency cues to the other. Perhaps a listener could summate the two types of signals and have prosodic and intelligibility cues simultaneously or independently, depending upon the needs of a particular listening situation.

In addition to the previous examples, the importance of prosodic cues to quality judgments and to the acceptance of hearing aids by a listener needs further study. Individuals often appear to overemphasize speech intelligibility through hearing aids at the expense of determining which aids are comfortable in varying listening conditions and have acceptable quality of reproduction for the listener. Whether or not these subjective evaluations are amenable to positive change via auditory training procedures and/or experience in listening through the aid(s) during trial periods has not been subjected to objective appraisal (Bode and Oyer 1970).

CHARACTERISTICS OF NOISE

Just as speech signals have varying sound pressures, frequencies, and durations, noise contributes its own moment-to-moment fluctuations, complicating the task of an impaired listener attempting to use a hearing aid in a changing noise background.

Many problems with hearing aids and their selection would be dramatically reduced if they were only to be used in "quiet" situations. Indeed, measurements of hearing aid electroacoustic characteristics over the years have, for the most part, reflected quiet listening conditions only. Impaired listeners have most of their reported difficulties understanding speech in noise conditions. It is to alleviate these problems that they seek personal amplification.

Most environmental noises, at least in those conditions where a hearing aid is needed and apt to be used, vary in both spectrum and duration. Frequency components in many noise conditions are typically confined to the low frequencies (below 1000−1500 Hz), with progressively lesser amounts in the higher frequencies. This low frequency range is the region where many impaired listeners have the most residual hearing. Hearing aids amplify and possibly distort both the desired speech signals and any environmental noises having components between the effective high and low frequency cut-offs of the hearing aid.

Hearing aid users have to adjust to the consequences of the fact that whatever speech-to-noise ratio (S/N) exists from moment-to-moment at the face of a microphone diaphragm, also will exist in their ear canals, except at higher levels for *both* the speech and noise. Aids with high frequency emphasis and peak clipping may even worsen the existing S/N. These are potential problems that only recently have been described (Bode and Kasten 1971). Perhaps worsened S/N ratios explain a major portion of the problems experienced and reported by hearing aid users. This effect in many experiments and in everyday hearing aid use may be further compounded by alterations in speech-to-noise ratios *within the listener* due to distortions resulting from his own unique hearing impairment.

Because of these complex interactions, and to add face validity to test procedures, audiologists have long recognized the importance of using some type of noise or competing speech background during hearing aid evaluations (Tillman and Olsen 1973; Goetzinger 1978; Tillman *et al.* 1970). Many objectives can be achieved by such testing. First, the speech understanding task is made more difficult than tests in "quiet," thus potentially sensitizing the task to subtle differences as test conditions are varied. Second, face validity is added to the testing protocol in that realistic listening environments are simulated. Third, if a particular hearing aid has greater distortion than others being evaluated, the resulting speech-to-noise ratio could be worsened with a concomitant reduction in the criterion speech understanding score. Fourth, given a differential interaction between aids and an individual listener's unique speech-noise processing abilities, the consequences cannot be realistically assessed by testing in quiet. For these reasons, many professionals engaged in hearing aid research and clinical evaluation are increasingly making use of some form of background competition.

Agreement has not been reached regarding the type of noise, overall levels, and speech-to-noise ratios to use for research and clinical purposes. The types of "noise" employed have included: (1) white noise (equal spectrum level at all frequencies within the pass-band of the earphone or loudspeaker); (2) saw-tooth noise (a low-frequency fundamental with odd harmonics); (3) "speech" noise (equal spectrum levels at all frequencies up to about 1000 Hz and then 6−12 dB per octave decrease in levels above 1000 Hz, i.e., a spectrum simulating the long-term average for real speech); (4) recordings of one or more talkers producing speech; (5) cafeteria and/or traffic noises (to achieve some face validity and also to add moment-to-moment fluctuations in levels and durations); and (6) white noise that is modulated and/or interrupted.

Given the variety of possible noise backgrounds, the differences of opinions among professionals regarding *the* best noise(s) to use, and the various noise and speech interactions reported in the literature, it is no surprise that controversy surrounds this topic.

Currently, individual researchers and clinicians must make well-considered but tentative decisions, such as: (1) *This* specific noise will be used for *this* specific purpose; (2) Levels will be calibrated so that speech-to-noise ratios that exist during testing will be known; (3) Normal listeners will be tested first in the specific conditions in order to establish and maintain normative limits; (4) Reconsideration of these decisions will be made at reasonable intervals; and (5) Efforts being made to standardize testing conditions among clinics will be supported.

SPEECH-NOISE INTERACTIONS

Critical Ratios and Effective Masking

The "critical ratio" in dB, and the "critical band" in Hz (Scharf 1970) have been of great practical and theoretical value to audiologists. Knowing, for example, the critical ratio associated with each audiometric frequency and the spectrum level (or level per cycle) of a given noise, one is able to predict average pure tone thresholds for normal and many impaired listeners in this noise.

The formula for a critical ratio is:

$$\text{(a)} \quad CR(dB) = T(N) - LPC$$

where T(N) is the established threshold in noise of the signal, and LPC is the level per cycle, or spectrum level, of the wide-band noise. It follows then that:

$$\text{(b)} \quad T(N) = LPC + CR(dB) = EL \text{ (Effective Level)}$$

The calculation of spectrum level is:

$$\text{(c)} \quad LPC = OL(N) - 10 \log BW$$

where OL(N) is the measured overall SPL of the noise and BW is the band-width of this same noise.

For example, given an OL(N) of 80 dB SPL and a "conventional" audiometric earphone having an approximate band-width of 10,000 Hz, and by substituting in formula (C) above, we obtain a LPC of 40 dB. Then, given a CR(dB) of about 30 dB for speech material (50% response level) we are able to use formula (b) above and predict a T(N) for this example of 70 dB. Most normal listeners and many impaired listeners (given that they do not have a threshold for speech in quiet of greater than this level) should be expected to demonstrate a 50-percent speech threshold of about 70 dB SPL, i.e., at a -10 S/N.

Understanding the above concepts, and having the appropriate CR(dB) values for speech and for pure tones, allows the audiologist to calculate and calibrate his testing system so that he knows the T(N) or "effective level" of the noise he is using, whether for masking the nontest ear or for determining the levels he wishes to employ during a hearing aid evaluation procedure.

Both the effective level (EL) and the T(N) of the above example is 70 dB SPL. The definition of effective masking level (EML) takes into account the threshold in quiet, T(Q), in the following formula:

$$(d) \quad EML = EL - T(Q) \text{ or}$$
$$= T(N) - T(Q)$$

This formula expresses a basic definition of psychoacoustic masking, the shift in threshold of audibility of a signal in the presence of another sound.

The above concepts and calculations can aid the audiologist in understanding what is happening during many of his clinical test procedures. They are also helpful in comparing normal and impaired performance in "simple" listening conditions, i.e., speech materials in broad-band, equal energy per cycle noise.

Normal and Impaired Perception in Noise

The CR(dB) concepts developed in the previous section should be viewed primarily as capable of predicting performance of normal listeners. However, many impaired listeners *probably* will perform close to the normal levels in noise. This is why you will hear some audiologists and psychoacousticians refer to noise as the "great equalizer." That is, although the EML will differ among listeners because T(Q) varies depending on the absolute sensitivity of the listener, the EL of noise will be similar for most listeners.

Much more research is needed before we can understand and predict the impaired listener's behavior even in simple noise environments. Though impaired listeners can differ dramatically from "normal" in quiet conditions, the separation between populations seems to be quantitatively much less during listening in noise environments (Bode 1978). For example, an impaired listener might show a 40 dB deviation from a normal listener during tests in "quiet" but less than a 5 dB difference in noise. We are not saying that the hearing-impaired listener would not have a substantial handicap relative to his normal hearing peers. Rather, we are saying that the *quantitative* difference in noise appears to be much smaller than usually assumed. Thus there is a continuing need for reliable and valid speech tests in noise. We have investigated and proposed such procedures using adaptive tests (Bode and Carhart 1973, 1974, 1975).

Binaural Unmasking: MLDs and Release from Masking

An interesting phenomenon that has excited students of human hearing for several decades is called binaural unmasking, masking level differences (MLDs), or release from masking. Reviews of binaural hearing and MLDs provide excellent background and summary information (Green and Henning 1969; Levitt and Voroba 1974).

Basically, an MLD is obtained whenever a phase, time, and/or level difference between either signal (S) or noise (N) exists between the two ears during dichotic stimulation with both the signal and the noise. One of the simplest binaural conditions is conventionally designated NOSO, wherein both noise and signal are each *identical* at two ears; that is, all noise components in one ear are *exactly the same* in all respects as the noise in the contralateral ear, and the signal is exactly the same in each ear. This general condition is called *diotic* stimulation as opposed to *dichotic* listening, which exists when there is *any difference* in signal or noise presented to the two ears.

Typically the NOSO condition is used as a reference in the systematic study of changes that occur in listener performance as time, intensity, and/or spectral differences are introduced between ears. A dramatic improvement in thresholds can be obtained if specific conditions exist at the two ears. It has been found consistently that NOSπ or Nπ SO conditions result in the greatest improvement, i.e., a "release from masking" in signal detection. The subscript π means that the signal *or* noise is out-of-phase *between* the ears by 180 degrees; intensity levels between ears are the same for the signal and for the noise. The improvement in detection thresholds (the MLD), relative to the NOSO condition, can be as much as $15-20$ dB for low frequencies (around $250-500$ Hz) and $3-4$ dB for higher frequencies ($1500-2000$ Hz upward) with intermediate changes between these regions.

Most of the work with MLDs has been done with pure tone signals but some investigations have been devoted to the use of speech stimuli (Levitt and Rabiner 1967; Carhart *et al.* 1967, 1968a; Carhart *et al.* 1968b). Here the findings have shown about a $6-8$ dB improvement in intelligibility thresholds for spondee words (low-frequency cues) and about 3 dB for monosyllabic words (high frequency cues) when either NOSπ or Nπ SO conditions are compared to the NOSO condition.

Laboratory studies have generated interest in applying these data to the study of impaired hearing under specific conditions of binaural listening (Schoeny and Carhart, 1971; Briskey 1978). It is impossible to review all of the MLD data here, but the reader is encouraged to review the above references especially for familiarization with the clinical applications of the MLD data. Better understanding of normal and impaired binaural hearing in noise, maximal benefits of various binaural conditions, and realistic goals for binaural hearing aid fittings will be valuable rewards for the serious student of audiology and, ultimately, for hearing-impaired listeners.

Applied research in MLDs and exploration of clinical applications is needed at this time. Most of the previous work has been done under careful laboratory conditions with earphone listening. Sound-field studies specifically and hearing aid research generally are open territories for investigation and clinical application.

SOURCES OF DISTORTION

Many types of distortion can exist between talker and listener, with distortion here referring to *any change* in an original speech signal in its path from a talker's mouth to eventual peripheral analysis in a listener's cochlea. Linguistic distortion within either the talker or listener (or both) is not considered in the present context. In the following are mentioned major sources of distortion.

Talker Variability

A talker's production of speech can distort the resulting acoustic signal either through inadequate or inappropriate generation and propagation of the acoustic signal. Distortion at the source (including visual cues) can increase the difficulty of an impaired listener's perception of the intended message.

Reverberation

In many listening environments a speech signal can be distorted by damping and/or introduction of energy not present in the original speech. An example is any hard-walled, reverberant condition in which the original speech is complicated by the addition of reflected frequencies. Typical classrooms and hallways, and other structures with high reflecting surfaces, can add potentially serious distortion to a transmitted speech signal (Ross 1978).

Talker-Microphone Distance

A major problem facing a hearing aid user is the often uncontrollable distance between the talker and the hearing aid microphone(s). In general, as this distance increases, the overall level of the speech decreases with high frequency components showing the greatest potential decrement. This is due to the ease with which high frequency sounds are reflected back toward the source by obstacles in the environment. Further, given that environmental noise often remains relatively constant in level, while the level of the speech decreases as a function of distance, the S/N ratio at the microphone can progressively worsen (Niemoller 1978).

Directional and Head Shadow Effects

Depending on talker and microphone location, differences in spectral components at the microphone can occur. For example, if a talker is directly to the *right* of a listener (90° azimuth) and the microphone is on the *left* side of the listener's head, then several changes in spectrum can exist. First, there can be about 0.8 millisecond time difference between the two sides of the head; second, speech at the aided side can be about 6.5 dB less intense than on the unaided side; third, due to head reflection and diffraction effects, component high frequencies can be attenuated more at the aided than at the unaided side. Interest in binaural hearing aids and in the various CROS aids has increased in an effort to eliminate or reduce, and in some instances, to utilize these effects (see Chapter 7; also Harford and Dodds 1974). Effects of the presence or absence of the pinna also have been investigated. Some evidence suggests that the pinna is important for localization of front-to-back and elevation (Freedman and Fisher 1968).

Hearing Aid Distortion

A considerable amount of time and energy has been expended by audiologists and hearing aid engineers in the study of the effects of hearing aid electroacoustic distortions on speech perception (see Chapter 2). Frequency response, bandwidth, harmonic and intermodulation products, and transient response have been studied with equivocal results, due probably to the traditional difficulty of isolating one "cause" while controlling effects of the other possible sources of distortion (Bode and Kasten 1971; also, Chapter 2).

Coupling between Aid and Ear

How the aid is coupled to the ear canal of a listener can have dramatic effects on the performance of the hearing aid and the listener (see Chapter 3). Open, closed, vented, tubular ear molds, and use of inserts have been studied. In recent years studies have indicated (1) the importance of knowing what negative and positive effects result from specific types of coupling; and (2) the inadequacy of typical coupler measurements of a hearing aid's electroacoustic characteristics in predicting what acoustic energies actually exist in a listener's ear canal (see Chapter 2).

Distortion Within A Listener

An impaired listener's unique difficulties in processing speech continues to warrant study. Reduced sensitivity at different frequencies can distort an incoming speech signal by frequency filtering. Further, depending on the location and specific pathology, impaired discrimination among phonemes at comfortable levels above threshold can reflect a combination of other sources of distortion, such as bilateral asymmetries in sensitivity, aural harmonics, inefficient spectral analysis within the cochlea, abnormal masking effects, loudness recruitment, impaired temporal integration, and processing deficiencies in the central nervous system. One can easily see why the task of hearing aid selection and use is complicated and why solutions to these problems require extensive knowledge and skill on the part of various disciplines.

Complex Interactions of Distortion

Briefly stated, given all of the above *possible* sources of distortion, it is impressive that so many impaired listeners do so well with hearing aids. The expectation is that they should not have satisfactory experiences. We typically are placing low-fidelity amplification on ears, which can further distort the speech signal, and then expecting the listener to show substantially improved performance!

Those listeners who are successful with hearing aids seem to have minimal distortion in the pathway from talker to listener and those who are unsuccessful have greater total distortion. The clinician has a great deal of detective work to do in order to move a given listener from the unsuccessful to the successful population. Sometimes the solution is relatively easy, more often it is not. Given the complexity of the topic, and the associated difficulties of impaired listeners, one need not apologize for the absence of simple solutions.

PRESCRIBING AIDS AND PREDICTING PERFORMANCE

Prescription of any remedial procedure implies that prediction of probable outcome is possible. In general, the state of the art in hearing aid evaluations is such that audiologists are not able to predict performance, i.e., given that we have unaided measures with a particular listener, we are not able to prescribe a specific set of hearing aid characteristics that invariably will be appropriate for this listener. We sometimes do this as a general recommendation, but I believe many of us feel uncomfortable doing this and prefer to have clinical data (objective and subjective) that confirm our generalizations.

We have examined data from routine clinical hearing aid evaluations in an effort to assess possible predictive interactions among conventional tests (Bode *et al.* 1972; Dodds and Bode 1972). Results were obtained from representative and similarly conducted evaluations with 68 patients seen in the Northwestern University Hearing Clinic. Intercorrelations among 26 aided and unaided tests were computer analyzed, with one of our primary objectives being the identification of "factors" that influence test performance of hearing-impaired listeners. All persons had been tested in "quiet" and against "competing messages" both unaided and aided.

In viewing the results, five factors appeared to account for test performance: (1) aided monosyllable discrimination; (2) test ear sensitivity; (3) nontest ear sensitivity; (4) inter-ear high frequency response; and (5) aided SRT.

One of the intriguing results, in addition to the identification of the five factors, was the statistical independence of these factors. In other words, knowing the patients' performance on those tests involving one factor did not provide predictive information regarding their performance on tests associated with any of the other factors. Perhaps most importantly, knowledge of either (A) unaided sensitivity in the test ear; (B) unaided sensitivity in the nontest ear, or (C) the unaided high frequency response in either ear did not allow prediction of how the individual listener functioned with hearing aids. This conclusion applied whether we were attempting to predict aided speech reception threshold or aided monosyllabic discrimination (either in quiet or in competing speech conditions). Apparently, the only way to determine performance of impaired listeners with hearing aids is to conduct a clinical hearing aid evaluation. Recommending personal amplification on the basis of unaided performance does not seem to be a reasonable procedure.

Further, since *aided* speech reception threshold and aided monosyllabic discrimination appeared to be independent factors influencing test performance, predictions from one type of test result to the other were not feasible. That is, knowing a patient's speech reception threshold with a hearing aid did not provide reliable information regarding his speech discrimination score with this hearing aid, either in quiet or in the competing speech conditions. Granted, knowledge of aided SRT and of the intensity level of speech stimuli impinging upon the aid allows specification of the sensation level of the speech, but this knowledge does not enable us to predict discrimination of speech materials. The monosyllabic discrimination factor apparently underlies many types of monosyllabic speech tests (Carhart and Tillman, 1972).

Competing message testing in our studies provided realistic information regarding the impaired listeners' performance with hearing aids, information that was neither obtained nor predicted by discrimination testing in quiet. This conclusion was related to the fact that the mean difference between best and worst aided performance in quiet was only 6 percent while competing message testing showed an average 15 percent difference between conditions. Clinical decisions regarding which hearing aid to recommend, of course, are enhanced when the differences among aids are maximized.

These perspectives have perhaps been considered during traditional hearing aid evaluations. The results of these studies provide validational support for these considerations and highlight the practical importance of attempts to explain and predict performance of clinical patients on a variety of tests. Further refinement of our measures of each factor should considerably increase our ability to estimate and/or predict the performance of impaired listeners with hearing aids.

The search for underlying factors that account for, or explain, test results with clinical patients is a continuing need, one that has been only minimally explored. The potential for reducing a large variety of test results to a few factors that explain listener performance is one of the objectives. Achievement of this goal might reduce the number of constructs needed to understand the complex auditory behaviors encountered in clinical testing situations and in everyday life.

CONCLUSION

I have attempted to suggest answers to the two problems posed at the outset: Why hearing aids typically do not restore hearing to normal, and why at present we are not able to prescribe hearing aids with any degree of confidence.

The answer to the first question is that one cannot expect low-fidelity hearing aids to interact with damaged, distorting hearing mechanisms in such a way that the listener with sensorineural impairment will function similarly to his normal hearing peer. The practical goals, given present status of hearing aids and the limits of our knowledge, is rather to reduce or overcome the speech sensitivity impairment as much as possible, to provide maximum discrimination and understanding of speech delivered in "noise" to the hearing aid, to provide prosodic cues when possible, and to achieve all of this with maximal comfort and minimal adjustment on the part of the listener. This entire book, of course, is addressed to current procedures and issues involved in accomplishing these goals.

The answer to the second question, regarding prescription of hearing aids, has been only partially suggested here. However, the issues discussed here and throughout this book, particularly in Chapter 9, should convince the reader that though the question is simple, the answers are not. Given the wide variation in complexities of speech signals, in the pathway and noise interactions existing in everyday life, in the many electroacoustic characteristics of hearing aids, in the idiosyncratic nature of various sensorineural pathologies, and in the generally unknown features and dimensions of speech perception, we can be sure that our work has only just begun. A variety of activity is currently underway, including applied research, sophisticated clinical testing, relevant legislative and professional action, and cooperative standardization efforts. These facts, as well as the increase in the number of dedicated individuals attacking present problems, serve to excite and encourage those of us who seek to understand the interactions of speech signals and hearing aids and to implement means by which the deleterious effects of these interactions can be minimized.

ACKNOWLEDGMENT

I wish to thank two individuals for their constructive comments regarding an earlier draft of this manuscript: Dr. Sally Revoile, Sensory Communication Research Laboratory, Gallaudet College; and Dr. Jerry Punch, Biocommunications Laboratory, University of Maryland.

BIBLIOGRAPHY

Bode DL, Oyer HJ: Auditory training and speech discrimination. J Speech Hear Res 13:839—855, 1970

Bode DL, Kasten RN: Hearing aid distortion and consonant identification. J Speech Hear Res 14 (1971) 323—331

Bode DL, Dodds E, Carhart R: A factor analysis of competing message testing in hearing aid evaluations. J Acoust Soc Am 52:184(A), 1972

Bode DL, Carhart R: Measurement of articulation functions using adaptive test procedures. IEEE Trans Audio Electroacoust AU-21:196—201, 1973

Bode DL, Carhart R: Stability and accuracy of adaptive tests of speech discrimination. J Acoust Soc Am 56:963—970, 1974

Bode DL, Carhart R: Estimating CNC discrimination with spondee words. J Acoust Soc Am 57:1216—1218, 1975

Bode DL: Adaptive speech testing applied to hearing impaired listeners. Annual Convention, American Speech and Hearing Association, 1978

Boothroyd A: Statistical theory of the speech discrimination score. J Acoust Soc Am 43:362—367, 1968

Briskey, RJ: Binaural hearing aids and new innovations, in Katz J (ed): Handbook of Clinical Audiology (ed 2). Baltimore, Williams & Wilkins, 1978, pp 501—507

Carhart R: Factors affecting discrimination for monosyllabic words in background noise. Paper presented at the Annual Convention of the American Speech and Hearing Association, 1967

Carhart R, Tillman TW, Johnson KR: Release of masking for speech through interaural time delay. J Acoust Soc Am 42:124—138, 1967

Carhart R, Tillman TW, Johnson KR: Effects of interaural time delays on masking by two competing signals. J Acoust Soc Am 43:1223—1230, 1968a

Carhart, R, Tillman TW, Dallos PJ: Unmasking for pure tones and spondees: Interaural phase and time disparities. J Speech Hear Res 11:722—734, 1968b

Carhart R, Tillman TW: Individual consistency of hearing for speech across diverse listening conditions. J Speech Hear Res 15:105—113, 1972

Danaher EM, Osberger MJ, Picket JM: Discrimination of formant frequency transitions in synthetic vowels. J Speech Hear Res 16:439—451, 1973

Danaher EM, Pickett JM: Some masking effects produced by low-frequency vowel formants in persons with sensorineural hearing loss. J Speech Hear Res 18:261—271, 1975

Dodds E, Bode DL: Evaluation of clinical hearing aid selection procedures. ASHA 14:473(A), 1972

Freedman SJ, Fisher HG: The role of the pinna in auditory localization, in Freedman SJ (ed): The Neuropsychology of Spatially Oriented Behavior. Homewood, Ill., Dorsey Press, 1968, pp 135–152

Gengel R: Auditory temporal integration at relatively high masked-threshold levels. J Acoust Soc Am 51:1849–1851, 1972

Goetzinger CP: Word discrimination testing, in Katz J (ed): Handbook of Clinical Audiology (ed 2). Baltimore, Williams & Wilkins, 1978, pp 149–158

Green DM, Henning GB: Audition. Annu Rev Psychol 20:105–128, 1969

Harford E, Dodds E: Versions of the CROS hearing aid. Arch Otolaryngol 100:50–57, 1974

Hirsh IJ: Information processing in input channels for speech and language: The significance of serial order of stimuli, in Brain Mechanisms Underlying Speech and Language. New York, Grune & Stratton, 1967, pp 21–38

House AS, Williams CE, Hecker MHL, et al: Articulation testing methods: Consonantal differentiation with a closed-response set. J Acoust Soc Am 37:158–166, 1965

Levitt H, Rabiner LR: Binaural release from masking for speech and gain in intelligibility. J Acoust Soc Am 42:601–608, 1967

Levitt H, Voroba B: Binaural hearing, in Gerber SE (ed): Introductory Hearing Science. Philadelphia, W.B. Saunders, 1974, pp 187–206

Liberman AM, Cooper FS, Shankweiler DP, et al: Perception of the speech code. Psychol Rev 74:431–461, 1967

Liberman P: Speech Acoustics and Perception. Indianapolis, Bobbs-Merrill, 1972

Niemoeller AF: Hearing aids, in Davis H, Silverman SR (eds): Hearing and Deafness. New York, Holt, Rinehart and Winston, 1978, pp 293–337

Picard M: Effects of selective amplification upon consonant intelligibility in normal and sensorineural listeners. Unpublished doctoral dissertation, University of Illinois, 1974

Ross M: Classroom acoustics and speech intelligibility, in Katz J (ed): Handbook of Clinical Audiology. Baltimore, Williams & Wilkins, 1978, pp 469–478

Sanders D: Aural Rehabilitation. Englewood Cliffs, N.J., Prentice-Hall, 1971

Scharf B: Critical bands, in Tobias JV (ed): Foundations of Modern Auditory Theory, vol 1. New York, Academic Press, 1970, pp 159–202

Schoeny ZG, Carhart R: Effects of unilateral menieres disease on masking-level differences. J Acoust Soc Am 50:1143–1149, 1971

Stevens KM, House AS: Speech perception, in Tobias JV (ed): Foundations of Modern Auditory Theory, vol 2. New York, Academic Press, 1970, pp 3–62

Tillman TW, Carhart R, Olsen WO: Hearing aid efficiency in a competing speech situation. J Speech Hear Res 13:789–811, 1970

Tillman T, Olsen WO: Speech audiometry, in Jerger J (ed): Modern Developments in Audiology. New York, Academic Press, 1973, pp 37–74

Kenneth W. Berger

9
The Search for a Master Hearing Aid

In his second contribution to this book, Ken Berger presents what many have considered an attractive alternative to traditional hearing aid selection and fitting procedures. Besides tracing the history of master hearing aids, Ken presents some insightful recommendations for an idealized unit, suggesting areas of much-needed research. He also compares the clinical use of the master aid with traditional selection procedures. A careful reading of this chapter should give you reason to constructively question many of the aspects of hearing aid selection and fitting. It should also stimulate significant questioning and discussion among the hearing—health team.

MCP

Traditional or modified hearing aid evaluations as performed in audiology clinics could undoubtedly be facilitated if a standard instrument were available to simulate various gain, output, and frequency response patterns. The fitting of hearing aids by hearing aid dealers would likewise be made easier by such an instrument. Although a number of so-called master hearing aids (or pressure-measuring instruments) have appeared on the market, their use does not yet appear to be widespread in clinics. *Nor are there good data to support the assumption that patient performance, as determined with such an instrument, can be used predictively in choosing a wearable hearing aid.*

The search for an acceptable and standard master hearing aid is alluring. Such an instrument would permit speech audiometric testing under various gain, output, and frequency response settings that simulate hearing aid characteristics. The time and endurance of both the client and the tester can, theoretically, be improved by using a single device rather than laboriously changing from one hearing aid to another during comparative testing. Furthermore, the master hearing aid could drastically reduce the huge stock of aids now on loan to clinics by manufacturers or by dealers.

In one survey of 308 facilities maintaining hearing aids for evaluation purposes, it was found that the number of different models in inventory ranged from 1 to more than 40, with a median in the range of 10−20 instruments (ASHA Reports 2). It can easily be seen that the hearing aid industry has a burdensome inventory of instruments on loan to clinic facilities. Not only does this large inventory of instruments represent a substantial investment by the manufacturer and his dealer, but many audiologists and clinics strongly prefer that their inventory of loaner instruments for evaluation purposes be much smaller than it is at present.

Thus, a true master hearing aid would be the solution to the present large inventory of aids in clinics and it would facilitate fitting or evaluating hearing aids in individual cases. Despite these obvious advantages, it seems curious that neither the hearing aid industry nor the audiologists have shown more than a moderate interest in the development of a standard instrument of this type.

The typical textbook of audiology mentions only briefly, if at all, the master hearing aid. The instrument seems to be used little in audiology clinics, but the number of such instruments in the offices of dealers in hearing aids is probably substantial (Nunley 1972). Although a number of hearing aid manufacturers make such an instrument available to their dealers, the purpose of using the instrument seems to be almost solely to sell their own specific brand product.

EARLY HEARING AID FITTING INSTRUMENTS

Although the so-called master hearing aid was relatively unknown and unused until about 1960, a number of prototypes date back to the carbon hearing aid era. In 1905 Miller R. Hutchison received patent No. 789,915 for a "method of determining degree of deafness." The device was designed to measure hearing in such a way that an aid could be fitted by selecting an appropriate transmitter and receiver from a series. Hutchison is better remembered as the inventor of the first electric hearing aid (see Chapter 1). In 1913 Eric T. Hincks of England received British patent No. 10,000 for a similar device for selecting components of hearing aids for individual needs. Both the Hutchison and the Hincks patents can be classified as master hearing aid units, but there is no evidence that either instrument was actually manufactured.

The first known hearing aid fitting instrument manufactured was that made by the Radioear Corporation in 1935 and originally called the *Select-O-Phone*. Subsequently it was learned that this name was copyrighted by another firm and the instrument was renamed the *Selex-A-Phone*. A second generation Selex-A-Phone is shown in Figure 9-1. Sam F. Lybarger received a patent for the Selex-A-Phone in 1938 (Patent No. 2,112,569).

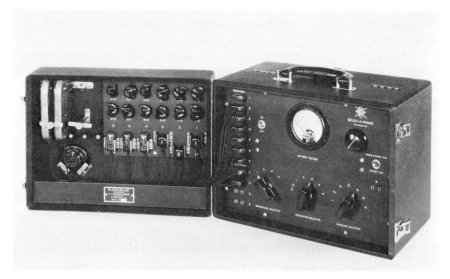

Fig. 9-1.   Selex-A-Phone.

From Figure 9-1 it may be seen that the second Selex-A-Phone provided for trials of four carbon test microphones (the original instrument had three) which differed in their frequency responses. For receivers, the client could try three different air conduction versions and three different bone conduction vibrators, in addition to an earphone. Six pairs of stock earmolds were available for the air conduction receivers to diminish acoustic feedback during trial. In addition, the client could try an amplifier, called an *intensifier* by Radioear. The instrument was powered by a battery and there was a battery test switch on the right of the main part of the carry-case.

The idea behind the Selex-A-Phone was that the local hearing aid dealer could, at his office or in the client's home, give the client a trial under amplification with an assortment of microphones and receivers. Whatever combination worked best was then ordered from the factory.

The Selex-A-Phones were owned by Radioear Corporation and sent out on consignment to their dealers. After the carbon hearing aid era passed, the instruments were recalled by the company. When the firm moved to a new location, evidently all of the existing models were destroyed and only photographs remain of this first master hearing aid. The Selex-A-Phone was a popular fitting instrument with Radioear hearing aid dealers, and by 1936 more than 65 local offices were using it.* Radioear publicity referred to this method of fitting as "Laboratory made-to-order Radioears."

The Selex-A-Phone was followed by the Aurogage of Dictograph Products,

*"Hearing Ears Again," Radioear Corporation, September 1937

Inc. (Acousticon tradename). The Aurogage was introduced at the American Academy of Ophthalmology and Otolaryngology meeting held in New York City in the fall of 1936.* The Audioscope was released by the Sonotone Corporation in 1937. These instruments were all somewhat similar in design and had similar purposes. Soon thereafter a slightly more cumbersome device was made available by the American Earphone Co. of New York City.

A fifth hearing aid testing device was advertised by a hearing aid office in Boston in 1938. This was called a Trutonometer and was described as "an exclusive new invention [that] selects the aid best suited to your individual requirements."† From this brief notice it seems evident that the device was a master hearing aid unit, and it is probable that the instrument was manufactured by or for Trutonophone, Inc., of New York City, an importer of German hearing aids. In some respects these early devices more accurately meet the concept of a master hearing aid than their descendants, although it is recognized that microphone, amplifier, and receiver alternatives were fewer in the carbon hearing aid era.

Hayden (1938a) pictures the Audioscope. In a subsequent report Hayden (1938b) may have been the first to employ the term *master hearing aid*, which he used "for want of a better generic name."

The first master hearing aids for carbon instruments were but a year or two old when Arthur Wengel introduced his Wengel Test Auditor (Wengel 1938). This was a vacuum tube instrument with crystal microphone. It was capable of serving as a pure-tone audiometer but also included filters so that speech testing could be accomplished under four different frequency responses.

Wengel worked closely with Robert West, Ph.D., who at that time was at the University of Wisconsin. Wengel proposed that "correct" hearing aid fitting, a science which he proposed be called *auralometry*, be determined by the client's understanding of speech under the several frequency responses. For this purpose lists of phonetically similar word pairs were to be used in testing. These same word pair tests appear in the pioneering publication on hearing aid evaluation by West (1938).

Wengel, an engineer with Ray-O-Vac battery company, held at least three patents on hearing aid amplifiers. He is also to be credited with manufacturing the first wearable vacuum tube hearing aid in the United States. To carry on his work in hearing aids, Wengel Laboratories, Inc., was established in Madison, Wisconsin. His hearing aids and the Wengel Test Auditor were available only through physicians and speech clinics. Despite Wengel's unique contributions, and for reasons unknown, his firm disbanded a few years later. Evidently Wengel's Test Auditor was later modified as The Analyzer (West 1950). The Analyzer was manufactured and marketed by Hearing Research Laboratories of Milwaukee, Wisconsin. No further details could be found on this apparatus.

*The Dictograph Flash, 1. December 1936, p. 7
†The Guilder, Boston, Massachusetts, 13. May 1938, p. 5

WARTIME RESEARCH IN ENGLAND AND THE UNITED STATES

At the close of World War II, reports appeared almost simultaneously on the subject of hearing aid design from laboratories in England and the United States. Apparently neither laboratory was aware of the work of the other group, but each employed what they called master hearing aids as part of their research and their conclusions were similar.

In 1947 The Committee on Electro-Acoustics of the Medical Research Council (MRC) published their findings relating to hearing aid and audiometer recommendations (Medical Research Council 1947).* This committee was given the task of making recommendations to the British government about hearing aid electroacoustic design. The recommendations were subsequently used in the manufacture of hearing aids for the government. These hearing aids, commonly referred to as Medresco hearing aids, are given at no charge to qualifying persons under the British Health Service program.

The committee on electroacoustics of MRC studied designs for hearing aids and made a number of comparisons. To arrive at their conclusions and recommendations, the committee commissioned the construction of two master hearing aid units, which were built for them by the Post Office Research Station at Dollis Hill, London. One master hearing aid was placed in the Department of Education of the Deaf at Manchester University in the Spring of 1945. The second unit was placed in the Otological Research Unit at the National Hospital, Queen Square, London. Aspinall (1951) published a short description of the MRC master hearing aid.

A total of 228 hearing-impaired subjects was tested using one of the master hearing aids. Based upon results obtained, the committee finally recommended that the government manufacture one of two body-style hearing aids, one with a crystal receiver and the other with a magnetic receiver. Both hearing aids were to have three vacuum tubes, a separate battery pack, and both included a tone control switch that permitted either a gradually rising or a flat frequency response.

A few years later, further research with a new master hearing aid was reported (Post Office Engineering Department 1953). This later report was concerned primarily with research on low- and high-frequency cut-off variations and with peak clipping and automatic gain control variables. A supplementary report in 1954 added data relating to bone conduction-type hearing aids.

In the United States a similar project was completed at the Psycho-Acoustic Laboratory (PAL) at Harvard University (Davis et al. 1947). The report of this

---

*Earlier, about 1939, the MRC sponsored limited research at the Liverpool School for the Deaf. A vacuum tube amplifier was used, designed to examine the effect of various frequency responses (Marchant and Turney, 1940).

work is the so-called Harvard Report, which is probably the most quoted and least read of all audiologic literature.

The research groups in England and in the United States proceeded along quite similar lines. Each had built master hearing aids of rather monstrous dimensions, each used a population of hearing-impaired subjects in their research, and each master hearing aid unit had filters that permitted subject performance to be evaluated under falling, flat, and rising frequency responses. In addition both groups concluded that a flat or slightly rising frequency response would serve most hearing-impaired persons in need of a hearing aid.

The PAL group used a master hearing aid with five basic frequency responses: (1) falling 12 dB per octave above 200 Hz, (2) falling 6 dB per octave above 200 Hz, (3) flat from 100 to 7000 Hz, (4) rising 6 dB per octave, and (5) rising 12 dB per octave. It is interesting to note that hearing aids with frequency responses this wide did not appear on the market until about a quarter of a century later.

The PAL group concluded that the "ideal" electroacoustic specifications for hearing aids could be served by two or three models, differing in respect to acoustic gain, maximum output, and one of three frequency characteristics: flat, rising 3 dB per octave, or rising 6 dB per octave. Since the 3-dB-per-octave rise was not included in the tests, it must be assumed that the recommendation was based upon some interpolation of the data.

The Harvard Report, and to a lesser extent the MRC report since it was not as widely publicized, greatly dampened the enthusiasm of those who used and believed in selective amplification. Although never stated, one can sense that in some respects the Harvard Report was attempting to dispute the need for the more time-consuming hearing aid comparison procedures which had only recently been published by Carhart (1946a, b, and c). Interestingly, the bibliography of the Harvard Report does not include any of Carhart's publications but "Captain Carhart's method" is mentioned within the report.

Although the present chapter was designed to deal with the development and operation of master hearing aids, I do not wish to let the opportunity pass to comment that the Harvard Report and the MRC report were by far the most complete and scientific documents then available on hearing aid acoustic responses and on the application of amplified sound to hearing-impaired individuals. On the other hand, it should be stressed that these reports, if viewed in comparison with the more rigorous and sophisticated experimental designs commonly employed today, leave much to be desired.

Both the PAL and MRC conclusions were based upon subject performance while using vacuum tube master hearing aids of broadcast quality, using external broadcast-type microphones and high-fidelity earphones. Earmold effects were not considered. Apparently neither group used counterbalancing procedures or had more than minimal subject qualifications. A number of different speaker-experimenters were involved with testing the subjects, and in the case of the PAL group, live voice testing was done with word lists that many audiologists criticize as having less than adequate reliability or validity. The PAL group tested relatively few subjects under all five frequency response conditions. Perhaps most important, 65 percent of the MRC subject group had conductive losses (presumably including mixed losses), whereas among the PAL subject group, 3 had conductive hearing losses, 7 had mixed losses, 5 had sensorineural losses, and medical history and audiograms were not available on 3 subjects. These subjects may have represented a typical clinical hearing loss population in the late 1940s. Today the problems of fitting hearing aids relate primarily to persons having sensorineural hearing losses, which would seem to place in doubt the applicability of most of the findings by either the PAL or MRC experiments.

HAIC MASTER HEARING AID

In the summer of 1953 the American Hearing Aid Association (AHAA) met at the Hotel Commodore in New York City with the New York hearing aid dealers and discussed a number of subjects. Among the proposals discussed was "generalized master hearing aid units which might be supplied to public [hearing] aid clinics."* Evidently nothing more came of this suggestion, and in 1955 AHAA disbanded.

Late in 1955 many of the functions of AHAA were taken over by the newly organized Hearing Aid Industry Conference (HAIC).† It is not surprising that the concept of a master hearing aid was resurrected. Stutz (1968) reports that the master hearing aid idea was again brought forward when Lee Watson was vice-president of HAIC. Since Watson became president in 1958, HAIC must have begun discussion on the instrument about 1957. The motives for developing such an instrument were twofold. First, it was to serve as a fitting device, and second it was to be placed into hearing clinics so that the rather large stock of hearing aids maintained in the clinics by manufacturers could be drastically reduced.

The prototype of the first HAIC master hearing aid was presented to their board of directors at a meeting in the Palmer House in Chicago on June 9, 1959. Many members of HAIC assisted with the design of the master hearing aid, but special credit should go to Hugh Knowles of Knowles Electronics for carrying through with the project. Knowles, through a subsidiary, Industrial Research Products, Inc., supervised the work of an engineering student, Harold Ludtke, who did much of the circuit design and acoustic measurements of the instrument. On June 15, 1959 Lee Watson reported to the directors of HAIC that the cost to date had been $1500 and that a meeting of interested industry members would be called in July for further discussion of the project. It was anticipated that once

*Audecibel, 2. Fall 1953, p. 14
†Since 1977 called Hearing Industries Association (HIA)

final specifications and modifications of the prototype were approved, from 6 to 15 units would be built initially and placed in selected audiology clinics.*

Meanwhile, an ASHA Ad Hoc Committee on the Master Hearing Aid, under the chairmanship of Moe Bergman, met with the Master Hearing Aid Committee of HAIC in New York City on April 27, 1959. Members of the ASHA committee were Martin Cohen, William G. Hardy, Kenneth O. Johnson, Donald M. Markle, and Howard Ruhm. The prototype master hearing aid was not then available, and the ASHA committee received only a description of the expected characteristics of the instrument. A number of questions were raised by the ASHA committee: Would the measurements made on the master hearing aid be applicable to commercial hearing aids? What important acoustic factors of hearing aids might not be available on the master aids? What would be the effect of the introduction of new hearing aid models by manufacturers on the continuing validity of the master hearing aid's responses? How would the selection of a commercial hearing aid model be accomplished after desirable performance characteristics had been indicated from the master hearing aid? and how would the applicability of the master hearing aid be evaluated? (ASHA 1959). These questions remain pertinent and largely unanswered some 20 years later.

Early in 1960 six master hearing aids were produced and placed in selected audiology clinics. HAIC records as to which clinics received units and what the responses from the clinics were cannot be located. It is known that one master hearing aid, probably a prototype rather than one of the six later versions, was placed at Wayne State University. Apparently the clinics using the master hearing aids did not find them satisfactory.

There are a number of possible reasons for the failure of the master hearing aids at that time, and Stutz (1968) gives several: (1) The idea was premature, (2) audiology clinics might have felt that such an instrument "threatened their most important source of revenue, that is to say, hearing aid evaluation," and (3) to be useful the major manufacturers must have their hearing aid models keyed to the master hearing aid. Stutz' first possible explanation may have some validity, but it should be noted that several hearing aid manufacturers placed their own master hearing aids on the market before or at about the same time as the HAIC units were placed out for trial. Since in most audiology clinics hearing aid evaluations are a minor part of the clinic load and, hence, clinic revenue, the second possible explanation must be dismissed either as sour grapes or a lack of knowledge as to typical clinic schedules. Rather, the fact that test results, based on measurements under the master hearing aid, could not be readily applied to various brand and model recommendations seems to have been the decisive and weak link to the master hearing aid concept. Intraindustry jealousies may be considered strongly suspect in preventing the application of master hearing aid data to various brand models. The hearing aid industry has always been strongly

*Letter from Lee Watson to directors of HAIC, June 15, 1959

brand-conscious, and certainly industry members would be reluctant to admit that performance data obtained under a master hearing aid could be applied to brand Y as well as to brand Z.

The production models of the HAIC master hearing aid provided for gain settings from 20 through 70 dB in 5-dB steps (the prototype model was only in 10-dB steps), output settings of 110−140 dB in 5-dB steps, and four frequency response settings. The circuit contained a three-transistor amplifier plus a push-pull output stage powered by a 3.9-V battery. After trial in the clinics, some reports began coming back to HAIC and minor modifications in the instruments were in the planning stage.* However, the enthusiasm of the HAIC members seems to have waned and, lacking positive support by the audiologists, the project was disbanded before further modifications were actually made.

COMMERCIALLY MADE MASTER HEARING AIDS

In 1947, long before HAIC considered a master hearing aid, Beltone Hearing Aid Co. introduced their Audio Selectometer.† In its original version this instrument was quite primitive, but the 1952 model was a binaural unit much like similar master hearing aids today. About 1947 or perhaps earlier, Alladin Hearing Aid Co. (later renamed Goldentone) made a master hearing aid device. This was described as "a portable hearing aid with different combinations of tone, power, and volume control" (Johnston 1948). The device was called Tone Tester.

Early in 1959 Vicon introduced their Metricon,‡ and on May 29, 1959 at a meeting of dealers a prototype of Audiotone's Auricon was presented by Byron Langford.§ The Qualitone Company has incorporated a master hearing aid circuit or unit in their audiometers since around 1960. Maico introduced their Precision Ear in April 1963 and a modification, model II, was introduced in February 1968. These were the earliest electronic master hearing aid units released by various manufacturers. Their mention is not intended as an endorsement of them and the omission from this discussion of other master hearing aids subsequently introduced is not intended as a criticism of other such units.

There has been some effort on the part of the hearing aid industry to popularize the term *pressure measuring instrument* (PMI) as a replacement term for master hearing aid. Since, unlike the speech audiometer but like hearing aids,

*A number of suggested modifications and also further acoustic measurement specifications are contained in reports from Industrial Products, Inc., to HAIC, dated June 22, August 1, and September 1, 1960.

†The Selectometer, Radio News, vol. 9, November 1947, p. 22−23

‡The Metricon was announced in an advertisement in Audecibel February, 1959 p. 2

§Audecibel, June 1959, p. 21. An advertisement picturing the first commercial version appeared in the same journal in January 1969, p. 18

these instruments are built to the sound pressure standard of 0.0002 dyne/cm²
there is considerable logic in the term. However, long use of the term *master
hearing aid* is difficult for many to relinquish, including the present author.
Pressure-measuring instrument describes what the device does and master hearing aid describes the purpose of the device.

The various pressure measuring instruments available on the market have a
number of features in common, but also a number of differences. The Metricon,
model 300B, has a gain control variable in 5-dB steps from 100 to 130 dB. There
are five frequency responses: (1) 3 dB per octave rise from 500 to 1000 Hz and 8
dB per octave from 1000 to 2800 Hz, (2) 3 dB per octave rise from 500 to 1000
Hz and 0 dB per octave from 1000 to 2000 Hz, (3) 12 dB per octave rise from
500 to 2800 Hz, (4) 12 dB per octave rise from 500 to 1000 Hz and 2 dB per
octave from 1000 to 2800 Hz, and (5) 0 dB per octave rise from 500 to 1000 Hz,
and −5 dB per octave from 1000 to 2800 Hz. The VU meter is calibrated so that
0 dB is 65 dB SPL.

The Metricon 500, manufactured by the Vicon Instrument Company, is a
third generation instrument of that firm. This instrument is pictured in Figure
9-2.

The Metricon 500 contains controls much like earlier pressure-measuring
instruments, but it is unique in that the entire apparatus is contained in binaural
earphone housings. Therefore, amplified ear-level hearing can be simulated more
accurately. In Figure 9-2 the top dial is marked RESP and is the frequency
response control, which can be set to one of five frequency slopes. The center

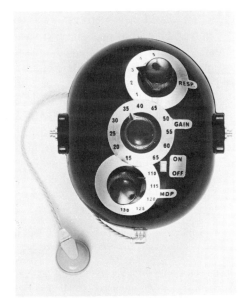

Fig. 9-2.   Metricon 500.

dial is the gain control, marked GAIN; this is calibrated in 5-dB steps from 15 to 65 dB re. 1000 Hz. The lower dial controls the maximum output (called maximum deliverable pressure by Vicon); this control is calibrated in 5-dB steps from 100 to 130 dB SPL. To the right of the lower dials is the on-off switch, which in later models became part of the maximum output dial. The hearing aid-type external receiver may be seen in Figure 9-2, which is the three-terminal variety, and the receiver receptacle is at the bottom of the ear muff. The microphone port is at the top of the ear muff and cannot be readily seen in the figure. The instrument is powered by two 401 batteries. The five frequency response patterns mentioned above are specifically:

	500−1000 Hz	*1000−2000 Hz*
1.	− 6 dB	+ 6 dB
2.	− 3	0
3.	−12	+10
4.	− 9	+ 2
5.	+ 5	− 5

The Auricon AR4 is available in a console model or combined with a pure-tone audiometer. It has a single VU meter and a white noise masking control. Maximum output is controllable from 75 to 130 dB in 5-dB steps, and there are five frequency responses. These frequency responses are illustrated in Chapter 2.

As may be seen from that figure, the Auricon provides a frequency response of low-frequency extension, and also various gradations up to a high-frequency emphasis response. This instrument also has a curvilinear AGC (called ACLC by Audiotone) output control in five steps of 5 dB each. The VU meter is calibrated so that 0 is 60 dB SPL.

A recent modification of Audiotone's master hearing aid is their model AR-11 (Fig. 9-3), which also comes in a console model called AR-12T. The AR-11 includes two electret microphones, mounted in behind-the-ear hearing aid cases, thereby permitting a more realistic placement than most master hearing aids. In addition to the controls on their model AR4, the AR-11 includes a "function control," which permits testing under monaural or binaural modes, and also CROS to left or right, and BiCROS to left or right.

The PrecisionEar II is a combination audiometer and pressure-measuring instrument. It includes a gain control variable in 5-dB steps from 20 to 70 dB. It has a maximum output control variable from 90 to 135 dB in 5-dB steps and there are five frequency responses.

Another contemporary unit is the ZA-170 Auralyzer manufactured by Zenith Hearing Instrument Corp. This unit consists of a speech audiometer combined with a pressure-measuring instrument to simulate hearing aid amplification under HAIC standards. The Auralyzer is shown in Figure 9-4.

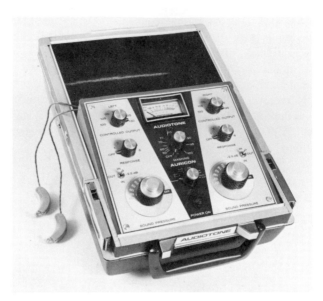

Fig. 9-3.   Audiotone master hearing aid AR-11.

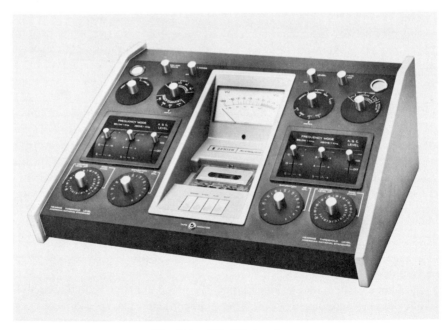

Fig. 9-4.   ZA-170 Auralyzer.

The Auralyzer permits either live voice or cartridge tape input and outputs to TDH-140 earphones, hearing aid receivers, or a receiver mounted in dummy behind-the-ear hearing aids. It is powered by alternating current. The size is 8 in. high, 21⅛ in. wide, and 16⅝ in. deep; weight is 24½ lb., plus carrying case.

In Figure 9-4 the microphone of the Auralyzer may be seen at the extreme top right. To the left of the microphone is the calibration control for the speech audiometer, and to its left is the calibration control for the tape cassette; both controls are related to the VU meter. Below the microphone is the output transducer selector, and to its left is the right-left−binaural output selector. Below the output selector dials, on the right, is the automatic gain control switch. Limiting levels of 105 or 115 dB can be selected; attack time is 7 msec and recovery time 20 msec. To the left of the AGC switch are two frequency mode selectors. It may be noted that the AGC and frequency selector lever switches are duplicated on the left side so as to permit binaural testing with independent settings.

Since the frequency mode selectors permit independent control over the frequency response from 500 to 1000 Hz and from 1000 to 2000 Hz, and each selector has five positions, 25 combinations of frequency response are possible. The specific possibilities are as follows:

500−1000 Hz	1000−2000 Hz
ELF*	+18 dB
0 dB	+12
− 6	+ 6
−12	0
−18	− 6

The dials at the lower extreme locations in Figure 9-4 are the hearing level dials for speech audiometry, which also serve as controls for HAIC gain. Continuously variable gain is available from 0 to 75 dB HAIC. The lower center dials are maximum output (or saturation) selectors, calibrated from 90 to 135 dB SPL. The two small controls at the upper left are the speech audiometer calibration control, for the left ear, and white noise masking calibration control. Below these small controls on the left is the on-off and on the right the input selector. A receptacle for a phone jack to plug in an earphone for monitoring the tape recording is located at the lower center of the Auralyzer.

Zenith has taken performance scores obtained with their hearing aid simulator a step further. By taking 18 points from critical band work found in earlier research and weighting the significant intensity values of vowels and consonants, a system was developed to classify any hearing aid into a fitting category. The HAIC gain and output curves of the various Zenith hearing aids were then transferred on a paper tape using an XY plotting system, and this paper

*Extended low frequency; 0 dB slope down to 150 Hz.

tape was fed into a computer. The curve data were then systematically compared to the stored reference curves which are representative of the Auralyzer. The computer at this point printed out lists of the hearing aids in a descending saturation output order with an evaluation of the frequency "fit" based on the weighted frequency and intensity selection. The computer printout is made available to hearing aid dealers in booklet form, and separate fitting data are shown based upon standard earmold, open earmold, with AGC, and with Zenith's Acoustic Modifier earmold.

THE IDEAL MASTER HEARING AID

From the brief description of several master hearing aid units given above, it seems clear that various existing instruments have much in common. On the other hand, differences between these instruments are also striking. Some units have a VU meter so that the inputs can be calibrated, while others do not. Zero on the VU meter may be 60 or 65 dB SPL, or unspecified. Some units employ earphones; some, external hearing aid-type receivers; and others, ear inserts. AGC and curvilinear AGC circuits are part of some units. Masking in both type and amount varies considerably. Although four or five frequency responses are common to most instruments, the terms used to describe these responses and the responses themselves vary considerably. *Furthermore, the frequency responses in the units may not represent frequency responses typically found in contemporary models of hearing aids made by the same manufacturer.*

The direction booklets which accompany the several master hearing aid units seem to include and discuss the respective specifications and technical data much less completely than do printed hearing aid data on hearing aids manufactured by the same companies. It does not seem unfair to state that the direction booklets accompanying master hearing aids are, for the most part, *sets of instructions to help the hearing aid dealer sell the manufacturer's product rather than to evaluate the client's performance or needs under amplification.* Similarly, it is rare to find a hearing aid dealer who cannot consistently and readily "prove" with a master hearing aid that virtually every client so tested performs significantly better under the binaural mode, whereas it is well known that differences between monaural and binaural amplification under highly controlled and objective test conditions are often extremely difficult to determine. For further discussion of monaural and binaural amplification see Chapter 7.

Despite present differences among commercially available master hearing aid units and the problems in applying resulting test data across hearing aid brands, the pressure-measuring instrument offers considerable promise as a hearing aid fitting device. If the master hearing aid is to play the important role of which it is capable, there will need to be general agreement among audiologists, hearing aid dealers, and hearing aid industry members as to what the instrument should accomplish and how it shall do so. Listed below are some of the control and design features that would appear to be essential in a flexible, and truly master, hearing aid:

1. *Binaural circuit.* The instrument should be easily and readily used in the evaluation of either ear or both ears, with complete binaural circuitry. All of the units previously mentioned have binaural circuits, so this feature seems to be one wherein there is agreement.
2. *VU meter.* Each circuit should have a VU meter, or a VU meter usable for each circuit, which permits calibration check of all inputs. A "0" VU level of either 60 or 65 dB SPL seems logical, but everyone involved should come to an agreement as to which of these levels will be used.
3. *Gain.* This should be variable in each circuit by 5-dB steps, perhaps from 15 dB to at least 70 dB.
4. *Output.* This should be a control separate from gain control and should be variable for each circuit in 5-dB steps, from 90 to 140 dB.
5. *Frequency response.* Six frequency responses might suffice: flat, high-frequency emphasis, high-frequency emphasis with low-frequency attenuation, extreme high-frequency emphasis, relatively flat response, and low-frequency emphasis. A statement on specific rise per octave of the various responses has purposefully been avoided here, but a general agreement should be reached by all involved and standard responses made available on the units. Ideally, flexibility in the frequency responses would be desirable so that there would be some permissible modification within each of the standard responses, such as a slight movement upward or downward in the frequency of the peak of the response.
6. An *AGC,* and hopefully also a curvilinear AGC circuit also, should be built into each unit. Several limiting levels and amounts of compression would be ideal.
7. *Receivers.* the unit should permit ready comparisons between typical hearing aid-type receivers and be so constructed that the client can wear a custom earmold during testing. Ideally the unit should also permit testing under open-mold (that is, "no mold") conditions, as well as under the several across-head arrangements available in contemporary hearing aids.
8. *Microphones.* Microphone type and placement are probably the most unrealistic aspect of past master hearing aids. Microphone placement needs to reflect body baffle or head shadow effects. It seems reasonable to expect the master hearing aid to be provided with plug-in microphones, which could be readily placed in dummy body or in behind-the-ear hearing aids, so as to more accurately simulate actual hearing aid wear. Ideally the instrument would have a switch to provide easy change from directional to omnidirectional microphone evaluation and another switch to permit testing under the several across-head signal routings.

Crucial to the above is the need for all manufacturers of master hearing aid units to come to a reasonable mutual agreement on each of the controls and calibrations as well as on quality standards. Unless the readings obtained by the hearing aid dealer or audiologist from the master hearing aid can be shown to be applicable to the typical standard brands and models of hearing aids on the market, the instrument will not serve a useful purpose in clinical testing. Unless the reliability and validity of hearing aid fitting with the master hearing aid can be improved to the point where data resulting from the PMI can be shown to be closely related to hearing aid needs, it will be but a gimmick to give an aura of the scientific method in hearing aid sales.

USING THE MASTER HEARING AID

The master hearing aid may be employed in lieu of actual hearing aids during traditional or modified hearing aid evaluations by the audiologist. In the first instance the master hearing aid merely serves as a substitute for an array of hearing aids that are typically evaluated one by one on the basis of speech audiometric scores. In using the master hearing aid, the audiologist can simply have the client manipulate the gain control while cold running speech is directed into the test room at conversational level. Next, a saturation sound pressure level (SSPL) can be determined either by the client manipulating the controls or by the audiologist doing so. Frequency response determination can be likewise obtained by asking the client which response seems most clear or natural, and then with the more objective determination of obtaining speech discrimination scores. It may be found that obtaining speech discrimination scores under several substantially different frequency responses will be helpful and, based upon the results of such tests, a decision made as to which other response or responses might be expected to produce better discrimination.

All of the tests that are done by the clinician with actual hearing aids can be done with the master hearing aid. The time required to change from one hearing aid to another, and making initial gain adjustments, is considerably reduced when using the master hearing aid. With increased use of the pressure-measuring instrument in clinics, research, and clinical reports should be expected to become available. At present, trial and error in the gain, SSPL and frequency response selection is the usual procedure.

In a modified hearing aid evaluation, many audiologists are primarily concerned with determining whether the client is likely to profit from amplification. The client is then sent to one or more reputable hearing aid dealers for more precise hearing aid fitting. In the modified hearing aid evaluation, the pressure-measuring instrument is also of value. By making a limited number of tests under one or more gain, SSPL and frequency response settings, the client's improvement or lack of improvement under amplification can readily be determined. The

client can then be directed to a hearing aid dealer for more specific electroacoustic fitting, with only a general statement by the audiologist to the dealer regarding
gain, SSPL, and frequency response recommendations.

Unfortunately, there have been few experimental reports on the master
hearing aid and, in fact, only a few clinical reports as well. Most reports on the
pressure-measuring instrument are quite general in nature (Greenbaum 1968,
Miller 1966, Nunley 1972, Selbst 1968, Victoreen 1968), but several studies
employing master hearing aids have appeared (Gillespie et al. 1965, Wasson
1963). Procedures using a master hearing aid are described by Lawrence and
Blackledge (1977), Lawrence et al. (1977), and Levitt et al. (1976). They
suggest determining speech discrimination scores after varying the frequency
response slope and breakpoint frequency of the master hearing aid. Thereby a
matrix of speech discrimination scores is developed and from this matrix the
combination of slope and breakpoint producing the best scores can be visualized.
There is a clear need for similar and more in-depth studies involving the master
hearing aid, and for comparison studies with the master hearing aid to other
evaluative procedures as well as to hearing aids purchased by the client from
master hearing aid data.

Despite certain advantages to using master hearing aids for the purpose of
selecting the desired electroacoustic response, such aids have the same weaknesses as "traditional" hearing aid evaluations. That is, speech audiometric scores
obtained under the master hearing aid, like a trial hearing aid, are not as reliable
on an individual basis as would be desirable. In addition, speech audiometric
scores seem insensitive to anything less than major changes in tone control
setting, the use of filters, or earmold modifications.

BIBLIOGRAPHY

ASHA Reports Number 2: A conference on hearing aid evaluation procedures, 1967
Aspinall E: A master hearing aid. J Br Inst Radio Eng 11:45−50, 1951
Carhart R: Selection of hearing aids. Arch Otolaryngol 44:1−18, 1946a
Carhart R: Volume control adjustment in hearing aid selection. Laryngoscope
     56:510−526, 1946b
Carhart R: Tests for the selection of hearing aids. Laryngoscope 56:780−794, 1946c
Davis H, Stevens SS, Nichols RH, Jr, et al: Hearing Aids: An Experimental Study of
     Design Objectives. Cambridge, Harvard University Press, 1947. Appeared in pre-
     liminary form in Laryngoscope 56:85−115, 135−163, 1946
Gillespie ME, Gillespie MR, Creston JE: Clinical evaluation of a "master hearing aid."
     Arch Otolaryngol 82:515−517, 1965
Greenbaum WH: The engineering of a master hearing aid. Natl Hear Aid J 21:7, 30, 32,
     1968
Hayden AA: Hearing aids from otologists' audiograms. J Am Med Assoc 111:592−596,
     1938a

Hayden AA: Audiometers and hearing aids. J Am Med Assoc 110:723–725, 1938b

Johnston WE: Letter to the editor. Natl Hear Aid J 1:7, 18, 1948

Lawrence DW, Blackledge VO: Protocol for evaluation of the effect of hearing aid electroacoustic parameters on perception of amplified speech. J Am Audiology Soc 2:197–201, 1977

Lawrence DW, Halladay H, Blackledge VO: Listener performance as criterion for setting frequency selective parameters of hearing instruments. Audiology Hear Educ 3:2, 26, 28–29, 1977; 3:3, 18–19, 28, 1977

Levitt H, White REC, Resnick SB: Prescriptive fitting of wearable master hearing aid: a progress report, in Rubin M (ed): Hearing Aids: Current Developments and Concepts. Baltimore, University Park Press, 1976

Marchant EW, Turney TH: A hearing aid for research and group use. J Scientific Instruments 17:149–155, 1940

ASHA. A master hearing aid, 1:140–141, 1959

Medical Research Council: Hearing Aids and Audiometers. Report of the committee on electro-acoustics. London, His Majesty's Stationery Office, Special Report Series No. 261, 1971

Miller A, Blackman B: Using a type of master hearing aid as an auditory trainer. J Speech Hear Disor 31:259–260, 1966

Nunley J: The birth of the new master hearing aid. Natl Hearing Aid J 25:8, 26, 1972

Post Office Engineering Department Speech Transmission System Type 3 (Master Hearing Aid). London: Post Office Research Station, Nov. 1953. Research Report 13156. Also addendum dated June 17, 1954

Selbst FE: A dealer looks at the master hearing aid. Natl Hear Aid J 21:9, 38, 1968

Stutz R: Whatever happened to the master hearing aid? Natl Hear Aid J 21:8, 28, 1968

Victoreen RR: The otometric hearing instrument. Natl Hear Aid J 21:10, 27, 1968

Wasson HW: A multifilter circuit simulating representative hearing aids suggested for hearing aid selections. J Audit Res 3:185–188, 1963 Reprinted in Audecibel 13:60–63, 1964

Wengel MW: Auralometry Explained. Madison, Wisconsin, Wengel Laboratories, 1938

West R: The Testing of Hearing Aids. Madison, Wisconsin, College Typing Co, 1938. Test answer sheets were available through The Volta Bureau

West R: The audianalyzer. Hear Aid 3:22, 1950

Derek A. Sanders

10

Hearing Aid Orientation and Counseling

It is a rare hearing aid user who can put on a new instrument and use it optimally without rather extensive counseling and orientation. This involves much more than simply showing the individual where the controls are and how to put the aid on and take it off. It includes discussions of the proper manner in which to adjust to the new and often abrasive sound of the aid, and to identification of and remediation of the tangential psychologic aspects of hearing loss.

This chapter systematically considers the various factors involved in helping a hearing-impaired person derive maximum benefits from a hearing aid. Each of the basic steps to hearing aid management is presented and discussed in a realistic manner. Derek Sanders also explores the personal adjustments the candidate for a hearing aid must be helped to make if he is to use the aid successfully. Derek's discussion of what a counselor should be and what his role involves is based on many years of experience. The approach described is humanistic in that it deals with the individual rather than the hearing impaired. The combination of a reality orientation and a real sensitivity to the often subconscious feelings of the hearing aid candidate makes this a valuable resource chapter for the reader.

MCP

While hearing aid technology continues to make impressive progress, the task of providing carefully planned, personalized counseling to the hearing aid user is, to a very large extent, a neglected one. Various groups wage political battles over who must assume this responsibility, each asserting its own particular competence to provide the service. Yet the truth remains that this aspect of the needs of the hearing-impaired person is not being provided effectively. The irony of the situation lies in the fact that even the most advanced technology is completely useless if, through ignorance, negative attitudes, or unrealistic expectations, the hearing aid is either improperly used or, as not infrequently happens, is not worn at all. The topic of hearing aid orientation and counseling is, therefore, of critical importance, since in most instances it will be the determining factor in the successful use of a quality hearing aid.

PROVIDING THE SERVICE

The question of who should provide hearing aid orientation and counseling seems to be arising with increasing frequency. It is a legitimate question, if the concern is to ensure that the client's needs are provided for by the person most qualified to offer this service. Unfortunately, the issue too often takes on the characteristics of a battle for territorial rights between conflicting parties, a problem that Smith discusses in Chapter 12. This generally results in attempts to prevent others from providing service rather than concentrating on ensuring the expansion of service coupled with raising standards. It is true that the audiologist is probably the person best equipped to meet the needs of the hearing-impaired person. The academic and practicum requirements established by the American Speech and Hearing Association for the certification of clinical competency in audiology are designed to ensure broad experience in the major aspects of managing the problems arising from impaired hearing. Characteristically, the training of other professionals is oriented to specialized aspects of the problem of hearing deficits rather than to total management. The otologist is generally fully occupied with the medical aspects of deafness, the hearing aid dealer's preparation seldom extends beyond fitting the aid, the primary focus of the teacher of the deaf is the special education of the child, whereas the speech therapist's exposure to hearing aids and the problems of hearing impairment will most likely have been limited. Thus, ideally, the major responsibility for counseling should be with the audiologist.

The reality of the present situation, however, is that most hearing-impaired persons who use hearing aids have not been in contact with an audiologist.

The situation as it involves children is far more favorable. Most hearing-impaired children are evaluated by clinical audiologists, who play the major role in the selection of appropriate amplification and, to a lesser degree, in preschool training. Nevertheless, it is my experience that the logistic and economic factors involved make it extremely difficult for the community center or hospital-based audiologist to provide the hearing-impaired child, in the normal school or special class, with the necessary ongoing training and counseling in the use of amplification. The growing subspeciality of educational audiology and the employment of audiologists in residential and day schools for the deaf bear witness to the difficulty the clinical audiologist experiences fully meeting the needs of the hearing-impaired school child.

The point I wish to stress is that counseling must be provided for the hearing-impaired person by the most qualified persons *available*. The accessibility of this help is as important as the sophistication of the counselor. It well may be that major responsibility for the ongoing counseling of a particular child will have to be assumed by a school speech therapist, a resource teacher, or an itinerant teacher of the deaf. It is the audiologist's responsibility to provide maximum support to these professionals, assisting them in their efforts to meet the needs of the children in their care. It is equally the responsibility of the person working with the child to increase his or her professional understanding of the problem and the capacity to deal with it. Similarly, it is of little avail to insist that the responsibility for counseling the adult lies exclusively with the clinical audiologist if 60 percent of the adults who wear hearing aids are not seen by him or her. Only through the integration of resources within a community can the services afforded the hearing-impaired person be extended. If appropriate orientation and guidance is to be available to the hearing-impaired population, efforts must be concentrated on ensuring that whoever is working with the client, whether an audiologist, hearing aid dealer, speech therapist or teacher, is cognizant of the need for counseling and of the major aspects of effective guidance. Smith's discussion of this issue (Chapter 12) emphasizes the responsibility of the clinical audiologist to assume the role of case manager. It is not essential that the audiologist, as case manager, should be the only person to assume a guidance role; indeed, as has been seen, he or she is often denied the privilege. It is, however, essential that he make every effort to ensure that such guidance is made available to the hearing-impaired child or adult, develop the most favorable relationships with other professionals on the rehabilitation team, and provide support and assistance in a manner which in no way belittles his colleagues' efforts.

UNDERSTANDING THE PROBLEM

It is important to realize that, while certain basic generalizations can be made about the impact of hearing impairment upon people, each individual may be expected to react differently (Meyerson 1963). The task of understanding the problem is, therefore, one that you and your client must share. It is unreasonable to believe that it is possible for a counselor to provide the client with a set of solutions to problems that the counselor has anticipated. To be effective, the solutions arrived at must be solutions to problems identified and described by the client. Such an approach during the earliest stages of rehabilitation permits you to communicate to the hearing-impaired person your true concern for the resolution of the particular difficulties. It allows you to communicate both acceptance of the validity of the client's anxieties or difficulties and your personal interest in assisting that client's efforts to reduce them. This requires considerable empathy. It necessitates rejection of the security of the authoritarian role of the specialist who knows what is needed. *Rather than impose solutions, your value lies in your ability to assist the client to identify and define problems and to find appropriate and acceptable ways of dealing with them. Your role is to facilitate the adaptation process, not to determine it.* To achieve this, it is necessary to have as complete an understanding as possible of the total impact a hearing deficit will have upon a person. It is helpful to read extensively about the psychology of deafness, but be prepared to listen to the client. So often we feel that our role as counselor requires that we provide direct guidance. Only the person with the hearing loss knows fully the particular anxieties the loss has created for him, the conflicts he experiences between wanting to obtain help and accepting the reality of the hearing loss. If you are prepared to let him express his feelings about these problems and other people's reactions to his "hard-of-hearing" behavior, the need to project the image of an expert who can provide solutions decreases. Seldom can solutions be provided by the counselor. Generally, the client must solve problems for himself. The counselor, through guidance and support, may be in a position to help the client to achieve this.

As audiologists, teachers of the deaf, or hearing therapists, we are particularly concerned with the effects of the hearing deficit upon a person's ability to communicate. Yet, as Ramsdell (1970) points out, this is not, as one might expect, the area of greatest impact of the hearing impairment. Ramsdell maintains that the most serious effects of impaired hearing, particularly a rapid loss of hearing, lie in the resultant reduction or loss of a "feeling of relationship with the world," which is maintained largely through auditory contact. This primitive hearing function, which permits the ongoing monitoring of events of daily living, provides the auditory background that gives a person the feeling he is a participant in the changing world around him. Reactions to these changes occur at a preconscious level:

> "The constant reaction establishes in us states of feeling that are the foundation for our conscious experiences, a foundation which gives us the conviction that the world in which we live is also alive and moving" (Ramsdell 1970, p. 438).

It is this primitive monitoring that serves as the coupler between the pattern of activity of our own personal system and that of the environment as a whole.

It is important, therefore, that you should be sensitive to the impact a reduction of the efficiency of this coupling may be expected to have on the hearing-impaired person. The severity of its effects will be greatest in cases of sudden or rapid hearing loss. In such cases, it may induce severe depression, which is cause for referral for psychiatric guidance. However, most of the people with whom you work will have experienced a progressive loss of hearing over a number of years, rather than a sudden loss. The progressive effects are insidious and therefore hard to recognize. Even the person who experiences a sudden onset of deafness will probably be unaware of the reason for his overwhelming depression which, Ramsdell points out, occurs even when a person is facing practical difficulties in a realistic way. It is reasonable to assume, therefore, that the person with slowly deteriorating hearing will be totally unaware of the origins of his feelings of progressive detachment and insecurity, his inner loneliness felt even when he is with his family. This feeling is deeper, less tangible, than those that can be explained by the problems of speech communication. As a counselor, you need to assist the hearing-impaired person to explore these vague feelings of insecurity. You can provide a framework for this process by discussing the role hearing plays in keeping an individual aware, at a preconscious level, that he is a part of things, explaining the impact impairment at this level is known to have on people. Explaining the role sound plays in localizing and identifying events around us and permitting us to behave appropriately will further help the client to realize the legitimacy of his feelings of insecurity and anxiety. Lack of understanding of such feelings often causes serious concern for the hearing-impaired person who does not identify the cause. Ramsdell states:

"Knowing the cause of depression does not remove it but fortunately the mere understanding of the reason for a feeling state does much psychologically to relieve its intensity" (p. 439).

The problem frequently is compounded by the hearing-impaired person's feeling that his inability to cope is a weakness. He is ashamed to admit the difficulties he is experiencing, the anxieties that beset him. Sometimes he may even repress his conscious concerns. Parents of deaf children frequently experience feelings of guilt and inadequacy. As a counselor, you must be aware of the likelihood that your client may be experiencing these feelings and be alert to the defensive behavior that results from them (Sandlin 1974).

In an article on the psychologic reactions to hearing loss, Rousey (1971) identified the most common patterns of defensive maneuvers an individual, including a hearing-impaired person, may use when under stress. These include regression, repression, reaction-formation, isolation, undoing, projection, turning against self, and sublimation. He stresses the role objective anxiety plays in provoking one or more of these defensive reactions. Objective anxiety arises from anticipation of being punished or penalized for the state of one's behavior. The client's perception of how others treat persons with handicapping conditions will therefore have a considerable bearing upon his pattern of adaptive behavior. His objective anxiety may result in modified self-perception sufficiently unacceptable as to cause him to deny the severity of his hearing handicap.

He may project the problems he is having onto others, accounting for his difficulty in hearing correctly by accusing others of mumbling, of deliberately cutting him out of conversations, or he may blame the room acoustics. When such projections can no longer be supported, a person will often begin to withdraw from threatening situations. He may give up a job, avoid group meetings, decline responsibilities that involve group discussions, withdraw from training programs, cease to attend plays or movies, or decline invitations to dinner parties. These defense reactions are frequently accompanied by self-deprecation. Since such adaptive behavior, negative though it may seem, is necessary to maintain the identity of the person, and since the real cause is either not recognized or not admitted, the person begins to lower his self-esteem to make it compatible with his behavior. This forced shrinking of one's life style may seriously shrink a person's self-image.

When the cause of the difficulties is consciously identified as the loss of adequate hearing the most common reaction, according to Rousey (1971), is one of mourning, a natural concomitant of loss. This, he points out, is related to Ramsdell's idea of separation of the invidivual from the world around him, a world that seems "dead", giving rise to depression or an all-pervading sense of sadness.

Roussey also explains that the loss of hearing frequently gives rise to a feeling of pain and mortification. He discusses mortification in terms of its two closely related derivatives, shame and self-esteem. He quotes Fenishel's description of shame as "constant fear of being criticized, ostracized or punished." Rousey (1971, p. 386) goes on to state, "It is probably certain that patients who express a conviction of shame over the need to wear a hearing aid or their hearing loss are struggling with some of these issues." These feelings are closely related to self-esteem.

As I will illustrate later, for many clients the need to accept the reality of a hearing loss and finally facing up to the need for help and for a hearing aid may constitute a real threat to their self image. To acknowledge this hearing loss, particularly by wearing a hearing aid, is a definite act requiring one to accept the fact that he is less than completely normal. This may be too great a step for a person to take without sympathetic support but to fail to do so will preclude satisfactory adaptation to the problem. Rousey draws our attention to the fact that the fear engendered by the threat to one's self-esteem may be handled by the development of varying degrees of arrogant behavior. This may be directed at anyone associated with the client's difficulties, whether a member of the family or a helping specialist, such as yourself. As a counselor, aware of such possible reactions, you will be less confounded by the apparently conflicting behaviors of aid-seeking and rejection-of-helper.

The basis of understanding the problem, therefore, lies in being aware of the fact that a change in our ability to continue to cope with the demands made upon us, whether that change be externally or internally induced, poses a threat to our psychologic stability. We may react to this threat in a number of ways, each of which has been discussed. Only when one has adjusted to the change in a manner that does not shrink life style and self-image can maximal adaptation be said to have occurred. It is a counselor's role to assist the client to achieve this goal. The success with which a client is able to maintain his normal life style, or with which a child successfully meets the emotional social and psychological challenges of development, will be the true measure of the effectiveness of a counseling program. Creating an emotional climate conducive to such growth in a hearing-impaired person and his immediate family will be your first task. How this may be achieved will be considered later.

I have suggested elsewhere (Sanders 1971a, p. 349) that counseling can be divided into two types: (a) personal adjustment guidance, the need for which has just been considered, and (b) informational guidance. I would like to emphasize that these two aspects of the counseling task are closely related. Much of the anxiety a person experiences in dealing with a new situation arises from his lack of information or, often, from erroneous information about the problem. *The goal of informational counseling is to permit the hearing-impaired person to obtain a realistic view of the problems resulting from his hearing impairment.* This will include not only an explanation of the type and degree of impairment, but also its impact on his ability to function in the various situations he encounters in everyday activities. Information about the effects of hearing loss often reduces anxiety by providing a logical explanation for an experience or behavior that may have been misinterpreted or misunderstood by the hearing-impaired person or his family.

Your role as a counselor permits you to explain the professional test results and evaluations to clients in a manner understandable to the nonspecialist. You have the ability to integrate the findings into a meaningful whole. *Informational guidance seeks to provide the hearing-impaired person with a clear understanding of the type of hearing problem he has, the effects such problems are known to have on a person's performance, and how those effects vary under different conditions.* The person should be advised of alternative ways of reducing the effects of the hearing deficit, what each alternative involves, and the prognosis for achieving significant improvement.

Informational counseling describes the objective realities of the situation, while personal adjustment counseling is concerned with helping the client to achieve a perception of the situation that is conducive to problem-solving. Since this perception is based upon the client's attitudes and feelings, it must result from his own personal insights reached through guidance by the counselor.

Approaching the Task

INFORMATIONAL COUNSELING

Although our major concern is with the person who is considering purchasing or has already purchased, a hearing aid, it is necessary to ensure that adequate informational counsel has been given that person about his type of hearing problem, whether his condition is reasonably stable or is a slowly deteriorating one, and, particularly, why medical treatment is not appropriate for him. The question of whether any previous counsel has been adequate is raised, not from doubts concerning the competency of other professionals, but because clients are often reluctant to admit that they do not understand something or to ask what they may be afraid is a silly question. *The adequacy of counseling is something only the client can evaluate.* It is important that you should have a comprehensive record of all previous test results, including the results of hearing aid evaluations. If you are an audiologist, you may have carried out these tests yourself. If not, then feel free to contact the audiologist who did, explaining that you are now working with his client and would like to be able to have the results in order to better understand the client's hearing status before and after amplification.

Your first task, therefore, is to provide information about the tests that were carried out, what the tests were intended to measure, what was found, and what the results suggest. At this point, it would be informative to explore with the client how far he agrees with the assumptions about to be made on the basis of the test findings. If a fairly accurate general picture of how such a hearing impairment can be expected to affect a person can be drawn, great strides can be made towards creating a feeling of confidence in the client. If your assumptions are denied by the client, then you have reason to assume that some unexpected factors are involved and it will be necessary to explore these.

As I have already pointed out, informational counseling concerning the role amplification can play will be successful only if the client's emotional state permits him to accept it positively. Before moving on to this aspect of counseling, it will be necessary to explore with the client his feelings about his loss, the extent of his difficulties, and his receptiveness to the idea of using a hearing aid. I will discuss this in the next section where the approach to the task of adjustment counseling is considered. For this discussion, assume that you have already reached a point where the client has a positive attitude towards amplification and is anxious to take advantage of it. Before realistic guidance in the effective use of a hearing aid can be given, an accurate picture must be obtained of the nature and severity of the communication difficulties the client is experiencing. This information is essential to avoid the mistake of underestimating the impact the hearing loss has on the hearing-handicapped person, or to avoid the error of applying generalizations that may hold true for groups of people but may be totally invalid assumptions when applied to any given individual. *The effects of a hearing difficulty are not readily represented by an audiogram.* A wide variety of factors influence how the deficit will impair a person's ability to continue to meet the demands of his environment. These will include, for example, the extent to which that person depends on understanding speech in his occupation or profession. A house painter or mailman will be less dependent upon hearing for speech than a salesman or a lawyer. Environmental conditions under which communication usually takes place will vary considerably. Many hearing-impaired persons can manage adequately in person-to-person conversation in reasonably quiet surroundings but have difficulty in noisy environments or in group situations. The extent to which a person's occupational environment is conducive to his hearing needs will influence the degree of difficulty he will have. Other factors include his familiarity with the situation and the people in it. His status will affect his ability to delegate difficult tasks to subordinates, such as having someone else take minutes at a meeting, asking a junior member of the staff to stand in for him, or having a secretary provide a summary of a discussion with a client. *The effect of the hearing deficit will therefore be determined by the special demands placed upon a person in his daily living in occupational and personal life situations, and by his ability to adapt to these.* It is necessary to establish the nature of the special needs of a person in order to develop a realistic plan of management. Underestimating the impact of a person's hearing deficit will result in inadequate counseling, and may even deprive that person of the help he needs.

An example of how a client's need can be underestimated presented itself not too long ago in a clinic where I am a consultant.

Mr. Brown held a managerial position in a business. He sought advice concerning a communication problem he was experiencing in certain environmental situations. He had a high frequency hearing loss, with speech test results (obtained in a sound isolated room) bordering on normal limits. His speech reception threshold was 26 dB ISO, the PB discrimination score was 86 percent with approximately equal performance bilaterally. The client stated that he had been told by an audiologist in another clinic that his hearing was not poor enough to warrant the use of a hearing aid. Furthermore he had been told that it was extremely difficult to fit his type of hearing loss. It was therefore suggested that he might take lipreading lessons. Almost a year had passed before he sought our advice. He said that he knew he was wrong in thinking that an aid could help him, but he was really having difficulty in catching everything that was said in certain situations and wondered if he ought not to begin lipreading training. Audiometric evaluation showed very little difference between our findings and those obtained by the other agency. A preevaluation session was arranged to explore the nature of his communication difficulties more fully. In this discussion, it was determined that although Mr. Brown's hearing had not changed to any significant extent, his business life had. A promotion had brought greater responsibilities and involved him in more decision-making. He spent more time attending, and sometimes chairing, committee meetings. It was in these group situations in particular that he was experiencing problems of being uncertain that he heard what was said. He was becoming apprehensive about his ability to manage the situation. Similar difficulties were experienced in church, at social gatherings, and at the theater. He had accepted the fact that these were difficult environments in which to follow speech easily. It was quite clear that this gentleman needed help. He was feeling threatened in his work situation and had accepted a deterioration in the quality of his social life.

My colleagues and I agreed that such hearing losses as he had are not the easiest to provide with satisfactory amplification, but disagreed with the former audiologist's statement that amplification was inappropriate. His special needs were recognized and arrangements made to attempt to provide for them. This approach, facilitated by a cooperative relationship with a hearing aid dealer, assisted experiments designed to find the most suitable hearing aid with an open canal mold. An eyeglass aid was selected because the client wore bifocal lenses at all times. Also, he was carefully advised about the gains being sought. My colleagues and I explained that we would probably not be able to document benefit by significant improvement in test results and that we would have to depend upon subjective evaluation.

Mr. Brown did, in fact, derive a surprising amount of benefit. He felt that one aid made such a great difference to his sense of confidence at work that he inquired whether he might gain even greater benefit from two. The initial audiologist would no doubt have been horrified, for we agreed to try. Now Mr. Brown not only has binaural aids, he has two sets of eyeglasses, one with aids for business, church, and such social activities as he found presented difficulties, the other pair for use at times when amplification is not necessary.

In this example, audiometric findings led an audiologist to reach a decision that did nothing to alleviate any of the very real problems experienced by the client. A similar situation in which audiometric data could have been misleading involved a child.

Susan, an 8-year-old child, was referred for hearing evaluation. Audiometric results showed that she had a 45 dB sensorineural loss in the right ear and a 20 dB threshold level in the speech range in the right ear. She was having difficulty with language art subjects at school, was a grade retarded in reading skills, and was beginning not to like school. She was an attractive, cooperative child with above-average performance on the Wechsler Intelligence Scale for Children, in which her verbal scores fell below her performance scores.

Although her audiometric results (sound field SRT 18 dB, discrimination 98 percent) alone would contraindicate the use of a hearing aid, her needs in school demanded significant rapid assistance. Advantageous seating and lipreading would not provide an adequate solution. Susan related to my colleagues and myself in a very mature manner because we explained what the tests showed us, talked with her about school, and told her that we felt that the difficulties she was having did in fact arise from her not hearing easily in class. We expressed a desire to help but explained that we could not be sure we could solve her problems. We did tell her that we had seen other children with similar difficulties and asked if she would work with us in an experiment to see if a small hearing aid might be the answer to her problems. We hastened to explain that she would have to make the final decision, but that she would have her teacher, her parents, and us to help her. Her response was very positive. Susan really wanted to participate in the experiment.

With her parents and Susan, we outlined a plan to provide a mild gain, behind-the-ear, loaner aid made available by the cooperation of a local hearing aid dealer. With the teacher's assistance, we obtained a picture of Susan's ability to function in various classroom activities, identifying specific situations in which the teacher felt her behavior indicated that she was experiencing difficulty. We used a profile development procedure, which I will discuss a little later, to establish baseline behavior and performance.

Several sessions were spent explaining to Susan and her parents what an aid is, what it does, what problems it creates, how to use and take care of it. We then tried the aid in the clinic, using it in the sound room for listening to speech material, for playing listening games, and for some tutoring activities. We next moved to a large clinic room with good acoustics, to the waiting area, and then to the secretaries' office. After three sessions with the aid, Susan took it to school where, with great support from the teacher, she wore it in language art class, social studies, and in the small math group. We maintained frequent contact with the teacher and discussed Susan's experiences with her.

Counseling sessions explored Susan's feelings in relation to specific situations. The aid was worn nowhere but in school, in selected situations. After 3 months there was no doubt that the experiment was a success. Susan was very positive that the aid helped, her teacher was delighted by Susan's increased ability to pay attention, to participate in group and class discussion, and to learn from oral presentations. The parents also felt the aid was helping her. When their request for state financial assistance was denied at the time of a fiscal crisis, they put themselves through some hardships to purchase the aid for Susan.

My colleagues and I could have been wrong in our prediction that amplification might provide the solution to Susan's problems, but we could not make a mistake since the only decision we made was to evaluate the effectiveness of amplification in meeting special needs under special circumstances. *This approach, which involves making the client the focus of counseling decisions rather than audiometric results and traditional wisdom, is more likely to achieve satisfactory results.* It illustrates the fact that we must not let our intellectual prejudices prevent an experimental approach to a problem.

Explaining the Effects of the Hearing Deficit

In order to explain to the hearing-impaired person how hearing loss affects his ability to understand speech, it is necessary to have a basic knowledge of the acoustic structure of speech. Familiarity with the nature of complex sounds, how energy in voiced speech sounds is concentrated into energy bands called *formants*, and the role that these formants play in carrying information about how a particular speech sound was produced, and, therefore, which speech sound it is, are required. Awareness of the similarity between the first formant values of several sounds emphasizes how important the second formant information is to differentiation between sounds. Plotting the pure-tone audiogram on an appropriate formant chart (Sanders 1971, p. 57) will indicate how a high frequency loss can result in confusion between some sounds that are audible but cannot be discriminated and also between some words that depend upon that single phoneme differentiation for their identification. Helping the hearing-impaired person to understand why these confusions are occurring will reassure him that the difficulties he is experiencing can be explained logically and are not due, as many people fear, to a deterioration in mental capacity. A discussion of the acoustic structure of speech as it relates to hearing deficit will be found in the chapter by Daniel Bode (Chapter 8) and in my text (Sanders 1971).

It is also important to understand how each sound affects its neighbors acoustically and how the production transitions from one sound to the next contain information that may, in some combinations, be sufficient to permit the identification of a sound even when the second formant is not audible. Similarly, it is important to understand the role of linguistic structure on speech perception, to explain how each unit further limits the probabilities of what the next unit may be, and to explain to the client in lay terms how his difficulties arose and what benefits he can realistically expect from amplification.

Many potential users of hearing aids either have incorrect concepts of what a hearing aid can achieve or do not have any clear idea at all.

It will be necessary to explain that a sensorineural hearing deficit seldom involves a simple loss of loudness. Due to the complex structure of the hearing mechanism, most sensorineural losses result in varying degrees of signal distortion. A person with a hearing deficit is faced with a situation in which there is first an overall reduction in the normal loudness of a signal and then a distortion of the signal because the complex speech signal is not uniformly affected across the range of frequencies it contains. Finally, an additional distortion arises because the normal neurophysiologic function of the sense organ of the ear has been irreparably damaged. The hearing aid can only overcome one of these factors; it can make sound loud enough. However, even the usefulness of the power it can provide is frequently limited by the fact that the amount of residual hearing that must be reached is limited. The upper physiologic limits of tolerance restrict the amount of power that can safely be provided. Thus, too frequently, in cases of severe deafness the sound level becomes unpleasant before the speech signal can be made loud enough to be useful. When recruitment is present, the situation becomes even more difficult. It is particularly important to explain these limitations of the potential benefits amplification may provide when the deficit is great or recruitment is present.

The client should be told that the aid can provide the necessary power within the limits of the ears' ability to use it. By making certain modifications in the aid, it may be possible to cut back on the power across "pitch ranges" where it is not needed as much, thereby increasing the chance of providing more energy in the range where it is needed. To some extent, this can be a successful procedure.

The most important point to get across, however, is that no hearing aid can correct the hearing deficit; no system of amplification can compensate for the loss of function of some of the components of the organ of hearing. The client should be told that what the hearing aid does is to make more of the signal available to the hearing that remains. Making more information available may significantly increase a person's ability to understand speech, but it does so by permitting maximal use of the hearing that remains. It does not restore hearing in any way. This point should be made because some persons, particularly the parents of hearing-impaired children, have the impression that a hearing aid is a corrective device and that after a period of use it will no longer be necessary to wear it. A question frequently asked is : "Will he not become dependent upon the aid?" This question is evidence of the same type of faulty reasoning. The answer is, of course, "We hope so," that is to say, we hope that amplification will permit a level of communicative behavior that otherwise would not be possible. The dependency is on the higher level of functioning that the aid makes possible—a very worthy goal to strive for.

Perhaps the most common incorrect assumption made by the potential hearing aid user is that in some way the hearing aid is selective and only amplifies speech. This concept may not be specifically expressed, but the reaction of clients to the noise of amplified nonspeech sounds is evidence that their expectations do not coincide with reality. This aspect of amplification must be discussed quite carefully to avoid hasty rejection of the aid. Also arrangements must be made to minimize the effects of environmental noise in early experiences with the aid. The problem of adjustment to noises in the world, even to one's own voice if it has not been at normal loudness for several years, is one of perceptual patterning. It is not infrequent for persons who have had their hearing restored to near-normal by a stapedectomy operation to experience a difficult period of adjustment. Occasionally, a person will state that they wish they had not had the surgery performed.

Von Senden (1960) reported similar reactions by his subjects to the restoration of sight following cataract removal. The problem arises from the discrepancy between the established perception of the auditory or visual world, and the sudden change in the information received after surgery or amplification. This discrepancy may be sufficiently disturbing as to threaten the client's stability, a situation not dissimilar to the effect of a sudden onset of deafness. It is the overwhelming feeling of being unable to cope with the changed situation that threatens and causes a person to reject that situation rather than adapt to it. This situation can and should be prevented by counseling the hearing aid candidate.

The nature of the situation should be explained, emphasizing that the person not only has been shut off from normal speech perception for a long time but also has been effectively cushioned against the constant noise background that once pounded away at him everyday with increasing loudness. People learn to identify the components of this noise so that they are able to accept it as normal despite its unpleasantness. To a degree, they become only partially aware of it. When a person has grown accustomed to relative quiet, sudden exposure to environmental sounds at near normal levels of loudness can be a very negative experience. It will take time for that person to adjust, because the process involves subconscious reassessment of the relative loudness of common sounds. By being aware that this is to be expected, the audiologist may gain the client's agreement not to make a hasty decision to reject amplification. Hearing aid evaluation informational counseling attempts to help the client to increase his objectivity in assessing the value of a hearing aid. It also helps to keep his observations and his feelings in two clearly identified categories. To further the task of assessing the value of the hearing aid objectively, it will be useful to develop a profile of the person's specific needs for amplification.

Defining the Need for Amplification

The criterion for carrying out a hearing aid evaluation is an assumption that amplification will provide the person with the potential for a higher level of adaptive behavior. It is advisable to define the needs before evaluating the person's performance with an aid or aids. Even with no more information than that provided by audiologic tests, some general idea of the extent of the need can be obtained. While it is unwise to apply a rule-of-thumb criterion to individuals, some reasonable assumptions may help to keep things in proportion. The main interest is to form some impression concerning how much amplification might help.

Diagnostic test data for prognosis concerning the use of amplification and for generally predicting communication and social performance are by no means uncommon. The Social Adequacy Index (SAI) developed by Davis (1958) at the Central Institute for the Deaf integrates the speech reception threshold value with discrimination loss to produce a social adequacy quotient that can then be compared to a social adequacy threshold level (SAI 33) at which a person can just manage in occupational and social environments. Other reports (AMA 1961, Carhart 1945) have investigated different weighting levels applied to the loss at different frequencies in order to predict behavior limitations of the deficit.

More recently, the relationship between audiometric data and actual performance was studied by Koniditsiotis (1971). For the 9 subjects she studied, hearing sensitivity, as measured by pure-tone and speech-reception threshold, was the best index of actual performance.

Predictions based upon audiometric data will of course vary as a function of a number of variables. Assumptions will be guided and guarded by knowledge and experience.

In some instances, a rather significant improvement can be anticipated. For example, a youngish person with a relatively flat sensorineural impairment of about 60 dB and a PB maximum of 88 percent should anticipate rather marked improvement in his ability to follow conversation when wearing a well-fitted hearing aid. An older person, with a sloping loss averaging 70 dB and a PB maximum of 68 percent, may still be unable to follow conversation easily, even with amplification, but may feel that if it gives him a fighting chance in important social situations, it may be worthwhile. The expectancies in these two examples are different, the goals are different, and the clients must know this from the start. They must realize that if Mrs. Johnson functions much better with her aid, it is most probably because she had a problem more responsive to amplification and most *unlikely* that she has a better aid, no matter how much she may profess the latter is the case.

It is most important for the client to know and believe in the ultimate limitations his particular hearing problem places on the maximum benefit he might reasonably be expected to derive from amplification. This is particularly critical when counseling parents of hearing-impaired children. Parents do not wish to have their child deaf or hard-of-hearing. Thus, their expectations of the difference amplification will make often are unrealistically high. They anticipate a dramatic shift to normal speech and language behavior when the aid is fitted; they often are under the impression that the child will hear normally, providing he wears the aid, and they are unaware that a child may hear some sounds or some parts of words while not hearing others.

This initial broad assessment of need is helpful, but careful management of the use of amplification requires more careful documentation of need. For example, Koniditsiotis (1971), in her small sample study, found that speech discrimination scores obtained by her subjects correlated poorly with actual behavior performance, being nonsignificant at the 5 percent rejection level. High *et al.* (1964) and Noble and Atherley (1970) reported similar observations.

"Of the greatest interest is the emergence of SRT for di-syllables as probably the best single predictor of questionnaire scores. SRT has been devalued in the literature by the allegedly more valid discrimination measure" (Noble and Atherly 1970, p. 244).

I have already stressed the need for a type of counseling relevant to the particular needs of the individual. Since attempts are being made to overcome, or at least to lessen, the severity of certain difficulties arising from the hearing impairment, it is important to be quite specific in defining the role of amplification for each individual. This must be done in terms of particular situations in which a person experiences communication problems. Millin's comments (Chapter 4) regarding the audiologist's failure to establish valid, standard test procedures for identifying the most appropriate aid, coupled with his emphasis on the distinction between diagnostic and predictive tests, stresses the importance of obtaining data concerning the actual performance of the client in daily life situations. While it is always desirable to seek an objective, controlled, predictive test, the absence of one should not create the feeling that subjective assessments by a client are of little use as a substitute. The hearing aid user must function in his subjective reality; for him, that is the only reality that directly affects his behavior. Changing behavior is only possible if subjective reality can be modified. Millin (Chapter 4) pointed out that even in the formal hearing aid evaluation, most audiologists operate under the assumption that testing the aid and the person separately is not the same as testing a person wearing the aid. That is to say, a definite interaction factor exists. The interaction factor is even more evident when the variables of a person, a hearing deficit, a specific environment, and a specific hearing aid are considered.

Therefore, in attempting to assess the subjective reality of a person's communication difficulties, the development of individual profiles must be determined.

Developing Communication Profiles

The task of counseling the potential hearing aid user involves four aspects. *The first is to assess the person's communication needs.* This necessitates the development of an awareness of the specific demands his life style places on his ability to communicate effectively. The second aspect involves *the determination of the extent to which he is failing to meet these needs.* The third concern is for *the effects that failure to meet these needs has had and is having upon the person.* The fourth aspect concerns *how he has attempted to resolve these problems.*

The Need Profile

Ideally, this should be developed before hearing aid selection procedures are carried out. I feel very strongly that the practice of moving to a hearing aid selection process after taking no more than a brief case history of problems is most unwise. I concur wholeheartedly with Alpiner's (Chapter 5) emphasis on the need for conducting an assessment of communication function prior to test evaluation. Such a procedure serves three major purposes:

1. It provides a baseline against which perceived improvement may be measured.
2. It focuses attention upon the client's perceived performance in specific and differing real-life situations, which it is unlikely will ever be synthesized in a clinic testing situation.
3. It identifies particular problem situations and serves as a guide in planning counseling and management.

The development of the profile involves assisting the client in defining his own difficulties. The task will be to structure the activity and to guide him in this data collection. This provides an excellent opportunity for the establishment of rapport during a nonthreatening stage of rehabilitation. Since the data must be recorded, assessments should be kept as a diary, or log. Generally speaking, major environmental areas in which examination of communication performance should be conducted are (a) the home environment; (b) the employment environment; and (c) the social environment.

It is advisable to use a set of guide questions to aid in structuring the situation. However, encourage the client to identify other situations and environments in which difficulty occurs.

High *et al.* (1964) first developed and tested the hearing handicap scale, designed to assess the effect of hearing loss on the subject's performance in ordinary hearing situations arising in an urban environment. They used 2 tests of 20 questions related mainly to speech communication and to a lesser extent to audition of background noise and warning signals. The response was specified in terms of the frequency with which difficulty was encountered in each situation. The limitations of this tool, as has been pointed out by Giolas (1970) lie in the rather narrow homogeneous nature of the items. A number of important aspects, particularly vocational status and attitude toward the handicap, are not included.

Giolas in his 1970 article appeals for further investigation into tools that explore the effects of hearing loss upon everyday functions. In discussing this need he states:

> "While it is reasonable to assume that a loss in sound reception will effect some handicap, the nature of the handicap in the everyday life situation is unknown. This is pointed out by repeated encounters in the clinical setting with individuals demonstrating quite similar audiograms and quite dissimilar functional behavioral problems. Still another way to look at the ineffectiveness of threshold measures as indicators of special handicap is to recognize the implications of a stable audiogram. Even after successful aural rehabilitation where there is obvious improvement in communication skills, the audiogram is not expected to improve. This points out once again that the status of a given handicap cannot be meaningfully assessed from threshold measures."

Such a scale, as suggested by Giolas, was designed and developed by Noble and Atherley (1970). Their instrument, the Hearing Measurement Scale for Disability, includes 42 scoring items weighted to give a measure of disability. The questions used cover areas of speech and hearing ability in different situations, acuity for nonspeech sounds, localization, speech distortion, effects of tinnitus, and personal opinion about the effects of the hearing deficit.

In follow-up publications, Atherley and Noble (1971) and Noble (1972) discussed the effectiveness of the tool as tested with specific populations. They describe it as a workable device that can provide useful clinical information about individual hearing-impaired persons or about groups of persons with a hearing deficit.

The audiologist may wish to use one of the already tested scales or seek the flexibility of developing variants of these for his own use. Remember, in developing the scale, attempts are to be made to both identify the types of communication situations in which problems occur and the degree of difficulty.

The scales I suggest in Appendices A-D illustrate the type of approach that may be taken. Notice that after each question the person is asked to identify the frequency with which the situation is encountered. Each answer is rated on a scale ranging from +2 to −2; the frequency of occurrence is rated 1-3. This permits an average rating to be computed for degree of difficulty in communication situations in a specific environment. By multiplying the value of the answer by the value of a question, e.g., "I experience a fair amount of difficulty" (value −1) by the frequency of occurrence of the situation e.g., "very often" (value 3), a weighted value (−3) is obtained. The same difficulty experienced only seldom reduces the weighted value in this example to −1. The absolute value (a × b) indicates the level of importance that the communication situation has for the person. The sign of the value + or − indicates the extent to which the individual perceives himself as having difficulty in that situation. The algebraic summation of all weighted values for an environment, when divided by the number of questions, will produce a mean value of the impact of the hearing difficulty for a given type of environment.

The advantage of the numerical value is that it permits one to compare assessed performance before and after hearing-aid use or aural rehabilitation.

Appendices A, B, and C are illustrations of profile guides for home, business, and social environments. I wish to stress that they are illustrations, not standard forms to be used with all clients. Together with each hearing aid candidate, appropriate guides will have to be developed. Similar guides can be developed for use with the teachers of young hearing-impaired children (Appendix D), with parents of hearing-impaired children, or with preteen-age, teen-age, or college-age students. You should be involved in the development of these profiles, but in a cooperative rather than a directive manner. The profiles appropriate for a young housewife, a business man who serves as a representative for a major manufacturer, an elderly lady living in a nursing home, and a fourth-grade child will be very different, since the demands placed upon them by their daily activities differ so widely.

The log book should provide a record of specific problem situations as they arise. The person keeping the log should be asked to note, as soon after the situation as possible, such information as:

Where were you when the problem arose?
What, briefly, was the situation?
How many people were you with?
What was the nature of the communication?
Were you an active participant?
What were the room acoustics like?
Was there a lot of noise?
How far were you from the speaker?
How much difficulty did you experience?

These two methods of problem identification and definition should provide a fairly clear understanding of the nature and extent of the client's communication needs. With this information available, the audiologist should be in an excellent position to discuss the entire question of amplification with the client.

Assessing the Client's Attitudes Towards the Use of a Hearing Aid

It is unjustifiable to assume that the presence of a client in your clinic necessarily indicates his willingness to use a hearing aid. Clients often only seek consultation to satisfy the persistent entreaties of a husband, wife, or other close friend or relation. The person may be silently adamant about not wearing a hearing aid. Some even go so far as to purchase the aid, only to reject it as soon as they feel they have satisfactorily demonstrated that they cannot tolerate it. They frequently reject the aid because "it advertises my hearing loss." Parents of a young, deaf child not infrequently fail to allow their child to wear the aid when they take him shopping, on a trip to the park, or to a community event because "I don't want people to know my child isn't normal." Freedman and Doob (1968, p. 148), in a fascinating study of how a deviancy or stigma affects the behavior of people, indicate that if the problem is not known to others, people will attempt to conceal it, which often leads to avoidance of social contacts, so that life style shrinks, as described earlier. There is little point in proceeding with a hearing aid selection process until a client, or the parents of a child, are positively motivated towards its use.

> "If the parents of a deaf child reject the use of an aid their child will do the same. Therefore it is necessary that the consultant learn how the parents feel about amplification. It is possible that in some cases it may take as many as three or more sessions to modify the thinking of parents who are anti-hearing aids" (Shore 1972).

It is necessary, at this point in the discussion, to consider some of the aspects of personal adjustment counseling as they directly relate to the acceptance of the hearing aid. That acceptance is determined by complex feelings on the part of the potential hearing aid user, feelings he may find disturbing, ill-defined, and difficult to explain. Not infrequently, they arise from the person's reluctance to accept his hearing loss.

ACCEPTING THE REALITY OF HEARING LOSS

An example of the difficulty accepting the reality of a hearing problem occurred in our university clinic.

A good-looking, young, male college student sought to improve a deviant speech pattern that clearly arose from a congenital hearing loss. His response to the suggestion that a hearing aid might do much to improve self-monitoring his speech evoked strong rejection. His hearing, he assured my colleagues and myself, was not a problem; it was his speech that was holding him back in his attempt to study drama. We accepted his explanation and began speech improvement work. After rapport had been established, we began to talk with him about the hearing loss. He admitted that he did have trouble hearing and that he did, in fact, own an ear-level hearing aid but never wore it. It took several sessions before he volunteered that he did not wear it because he considered his hearing loss a weakness, a physical defect in what he *felt* was otherwise a physical identity of which he was proud. It was extremely hard for him to accept this blemish; to advertise it seemed folly. The hearing aid, therefore, became for him what Goffman (1963) refers to as a "stigma symbol." These are ". . . signs which are especially effective in drawing attention to a debasing identity discrepancy, breaking up what would otherwise be a coherent overall picture with a consequent reduction in our valuation of the individual.''

Until this young student was able, through counseling, to deal with the reality of the hearing impairment and to reassess its role in the determination of his self-identity, the hearing aid had to be rejected by him. He could not afford to accept it even though, as he subsequently became aware, he was more ''normal'' with than without it in terms of adaptability. He had resorted to the process of ''covering'' his handicap by a pattern of adjustment that sought to protect him from having to face up to his stigma. Goffman (1963, p. 104) illustrates such behavior with a condensation from Warfield (1948):

> ''Frances figured out elaborate techniques to cope with 'dinner lulls,' inter-missions at concerts, football games, dances, and so on, in order to protect her secret. But they served only to make her more uncertain, and in turn more cautious, and in turn more uncertain. Thus, Frances had it down pat that at a dinner party she should (a) sit next to someone with a strong voice; (b) choke, cough, or get hiccups, if someone asked her a direct question; (c) take hold of the conversation herself; ask someone to tell a story she had already heard; ask questions, the answers to which she already knew.''

The audiologist must decide for himself how to generate needed informa-tion. He should, however, seek information about both performance and at-titudes. Compare, for example, the outline I have suggested with the information obtained by the Denver Scale. Notice that although these two approaches seek to achieve the same goal, the Denver Scale approaches the task in a different manner. The information it generates is heavily weighted in terms of how the client feels about the effect of his hearing loss on his performance in communica-tion and how he feels others react to him. It provides valuable information for adjustment counseling that my outlines do not generate. On the other hand, the Denver Scale does not provide specific information about specific types of situa-tions peculiar to a particular person's environment. For this reason, I feel these two approaches are complementary, with only a small area of overlap.

Developing Realistic Expectations for Amplification

I have already pointed out the need to discuss with the client how his hearing deficit affects his ability to perceive speech. I also mentioned the importance of explaining the limiting effects of such factors as recruitment or reduced discrimi-nation performance. In discussing the need to explain the effects of the hearing deficit, I stressed the importance of explaining how the contribution of the hearing aid to the solution of hearing problems is confined mainly to the role of making more information available. I will again emphasize that *the ultimate success in the effective use of amplification lies in the amount and pattern of residual hearing, and the capacity of the auditory system to process the informa-*

tion made available to it. These factors should be assessed in terms of how they will limit the amount of improvement a hearing aid might realistically be expected to make possible. The most important factors to weigh are:

1. *The severity of the loss.* Remember that the limits of useable residual hearing are bounded by the threshold of detection and the intensity level at which the person feels he could *comfortably* listen to speech *over long periods of time* (most comfortable loudness level—MCL), not by the physiologic limits of discomfort. If this dynamic range of hearing is narrow, hearing aid benefits will be severely limited.

2. *The pattern of the audiogram.* If there is a sharp drop in sensitivity as frequency increases, it may be difficult to provide sufficient damping of energy levels in the range of frequencies where hearing is normal. It may not be possible to provide all the amplification desired in the high frequencies. Furthermore, the performance of hearing aids in reaching these high frequencies is somewhat limited. Unusual peaks in hearing sensitivity may also limit the contribution an aid can make.

3. *The maximum discrimination performance.* This is often the most important factor, for the fact that sound can be made loud enough is of little help if discrimination is sufficiently poor as to nullify the benefits of the loudness. Speech must be loud enough and of sufficient clarity to be useful.

Specific information concerning the relationship of these factors has been dealt with in other chapters. Your task is to use your understanding of the nature of amplification and hearing aid modifications to provide for special needs to assess the potential benefit available to each client. This must be done before an aid is tested, to ensure that the person from the start is evaluating the help the aid provides in terms of what he has been led to assume it should. If an aid can reasonably be expected to bring communication performance to within normal level in all but the most difficult listening situations, then the hearing aid candidate's demands may justifiably be set high. If, on the other hand, poor maximum discrimination determines that amplification can do little more than increase the person's ability to follow conversation in the most favorable listening conditions, and even then mainly because of the increased ease with which the person can interpret visible speech cues against the background of increased auditory information, then the decision to purchase an aid must be made on the basis of these limited expectations.

The aim is to forestall the disappointment that arises from expecting too much. Writing about the disappointment frequently expressed by new hearing aid users, Niemeyer (1973) states:

"As long as he carries on a conversation with a single person, in a quiet room that is, as long as he uses the hearing aid under similar acoustic conditions as those prevailing at the time of selecting the hearing aid on the basis of the speech audiometric results, his understanding is good and this

already means an important step forward to him: the interpretation of succeeding sound events, diachronous hearing, does not present any insuperable hurdles to him. However, when he wants to participate in group conversations, or when conversations take place in a noisy environment, his understanding falls off considerably; synchronous hearing, the perception of
acoustic events simultaneously presenting and the isolation of the speech
signal from the noise is poor. This particular handicap already distresses
most of the patients with internal ear deafness even before they use a hearing
aid and the situation is even, accentuated by amplification through the aid.
The hearing handicapped individual who places his hopes in the technical
hearing prosthesis again feels shut out and unable to share fully in group
conversations.''

With sensitive counsel and a fairly thorough understanding of the nature of the
task, the client will have the ability to make a wise decision about whether the
benefits he will derive from amplification are sufficient to warrant the use of a
hearing aid. Such a decision may, in some circumstances, need to be made
before the aid is purchased. However, it is hoped that the cooperative efforts of
the counselor and local dealers will permit aids to be subjected to a trial period
before purchase. Since extended trial periods are often difficult to arrange, the
importance of the aspect of counseling just discussed cannot be overemphasized.

When a young child is being fitted for amplification, the need for counseling
parents in terms of what to expect is, if anything, more critical than when an
adult is involved. Ross (Chapter 6) discusses this need and makes specific reference to the writings of McConnell (1968) and Luterman (1971). In addition, I
refer the reader to an article, *Early Intervention for the Young Deaf Child
Through Parent Training,* by Horton and McConnell (1970), available in reprint
from the authors at the Bill Wilkerson Hearing and Speech Center, Nashville,
Tennessee. For an in-depth treatment of the hearing-impaired child's use of
sensory information, I would suggest a recent text, *Sensory Capabilities of
Hearing Impaired Children,* edited by Rachel E. Stark (1974).

THE ROLE OF THE AMPLIFIED SIGNAL IN
COMMUNICATION

For those children and adults for whom completely normal auditory performance is not possible by amplification, it will be necessary to explain, in as
simple a manner as possible, that communication is a total process that is made
easier because it takes place within a context. Within the auditory channel, the
constraints of language limit how the speaker may put together speech sounds,
words, sentences, and phrases. The meaning content exerts further constraints,
which operate on the visible aspects of speech. Added to this are the cues
provided by the speaker's dress and gestures and the immediate environment so

that the situation is one in which the listener, unconsciously familiar with these factors, can afford to miss part of the acoustic signal yet still be able to perceive the message. *Counseling therefore should place the hearing aid within the larger context of the total communication event.* The hearing aid user should not assume either that all of the information must be perceived through the aid if speech is to be understood or that if the aid provides less than complete comprehension, it is not worth using. With auditory and visual communication, it may well be possible to close the communication gap. This type of information also will be of value to the adult user of a hearing aid, particularly when less than complete benefit from amplification is possible. It will help the user to understand that the successful use of amplification is not to be assessed as complete understanding of speech in most situations but rather as the degree of improvement it permits in overall communicative behavior.

INSTRUCTING THE CLIENT IN THE OPERATION AND CARE OF THE HEARING AID

A hearing aid user should be thoroughly familiar with the aid he is using. Informational counseling therefore must include an explanation of the type, make, and model of aid the client is to wear. Each of the accessible controls should be described, not forgetting to show how to turn the aid on and off. Explain the purpose of each control, demonstrate its use, and then have the client demonstrate his understanding. For example, in explaining the volume control on the aid, I point out that it is no different from the volume control on a radio. When the radio is turned on the level is adjusted to be comfortable for the environment the listener is in and is then left at that level. For convenience, the position on the dial that produced that comfort level may be noted, so that when the radio is again turned on the volume can be reset immediately. It is not necessary to constantly readjust the volume control. The same is true for the aid. It may be necessary to experiment with various volume settings until a person becomes adjusted to the relative loudness of sounds, but he should be encouraged to resist the temptation to turn down the volume when a louder than average sound occurs and then have to reset it for speech a few seconds later. If tolerance is a problem, an automatic volume control should have been included in the initial requirements for selection of an aid.

The tone or frequency control is another feature of many radios and record players. On a hearing aid it serves the same purpose, emphasizing the bass or treble to produce a sound the listener considers natural. On the hearing aid, the tone control helps to compensate to some degree for the pitch distortion resulting from the uneven pattern of hearing loss. You should illustrate for the client the effects of various tone control settings upon the quality of the sound. The letter or number of the appropriate setting should be written down for the hearing aid user. The telephone circuit setting on body-worn aids often is also included on the tone control. Its use should be explained and demonstrated; then the client should repeat the procedure to ensure that he has understood.

You should demonstrate how the battery is inserted, stressing the importance of matching the + sign on the battery to the + sign on the battery receptacle of the aid. Care in inserting the battery is important, lest the aid terminals be bent or the plastic socket in ear-level aids crack.

When a conventional body aid is worn, explain that the hearing aid cord is the lifeline from the amplifier to the receiver button in the ear. It is a very delicate component and must be carefully handled lest the hair-thickness wires be broken. The terminals at the ends of the cord should fit firmly into the socket in the aid and in the receiver button.

The purpose of the receiver button of the body-worn aid should be explained and the way in which it snaps onto the mold demonstrated.

When behind-the-ear or eyeglass-type hearing aids are to be worn, the demonstration will be simpler because the receiver is housed in the same casing as the microphone and amplifier. Nevertheless, the on-off switch, volume control, telephone position, and use of the aid with the phone must be demonstrated. Also, how the tubing carries the sound to the mold and how it is attached must be explained to the client.

Explanations for special aids, such as CROS and BICROS, should be made very carefully. I believe it extremely important that a hearing aid user be sophisticated in his knowledge of the instrument that is to become so very important to him. In the case of young children, parents should be given this information. Downs (1971) outlined and discussed methods for maintaining three cardinal principles, which she lists as:

1. Keeping the hearing aid on the child.
2. Keeping the hearing aid functioning on the child.
3. Using the hearing aid as an amplification device to aid hearing.

Downs identifies such practical problems as an earmold and receiver that will not stay in an infant's ear, a problem that may be solved by connecting them by a small tube molded to the ear so as to permit the receiver to be positioned behind it, or perhaps by placing the aid on the back of the child, thus keeping the cord away from his hands. For the child who keeps pulling the aid out, she recommends carefully rechecking the selected volume level, lest it be too high, and ensuring that the mold is comfortable. If these points check out negatively, then the child will need to be trained (Downs, 1966). Downs discusses the problem of feedback, pointing out the need for frequent new molds for growing children and emphasizing the need for frequent analysis of the performance of the hearing aid. She covers points of care and maintenance, which I will discuss later. This information must be simply, carefully, and, if necessary, repeatedly explained and demonstrated to parents. However, never underestimate the ability of school-age hearing-impaired children to become sophisticated hearing aid users. Paulos (1961) convincingly demonstrated the effectiveness of a program specifically designed to educate these youngsters in the nature of their hearing difficulty and in the role of amplification. It is the child's hearing problem; he has to wear the aid; he knows what it is like. I therefore treat a child with the same respect as I do an adult, for with such an approach, the child always manages to impress me with his or her competence. This experience can be an important step in personal adjustment counseling. Two publications, *Caring for a Child's Hearing Aid* by Charlotte Dempsey, available from Zenith Corporation, and *Tim and His Hearing Aid* by Eleanor Ronnei and Joan Porter (1965), also available in Spanish as *Pepe y su Audifon*, will be of additional help to you in working with parents and children.

A very important component of the hearing aid is the earmold. Have a lot of patience with the adult or child when you explain and demonstrate how to insert it so that it fits tightly yet comfortably. I like to stand behind the person and monitor his hand on the first attempts to fit the mold. Much support and encouragement is needed at this task, but remember these are the most important stages of developing a helping relationship designed for cooperative problem-solving. If the client's trust can be earned in dealing with these practical problems, the chances of success with problems involving personal feelings and behavior will be enhanced. Impatience or lack of empathy during early contacts may destroy the possibility of developing an effective helping role.

In addition to understanding the hearing aid, the audiologist will need to explain how to care for it. The most important aspects of care involve the following instructions:

1. Handle the aid gently; it is an expensive, delicate instrument. Avoid placing it where it will get hot, e.g., on a radiator, in the glove compartment of the car. Keep the aid dry and do not clean it with anything other than an almost dry cloth. Make quite sure that food and dust are not trapped on the microphone grill of the aid.

2. Remove the battery when the aid is not in use. The battery will continue to drain even if the volume control switch is off.

3. Ensure that the terminals of the battery socket and the battery contacts are noncorroded and clean. They may be gently roughened with the small end of an emery board used for shaping fingernails. The prongs of the cord should be kept bright in the same manner. Should corrosion have occurred, it may be removed by using a damp cloth sprinkled lightly with baking soda.

4. Use a voltmeter sparingly when testing batteries; remember it too consumes battery power. Buy and number two or three batteries at a time, rotating them each day. Wrap extra batteries in a plastic wrapping material and store them in the refrigerator. *Do not use a battery that appears to be leaking.*

5. Clean the earmold regularly, using warm, soapy water (nondetergent) and a pipestem cleaner, if necessary. Rinse thoroughly in clean warm water. Blow

out to clear the aid of bubbles, then push a pipe cleaner gently through it to dry. Dry the outside with cloth. It is adviseable to wash the mold at night, then stand it on a paper towel to dry completely.

6. Should the hearing aid get wet, immediate action may preserve it by:
    a. removing the batteries at once;
    b. draining all water;
    c. drying with absorbent cloth, and placing in a warm *but not hot* place. The low heat of a hairdryer could be used. A jar containing silica gel, available from your hearing aid dealer, will provide an excellent dry climate for the aid when it is not in use.

CHECKING THE HEARING AID AND IDENTIFYING PROBLEMS

When first fitted with a hearing aid, a person often finds that the sounds he hears are different from what he expected. This is a result of the combined filtering effect of his hearing impairment and the frequency characteristics of the aid. Adult hearing aid users will become accustomed to how speech and environmental noises sound through the hearing aid. This provides a norm against which a subjective judgment can be made as to whether the aid is functioning as expected. For young children, parents must make this decision. They should make a point of frequently listening to speech and noise through the child's aid in order to develop an auditory image of how it sounds when functioning well. They should routinely listen to the aid each day to check its function before putting it on the child.

From time to time, things will go wrong with the hearing aid. These malfunctions should be detected immediately in order that the hearing aid user not be deprived of amplification for longer than is absolutely necessary. When an aid is believed not to be functioning properly, the user or the parents of a child should be able to run simple checks to eliminate some basic causes before making a trip to the hearing aid dealer.

The following checks should be made routinely, either by the user, or on his behalf by a person with good hearing:

The Battery

Open the battery case and remove the battery. Using a simple battery tester, which every hearing aid user should have, test to insure that the battery is at the required voltage. Even a new battery should be tested before use. Discard or store old batteries in a box clearly marked *"used batteries."* Check that the terminals of the battery and the contact points of the aid are bright. If they are not, they can be cleaned with a pencil eraser or with a fine emery board. Insert the battery, making sure that the + and − signs on the battery match those marked on the hearing aid.

If the aid does not function at all, the prime suspect is a dead battery. Replacement of the battery in this case will make the aid functional again. Intermittent function of the aid may arise from a faulty connection between the battery and the contacts. When this is the case, it is often observed that tapping the aid lightly will cause it to function briefly, only to have it go off again very soon. Cleaning the terminals and connections should correct this.

Sometimes a hearing aid user is concerned that the battery appears not to last very long. This is not an unusual complaint after purchase of a more powerful aid, which places a heavier drain on the battery than did the previous hearing aid. A hearing aid wearer should be advised how many hours a battery should be expected to last (see Chapter 2). Once he has begun to use the aid regularly, the user or parents of a child should be encouraged to keep a log of the number of hours the aid is on each day. After 2 or 3 weeks, they will know the weekly average in-use hours, which can then be compared to the expected battery life.

The Earmold, Tubing, and Connections

The earmold should be kept free of wax. If the mold becomes completely blocked, the aid will appear not to function. When an aid is reported "dead," after checking for a dead battery, check for a wax plug in the mold. If it is dirty, remove the mold and clean it carefully as described above. Check the tubing, which on ear-level and glasses aids connects the mold to the hearing aid. This tube must be unobstructed to allow the sound to travel from the aid to the ear. If moisture forms and condenses in the tube, the passage of sound will be blocked. Similarly, if when the aid is inserted, the tube becomes kinked, the sound will be prevented from reaching the ear. Care must be taken to avoid this occurring when inserting the mold. Someone can be asked to check the tubing, or it may be possible for the user to check for himself by using a mirror. Sometimes kinking will occur if the tube is too long. In this case the hearing aid dispenser should be consulted. Stiff, discolored, or cracked tubing should be replaced. It is advisable for the hearing aid user to have extra tubes available as replacements and that someone be able to change a tube if the client is not able to do this.

Finally, check that the connections between the tubing, the earmold, and the aid are clean and unobstructed. If the connection on the hearing aid is blocked, consult the hearing aid dispenser.

The Controls

Improper setting of the controls is a not infrequent cause of apparent malfunction. Particular attention should be paid to the on-off switch, which must be in the on position for use, and to the M-T switch. When used normally, the aid must be switched to M for environmental microphone. When switched to the T (telephone) circuit position the environmental microphone will not operate. The telephone circuit enables the client to listen to a telephone conversation without distraction from amplified environmental sounds. The T setting is only appropriate for telephone use.

The tone control should be on the setting recommended by the dispenser. Expressed dissatisfaction with the quality of the sound of the aid may arise from the tone control inadvertently having been moved from the usual setting, thus changing the characteristics of the amplified sound.

The Quality of the Sound

It is difficult for a non-hearing aid wearer to listen to an aid unless he has his own mold. If someone (parent, spouse, teacher, or nursing home staff member) assumes responsibility for checking the aid, it is highly adviseable that he have a mold with which to do so. A stock mold may be purchased for this purpose from a hearing aid dealer. Otherwise it will be necessary to place the receiver or ear-level mold in the auricle of the ear, covering it with the palm of the hand.

Turn the volume control on and rotate it up and down, listening for scratchiness or dead spots. The loudness of the sound should grow smoothly as the volume control is turned more fully on. A sudden jump in loudness, or lack of control over loudness, indicates that the volume control is defective. The volume control should be neither exceptionally loose nor very stiff. Rotating the volume control gently up and down a half dozen times occasionally will overcome scratchiness caused by dirt. Intermittent function of the aid may originate in a faulty volume control. Similarly, check the on-off switch, turning it back and forth to check for loose contacts.

Check tone controls, listening for appropriate changes in pitch and quality of the sound. Check the telephone switch to ensure that speech over the telephone is amplified on the T setting while environmental sounds are not. If the sound is weak on the T setting, replacement of the telecoil may be necessary.

The Cord

Check for breaks in the cord of a body aid by rolling it back and forth between finger and thumb while listening for "cut outs." A faulty cord may result in intermittent sound or absence of sound. If in doubt, replace the cord. The firmness of the connections between the cord and the aid, and the cord and receiver button, should be checked. Terminal prongs should be straight and clean.

The Receiver Button

The receiver button should be inspected for cracks or chips in the plastic case. These are indicative of trauma to the receiver and often identify hidden damage to the internal components. It is advisable to have an extra receiver button as standby. The snap connection between the receiver and the earmold should be tight. A plastic washer should be used to ensure maximum seal.

Feedback

Feedback, which is caused by the amplification of sound leakage from the aid, will be recognized by its characteristic squeal or whistle. This most often results from an ill-fitting earmold. To check for the cause, remove the hearing aid and close the opening in the canal of the receiver by pressing your thumb against it. Now turn the aid on full. If the whistle no longer occurs, the fault is undoubtedly in the poor fit of the mold when placed in the ear. This can be confirmed if the feedback whistle can be stopped by pressing the mold more tightly into the ear when wearing the aid. In a body-worn aid, the mold should be disconnected from the receiver and the open nozzle of the receiver covered with your thumb to check whether the whistle can be stopped. If feedback cannot be stopped when you block the sound outlet from your aid with your thumb, the aid should be returned to the dealer.

Whistling will sometimes occur in ear-level aids if the wearer stands with his ear close to a reflective surface or if his hand is close to the aid as he adjusts it. This is normal and is not a cause for concern (Chapter 2).

It is most important that informational counseling be conducted in a serious but relaxed, friendly manner. Go over each point carefully, demonstrating procedures where appropriate. Try to avoid rushing the client as it is difficult to remember large amounts of information that is presented rapidly. It will help if short, concise, written synopses of what is told to the client are available. These may be kept in a folder, together with the client's log book. Follow the outline of these notes quite closely. Before he leaves, make sure that the client goes over the material to be sure he has understood all explanations.

I appreciate that you may feel an urgency to move to the stage of trying out the hearing aid. It is, however, very important to lay a firm foundation of understanding of, and to develop realistic expectancies for, that trial stage.

Before I discuss how to go about introducing the client to the user of the aid in his everyday life, I shall examine some of the misconceptions about hearing aids which, if they exist, should be corrected.

MISCONCEPTIONS ABOUT AMPLIFICATION AND HEARING AIDS

I have mentioned earlier in the chapter some of the misunderstandings that exist about what hearing aids can achieve. I pointed out that, contrary to the beliefs of some people, hearing aids can be extremely helpful to persons with sensorineural problems, but that they can in no way restore hearing. Nevertheless, amplification can often improve the effectiveness with which a person uses sound, sometimes to the extent of normalizing auditory competence. The opposite misconception, namely that everyone who has a hearing loss can or should wear a hearing aid, is equally untrue. I have emphasized that the need for a hearing aid can only be determined after careful profile development, since many variables beyond auditory sensitivity are involved. Informational counseling should correct misconceptions arising from the fact that there are so many different brands and models of hearing aids on the market. It is untrue, for example, that any one hearing aid is, by design, superior to all others. Most amplification needs can be provided for by any major manufacturer of hearing aids. A case can be made for the claim that there is a best set of specifications for a particular hearing problem, but as emphasized in other chapters, identifying these criteria is not easy. On the other hand, it is a misconception that a person can therefore buy any hearing aid on the assumption that they all do the same thing. How needs vary has been discussed. Other chapters explained design modifications developed to meet various acoustic needs. Careful assessment of need must be undertaken if appropriate modifications are to be made in a basic amplifying unit.

A valuable but rather depressing report on the problems confronting hearing-impaired persons seeking services contains a section (Part 2 of *Paying Through the Ear* (1973) entitled *"Consumers Guide."* In explaining misconceptions about hearing loss and hearing aids, it is stressed that as far as hearing aids are concerned, a one to one correlation does not exist between price and quality. The authors caution against the assumption that one should purchase the most expensive aid. They explain that new hearing aids, like new models of cars, involve, for the most part, style changes rather than major engineering improvements. Also like cars, if style is disregarded, a hearing aid is usable for as long as it is known to be operating as it originally was intended to. This cannot be determined definitely without subjecting it to technical performance evaluation. I recommend that an aid be checked for performance every year or so for adult users, and every 6 months for children (Downs 1971).

These are only some of the misunderstandings your client may have about his hearing problem and amplification. Informational counseling can anticipate these misconceptions, but that is not enough. You must create an atmosphere in which the client feels that no question he may have is irrelevant or stupid; you must, in other words, seek to satisfy all of the client's needs for information.

COUNSELING IN THE INITIAL USE OF THE AID

The initial use of the hearing aid frequently sets the client's future attitude towards amplification. My discussion of this point has centered upon preparing the client for this experience. I have emphasized the need to develop positive attitudes within a realistic set of expectations. The client should, by this time, understand the nature of his hearing problems, should be aware of the particular situations in which he has most difficulty, and should have a realistic appreciation of how much improvement to expect.

There are two schools of thought concerning the next stage—the task of getting used to the hearing aid. Some audiologists believe that maximum adjustment will be made only if the client wears the aid consistently at all times. It is felt that this forces the person to face up to the real auditory world. Experience with adjustment patterns to the use of bifocal lenses or the wearing of a dental bridge lends support to this approach. Denied the opportunity to delay the adjustment task, the rate of successful adjustment may be greater. However, the failure rate is not known. There are, without doubt, hearing aid users who make an extremely rapid adjustment by any approach. These, however, are not the users who concern us. I personally favor a more conservative approach. Using the profile of hearing difficulties, I recommend that the counselor identify situations in which the listening environment will be favorable and those in which the most favorable response to the hearing aid may be expected. These should comprise the initial experiences in hearing aid use. They should occur among people with whom the person feels comfortable and who, perhaps because of counsel, are sensitive to the feelings of apprehension and embarrassment the hearing aid user will naturally experience. This kind of environment will provide favorable acoustic experiences and will minimize *psychologic reactions to wearing the aid.* Referring to this consideration of the clients feelings about his aid, Newby (1964, p. 342) says: "Thus even the beginning hearing aid user should be successful with the aid, at home with members of his family."

The schedule of use planned for the client should be as individualized as other management procedures. Some clients are positively oriented towards the use of an aid even before they open the discussion of their hearing difficulty by stating, "What I'm really hoping is that I can wear a hearing aid so I will understand what people say." Even such a positive attitude should be handled gently lest the audiologist unwittingly expose the person to a greater stimulus complexity than his mind can immediately adjust to. In Niemeyer's (1973) words:

". . . the hearing aid novice must patiently acquire his skill in dealing with the confusion of varying and rapidly changing acoustic impressions. In the initial stages he needs encouragement, guidance, and instruction to enable him to master an adaptation and training program of increasingly difficult steps."

Schedules should be designed to control two parameters: (a) the environment in which the aid is worn, and (b) the duration of its use. The aim is to increase both.

As I have already stated, initial experiences with the aid are best made at home, where the noise level is low and reverberation is minimized by curtains, carpets, and upholstered furniture. Recommendations should be made that the aid be tried initially for two or three periods of about an hour each day, until the user feels comfortable with it. Since a perceptual adjustment will be involved, the person should experiment with different settings of the volume control, not simply to determine the appropriate level but to develop some concept of how the volume control affects the loudness of sounds. The client should be advised to see how his own voice sounds to him when he speaks at soft, normal, and loud levels. Reading out loud or conversing with a cooperative family member will help him to become accustomed to his "new" voice. Listening to the voices of children or grandchildren, whose natural levels of pitch are quite a lot higher than adult voices, may bring a lot of pleasure, providing the children are not shouting or all talking at once. The radio and television should be listened to when adjusted to comfortable loudness by a person with normal hearing. The volume control of the hearing aid may need to be adjusted for this actively.

The hearing aid user should gradually expand both his listening time and the range of things he listens to. Using his "home profile," he should begin to explore using his aid in situations that previously presented difficulty. The person can be helped to rank those situations by using the overall item rating score (degree of difficulty × frequency). Have the client keep brief notes of difficulties and successes.

Once the person feels fairly confortable using the aid around the home, he or she can begin to try wearing it in similar situations when visiting friends or relatives.

The schedule should then be expanded to incorporate activities that can be planned by reference to the profile sheets for business, social, or school environments.

During this period, hearing aid counseling should continue, preferably as part of a comprehensive program of management of the person's communication problems. Auditory and visual communication training sessions, speech improvement, and adjustment counseling should be part of the support program based on the client's needs.

After 2 or 3 months, adjustment to the aid will hopefully be demonstrated by the client's growing dependency on it as an aid to living the kind of life his hearing problem had previously encroached upon. It is hoped that the aid will become as natural to him as eyeglasses are to those who cannot function without them. This will be an appropriate time at which to reassess communicative performance, using the profile development charts. Comparison of scores, item by item or section by section, will reveal whether, in the considered judgment of the client, improvement has resulted from using the hearing aid. It will also identify situations in which further investigation and training may be fruitful. Wherever possible, it helps to have the same questions answered by the husband, wife, parent, boyfriend or girlfriend of the client. This parallel pre- and post-amplification evaluation by someone close to the client aids in objectifying the perceived effects of the hearing aid on actual communication performance.

Downs (1966) outlined a program to aid parents in establishing hearing aid use by their young child. She suggests that in many cases, counseling the parents to help them accept the child's hearing loss may be the first step. I have talked a little about this earlier and will discuss it more in the final section on personal adjustment counseling. Downs (1966) advocates the firm approach: ". . . we tell him what is going to be done, and we do it."

Starting early in the morning, Downs recommends showing the child the aid while pointing to the clock (e.g., 9:00 am) indicating a 5-minute time-span during which the aid will be worn. Using physical constraint if necessary, gently insert the mold with the hearing aid turned off. If the child accepts it without protest, occupy him for 5 minutes in a pleasurable manner. If he rejects the mold, constrain him for the 5-minute duration, talking reassuringly to him. It is recommended that this be repeated 4 times a day until the mold is accepted. At the next session, Down advises that the parent turn the aid on one-quarter volume and speak softly and soothingly into the aid. The aid may then be inserted into the harness, while the child is occupied pleasantly for 5 minutes. If he objects, he should be held firmly for that period.

The next stage (second week) extends the time to 15 minutes and expands the environment by walks around the house to help the child to relate the sounds he hears to the objects or events that make them. I have discussed the importance of this procedure in a chapter on auditory training in another text (Sanders 1971).

The third stage (third week), as described by Downs, increases the time the aid is worn to 4 30-minute sessions in which the mother draws attention to the sounds her daily home activities generate.

The fourth week extends the time to 45 minutes, with the aid set at the volume setting recommended by the teacher of the deaf or the audiologist. By the sixth to eighth week, the aid hopefully will be worn most of the day. However, Downs recommends three exceptions: (1) 3 10-minute breaks each day, (2) nap time, and, (3) rough play.

A program such as that outlined by Downs depends upon the support and guidance of parent counsel. Hearing-impaired children, even those with mild losses, should be under the constant supervision of an audiologist or a teacher of the deaf. In most cases these children will need an intensive training program in which effective use of amplification is a major goal.

The period of adjustment to the use of a hearing aid is, for both child and adult, one that demands both a perceptual and a psychologic adaptation. Adjustment to the aid is a vital component of a larger psychologic reality of being a hearing-impaired person. I would like, therefore, to remind the audiologist that, although for purposes of continuity I have separated informational and personal adjustment counseling, in reality they will need to be treated as interwoven components of the orientation and counseling process.

To this point, my discussion has mainly been concerned with informational counseling. To complete this chapter, the nature of the adjustment counseling task with which you will be involved must be examined.

PERSONAL ADJUSTMENT COUNSELING

The Counselor's Role

The most common view of a counselor is that of a person with the necessary training and experience to permit him or her to diagnose a problem, to determine what is needed to effect a solution, and to direct the client in a manner aimed at achieving the changes believed necessary. The problem with such a definition is that the burden of responsibility for success or failure lies with the counselor. Furthermore, the solutions arrived at are based upon the counselor's perception of the problem, which may only vaguely approximate the client's concept of his difficulties. Unfortunately, as a counselor, the respect that comes with being an "expert" and the power inherent in being perceived by others in this role may be found to be very rewarding. Great satisfaction may be derived from the knowledge that a client needs you, that he even may be dependent upon you. These are quite natural feelings, particularly for beginners in the field. To experience these feelings should not cause you to feel guilty, but you should recognize that they are self-gratifying no matter how well you rationalize them. As such, they will not aid the counseling process. *Such feelings on the part of a counselor may in fact hinder the growth process, since you are seeking to have the client achieve independence, not dependency, and to learn how to define and solve his own difficulties, not to have solutions provided for him.*

It will probably be helpful, therefore, to adopt a nondirective approach to counseling. This approach is aimed at helping the client find solutions. It also protects you from making inappropriate decisions, and inhibits the client from "blaming" you if he does not like the suggested solution or it does not work. It does not require that you be highly trained before you can offer help, thus increasing your usefulness to the client. It also absolves you from the responsibility of making decisions, since your role is to assist the client in making decisions rather than imposing decisions upon him. Your concern is to *create a climate in which solutions to problems can be found, rather than being concerned with the solutions themselves.*

Kodman (1966) identifies three conditions that the counselor must seek to achieve if success is to be facilitated: (a) accurate empathy, (b) unconditional positive regard, and (c) self-congruence or genuineness. Each of these is drawn from the Rogerian school of client-centered therapy.

Accurate Empathy

This involves listening very carefully, to the client's problems and feelings about his problems in order to obtain as clear a picture as possible of how the situation looks and feels to him. Rogers (1951, p. 34) states:

". . . it is the counselor's aim to perceive as accurately as possible all of the perceptual field as it is being experienced by the client, with the same figure and ground relationships, to the full degree that the client is willing to communicate that perceptual field; and thus having perceived this internal frame of reference of the other as completely as possible, to indicate to the client the extent to which he is seeing through the client's eyes.''

Thus, empathy is necessary if you are to be able to absorb the emotionally laden, poorly defined problem expressed by the client and reflect it back to him with an objective focus that may permit him to see his difficulty in a new light or, as Rogers (1951) says, ''with a new quality,'' facilitating his search for a solution.

For example, a client may express the feeling: ''I don't think I could wear an aid; I mean—I'd feel funny about it.'' An empathic helper might clarify the statement by saying: ''You feel the aid would in some way be degrading; that others would think less of you,'' encouraging the client to clarify his feeling with: ''Well yes, I mean it's like admitting to having a weakness.''

Thus empathy helps guide the client to explore his feelings. The process involves *active listening* on your part.

Unconditional Positive Regard

This involves accepting the client as he is. To quote Rogers (1951, p. 20) again:

''The primary point of importance here is the attitude held by the counselor toward the worth and the significance of the individual. How do we look upon others? Do we see each person as having worth and dignity in his own right? If we do hold this point of view at the verbal level, to what extent is it operationally evident at the behavioral level? Do we tend to treat individuals as persons of worth or do we subtly devaluate them by our attitudes and behavior? Is our philosophy one in which respect for the individual is uppermost? Do we respect his capacity and right to self direction, or do we basically believe that his life would be best guided by us?

Ask yourself if you will treat the client with a hearing aid that is being bought by the State Welfare Agency with the same respect as you will the private paying client. Will you react in the same manner to the unmarried mother whose fourth child is hearing-impaired as you will to a lawyer's child who is to wear a hearing aid? Will the hearing-impaired college graduate be treated with more respect than the high-school dropout? How well will you be able to empathize with persons of differing backgrounds and patterns of behavior?

Genuineness

This arises from empathy with and respect for a client, which permit you to feel at ease in the counseling situation, to feel unthreatened, and thus able to act in a manner congruent with your true self. It means not putting on the mask of professionalism. Genuineness is evidenced by rejection of the impressive jargon of a profession, by a relaxed, friendly manner, by an ability to accept suggestions from the client and even criticism if appropriate.

"The personality of the helper must play a vital part in any helping relationship. It is the helper's use of himself which makes the interaction whatever it is to become. If a helper's self is to have such a significance, it must be involved in the dialogue." (Combs *et al.* 1971, p. 57)

These three conditions of accurate empathy, unconditional positive regard, and genuineness have been shown to correlate with a high degree of counselor effectiveness (Kodman 1966).

The Problem

I have already considered this in some detail under the heading *Understanding the Problem,* and discussed the conflict that often arises between the need to seek assistance and the acceptance of the hearing loss that act involves. The feeling of being shut off from the world, which Ramsdell (1970) explained, and the loneliness, sadness, and depression often arising from that feeling, were discussed. I pointed out that the hearing-impaired person often feels ashamed of his inability to cope, and judges his inadequacy as a weakness. Ramsdell's description of the hearing-impaired person's feelings of threat to his self-esteem and the arrogant behavior that may be used as a way of handling this threat have been considered. I suggested that the idea of wearing a hearing aid brings these feelings into focus, since it requires not only acknowledging one's hearing difficulty, but a willingness to let others know about it.

Parents of hearing-impaired children face all of these problems, plus the acute feelings of responsibility that give rise to guilt. "What did I do to deserve this?" "If I had not caught German measles this would never have happened to my child." "I feel so guilty that I did not know she was deaf until she was almost 3 years old—how could I not have known?"

I also spoke of the affects these feelings often have on the individual, causing him to arrange his or her life or the life of the child so as to avoid threatening contacts. Sullivan (1956, p. 145) states:

"The awareness of inferiority means that one is unable to keep out of consciousness the formulation of some chronic feeling of the worse sort of insecurity, and this means that one suffers anxiety and perhaps even something worse, if jealousy is really worse than anxiety. The fear that others can disrespect a person because of something he shows means that he is always insecure in his contact with other people, and this insecurity arises, not from mysterious and somewhat disguised sources as a great deal of our anxiety does, but from something which he knows he cannot fix. Now that represents an almost fatal deficiency of the self system, since the self is unable to disguise or exclude a definite formulation that reads, 'I am inferior. Therefore people will dislike me and I cannot be secure with them'."

Such feelings are usually present to some extent in all hearing-impaired persons and in the parents of hearing-impaired children. Most can handle them with only minimal help, others will need a prlonged helping relationship, and still others will have problems of a severity necessitating professional psychologic guidance. Usually, this latter group of people have personality problems that the hearing difficulty aggravates.

The problem, then, is to create a climate in which a change in the client's perceptions of his difficulties can occur and in which the client can explore new ways of solving them. If behavior is to change, the self-concept must change.

"The most important single factor affecting behavior is the self-concept. . . . the beliefs that people have about themselves are always present factors in determining their behavior. (Combs, *et al.* 1971, p. 37)

You must seek, therefore, to establish a climate to facilitate change. The requirements of such a climate have been described by Combs, *et al.* (1971, Chapter 11). They include:

1. *Establishing conditions for the confrontation of the problems by the client.* This will be best achieved by offering guidance and understanding and by proceeding in a mutual exploration of the problem with the client's help.
2. *Bring the client into dialogue with some new experience,* a stage the authors describe as the informational phase. I have discussed this earlier, as it concerns problems created by a hearing deficit and by amplification. I would include, in this section, the help which may be afforded the client by group sessions with other hearing-impaired persons.
3. *The person must discover the personal meaning of the new information.*

To achieve this climate the client must be convinced that you and they are, as Combs (1971, p. 215) say, "partners in the helping encounter." This, they state, determines the direction of that encounter by serving as a model, by pointing the way to the most fruitful paths of exploration, and by suppressing or extinguishing less profitable routes. They then list (Combs *et al.* 1971, p. 220) four criteria for an atmosphere that permits growth, they explain that the client must feel: "(a) that it is safe to try, (b) reassured that he can, (c) encouraged to make the attempt, and (d) satisfied to do so."

Finally, Combs *et al.* (1971, p. 230) state:

"Freeing atmospheres provide the stage on which exploration of self and the world takes place. For effective practice, a large portion of the helper's attention and efforts will need to be devoted to the creation of atmospheres which make exploring possible and encourage students and clients to make maximum use of relationships. When this is done well, the need of the individual for adequacy can be counted on to supply the impetus for movement."

CONCLUSION

I began by stating that I believe orientation and counseling of the potential hearing aid user should constitute the hub of a program to ensure effective use of amplification. I hope that from the discussion of this topic, you will conclude that the task of meeting the needs of the hearing aid user extends well beyond the mechanics of instruction in the use and care of a hearing aid. How the client or the parents of a hearing-impaired child feels about the hearing problem may be aggravated by a recommendation that a hearing aid be worn. Support during the period of adjustment and acceptance of the aid will be, in many cases, the factor that ensures success.

You should not be dissuaded from becoming involved in counseling by a lack of formal training. If the task is accepted as one involving cooperative problem-solving in which both the counselor and the client together seek to define difficulties and devise solutions, situations that threaten a professional image should not arise. Basic requirements are a willingness to listen, a willingness and an ability to empathize, and a willingness to accept. Beyond these, clear thinking and practicability, supported by a knowledge of hearing impairment, should be sufficient to facilitate movement towards solutions.

Above all, remember that the hearing-impaired client is an individual. Success in providing effective service depends upon the ability to define and provide for each client's highly individualized needs.

BIBLIOGRAPHY

American Medical Association: The committee on medical rating of physical impairment. JAMA 177:489−501, 1961

Atherley GRC, Noble WG: Clinical picture of occupational hearing loss obtained with the hearing measurement scale, in DW Robinson (ed): Occupational Hearing Loss, London, Academic Press, 1971

Carhart R: An improved method for classifying audiograms. Laryngoscope 55:640−662, 1945

Combs AW, Avila DL, Purkey WW: Helping Relationships: Basic Concepts for the Helping Professions. Boston, Allyn and Bacon, 1971

Davis H: The articulation area and the social adequacy index for hearing. Laryngoscope 58:761−778, 1948

Downs MP: The establishment of hearing aid use—a program for parents. Maico Audiol Libr Ser 4:5, 1966

Downs MP: Maintaining children's hearing aids—the role of the parents. Maico Audiol Libr Ser 10:1, 1971

Freedman JL, Doob AN: Deviancy—The Psychology of Being Different. New York and London, Academic Press, 1968

Giolas TG: The measurement of hearing handicap. Maico Audiol Libr Ser 8:6, 1970

Goffman E: Stigma: Notes on the Management of Spoiled Identity. Englewood Cliffs, Prentice-Hall, 1963

High W, Fairbanks G, Glorig A: Scale for self-assessment of hearing handicap. J Speech Hear Disord 29:215−230, 1964

Horton KB, McConnell F: Early intervention for the young deaf child through parent training. Proc Int Congress Education Deaf (Stockholm) 1:291−296, 1970

Kodman F: Techniques for counseling the hearing aid client. Maico Audiol Libr Ser 4:8, 1966

Koniditsiotis CY: The use of hearing tests to provide information about the extent to which an individual's hearing loss handicaps him. Maico Audiol Libr Ser 9:10, 1971

Luterman D: A parent-oriented nursery program for pre-school deaf children—a follow-up study. Volta Rev 73:106−112, 1971

McConnell F: Proceedings of the conference on current practices in the management of deaf infants (0−3 years). The Bill Wilkerson Center, Vanderbilt University, Nashville, Tennessee, 1968

Meyerson L: The psychology of impaired hearing, in Cruickshank W (ed): Psychology of Exceptional Children and Youth, Englewood Cliffs, Prentice-Hall, 1963

Niemeyer W: Psychological aspects of hearing-aid fitting. J Audiol Tech 12:3, 1973. Reprinted in Maico Audiol Libr Ser 12:3 and 4, 1974

Newby H: Audiology (ed 2). New York, Appleton-Century-Crofts, 1964

Noble WG: The measurement of hearing handicap: a further viewpoint. Maico Audiol Libr Ser 10:5, 1972

Noble WG, Atherley GRC: The hearing measurement scale; a questionnaire for the assessment of auditory disability. J Audit Res 10:193−214, 1970

Paulos TH: Short-term rehabilitation program for hard-of-hearing children. Hear News 29:4−7, 1961

Pollack D: Educational Audiology for the Limited Hearing Infant. Springfield, CC Thomas, 1972

Public Citizen's Retired Professional Action Group: Paying Through the Ear, a Report on Hearing Care Problems, 1973, Public Citizen, PO Box 19404 Washington, DC, 20036

Ramsdell DA: The psychology of the hard-of-hearing and deafened adult, in Davis H, Silverman SR (ed): Hearing and Deafness (ed 3). New York, Holt Rinehart and Winston, 1970

Rogers C: Client-Centered Therapy. Boston, Houghton Mifflin, 1951

Rousey CL: Psychological reactions to hearing loss. J Speech Hear Disor 36:382−389, 1971

Sanders DA: Aural Rehabilitation, Englewood Cliffs, Prentice Hall, 1971a

Sanders DA: A case management approach to aural rehabilitation. Hear Speech News 35:4−7, 1971b

Sandlin RE: The psychology of the hearing impaired. Hearing Instruments 25:22−23, 1974

Senden M von: Space and Sight. The Perception of Space and Shape in the Congenitally Blind Before and After Operation. London, Methuen, 1960

Shore I: Hearing aid consultation, in Katz J (ed): Handbook of Clinical Audiology. Baltimore, Williams & Wilkins, 1972, p. 656

Stark RE: Sensory Capabilities of Hearing Impaired Children. Baltimore, University Park Press, 1974

Sullivan HS: Paranoid dynamism, in Perry HS, Gawel ML, Gebbon M (eds): Clinical Studies in Psychiatry, New York, Norton, 1956, p. 145

Warfield F: Cotton in My Ears, New York, Viking, 1948

APPENDIX A

Profile Questionnaire for Rating Communicative Performance in a Home Environment

1. a) In my living room, when I can see the speakers face, I have:

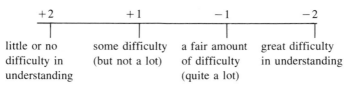

little or no difficulty in understanding | some difficulty (but not a lot) | a fair amount of difficulty (quite a lot) | great difficulty in understanding

   b) This happens:

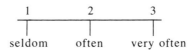

seldom   often   very often

2. a) If I am talking with a person in my living room or family room while the television, radio, or record player is on, I have:

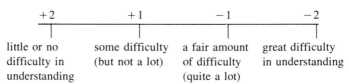

little or no difficulty in understanding | some difficulty (but not a lot) | a fair amount of difficulty (quite a lot) | great difficulty in understanding

   b) This happens:

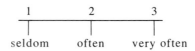

seldom   often   very often

3. a) In a quiet room in my house, if I cannot see the speakers face I have:

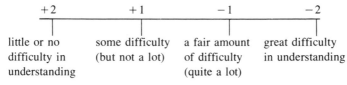

little or no difficulty in understanding | some difficulty (but not a lot) | a fair amount of difficulty (quite a lot) | great difficulty in understanding

   b) This happens:

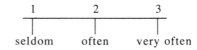

seldom   often   very often

4. a) If some one in my house speaks to me from another room on the same floor, I epxerience:

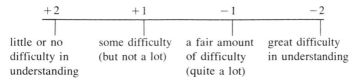

+2	+1	−1	−2
little or no difficulty in understanding	some difficulty (but not a lot)	a fair amount of difficulty (quite a lot)	great difficulty in understanding

   b) This happens:

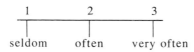

1	2	3
seldom	often	very often

5. a) If someone calls me from upstairs when I am downstairs, or from the window when I am in the garden, I will experience:

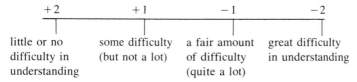

+2	+1	−1	−2
little or no difficulty in understanding	some difficulty (but not a lot)	a fair amount of difficulty (quite a lot)	great difficulty in understanding

   b) This happens:

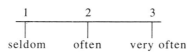

1	2	3
seldom	often	very often

6. a) Understanding people at the dinner table gives me:

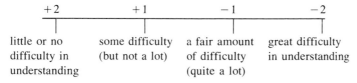

+2	+1	−1	−2
little or no difficulty in understanding	some difficulty (but not a lot)	a fair amount of difficulty (quite a lot)	great difficulty in understanding

   b) This happens:

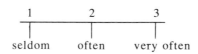

1	2	3
seldom	often	very often

7. a) When I sit talking with friends in a quiet room, I have:

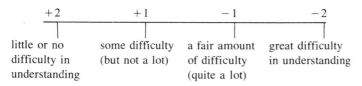

+2	+1	−1	−2
little or no difficulty in understanding	some difficulty (but not a lot)	a fair amount of difficulty (quite a lot)	great difficulty in understanding

b) This happens:

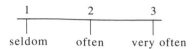

8. a) Listening to the radio or record player or watching TV gives me:

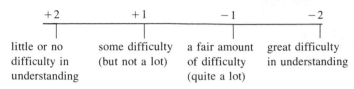

b) This happens:

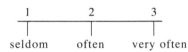

9. a) When I use the phone at home, I have:

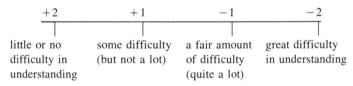

b) This happens:

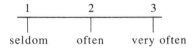

APPENDIX B

Profile Questionnaire for Rating Communicative Performance in an Occupational Environment

1. a) In talking with someone in the room where I work, I have:

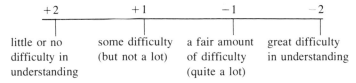

b) This happens:

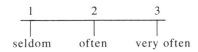

2. a) When I am in a room at work where there is noise, I have:

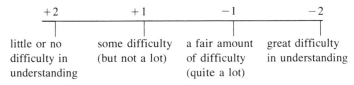

b) This happens:

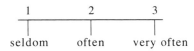

3. a) When I am at a meeting with a small group of people, around a table in a fairly quiet room, I have:

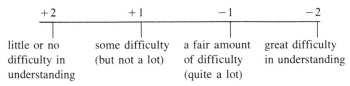

b) This happens:

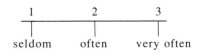

4. a) If I have to take notes by dictation in a fairly quiet room, I have:

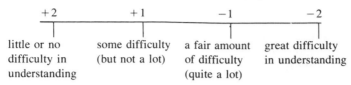

+2	+1	−1	−2
little or no difficulty in understanding	some difficulty (but not a lot)	a fair amount of difficulty (quite a lot)	great difficulty in understanding

b) This happens:

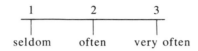

1	2	3
seldom	often	very often

5. a) If I have to make notes at a meeting, I have:

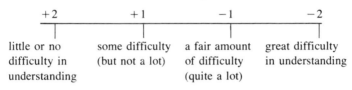

+2	+1	−1	−2
little or no difficulty in understanding	some difficulty (but not a lot)	a fair amount of difficulty (quite a lot)	great difficulty in understanding

b) This happens:

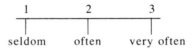

1	2	3
seldom	often	very often

6 a) If I have to use the phone at work, I have:

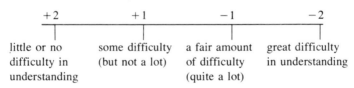

+2	+1	−1	−2
little or no difficulty in understanding	some difficulty (but not a lot)	a fair amount of difficulty (quite a lot)	great difficulty in understanding

b) This happens:

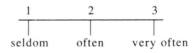

1	2	3
seldom	often	very often

APPENDIX C

Profile Questionnaire for Rating Communicative Performance in a Social Environment

1. a) If we are entertaining a group of friends, understanding someone against the background of others talking gives me:

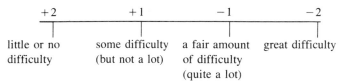

+2	+1	−1	−2
little or no difficulty	some difficulty (but not a lot)	a fair amount of difficulty (quite a lot)	great difficulty

   b) This happens:

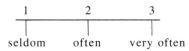

1	2	3
seldom	often	very often

2. a) If we are playing cards, understanding my partner gives me:

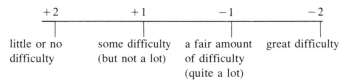

+2	+1	−1	−2
little or no difficulty	some difficulty (but not a lot)	a fair amount of difficulty (quite a lot)	great difficulty

   b) This happens:

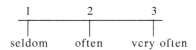

1	2	3
seldom	often	very often

3. a) When I am at the theatre or the movies, I have:

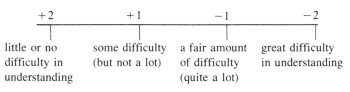

+2	+1	−1	−2
little or no difficulty in understanding	some difficulty (but not a lot)	a fair amount of difficulty (quite a lot)	great difficulty in understanding

   b) This happens:

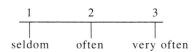

1	2	3
seldom	often	very often

4. a) In church, when the minister gives the sermon, I have:

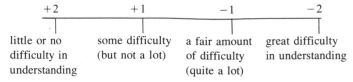

b) This happens:

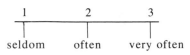

5. a) In following the conversation when we eat out, I have:

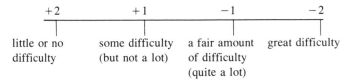

b) This happens:

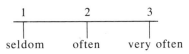

6. a) In the car, I find that understanding what people are saying gives me:

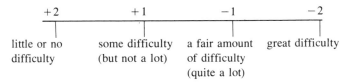

b) This happens:

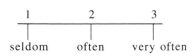

7. a) When I am outside talking with someone, I have:

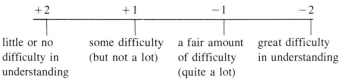

b) This happens:

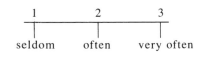

APPENDIX D

**Profile Questionnaire for Rating
Communicative Performance
in a School Environment**

1. a) When I am working with Mary, individually, at my desk, she is able to understand
what I say with:

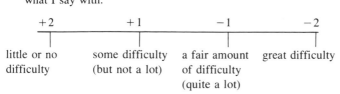

+2	+1	−1	−2
little or no difficulty	some difficulty (but not a lot)	a fair amount of difficulty (quite a lot)	great difficulty

b) This happens:

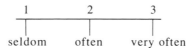

1	2	3
seldom	often	very often

2. a) When she is one of a small group of children in a learning situation, she understands what I say with:

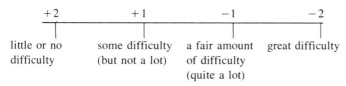

+2	+1	−1	−2
little or no difficulty	some difficulty (but not a lot)	a fair amount of difficulty (quite a lot)	great difficulty

b) This happens:

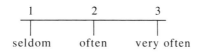

1	2	3
seldom	often	very often

3. a) In a small group she understands what the other children say with:

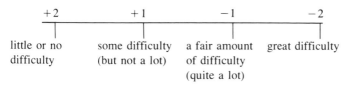

+2	+1	−1	−2
little or no difficulty	some difficulty (but not a lot)	a fair amount of difficulty (quite a lot)	great difficulty

b) This happens:

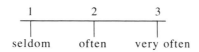

1	2	3
seldom	often	very often

4. a) When I speak to the class as a whole, Mary is able to understand with:

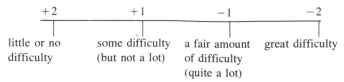

little or no   some difficulty   a fair amount   great difficulty
difficulty   (but not a lot)   of difficulty
                                           (quite a lot)

b) This happens:

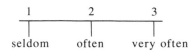

seldom   often   very often

5. a) When we watch a movie film, television program, or filmstrip, she seems to understand with:

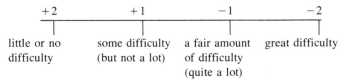

little or no   some difficulty   a fair amount   great difficulty
difficulty   (but not a lot)   of difficulty
                                           (quite a lot)

b) This happens:

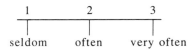

seldom   often   very often

6. a) In playground or gymnasium games or in activities, she is able to follow verbal directions with:

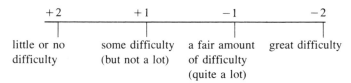

little or no   some difficulty   a fair amount   great difficulty
difficulty   (but not a lot)   of difficulty
                                           (quite a lot)

b) This happens:

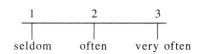

seldom   often   very often

7. a) In her contact with the other children in class, and in social activities during break periods, she seems to understand with:

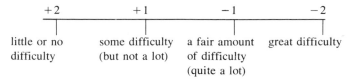

+2	+1	−1	−2
little or no difficulty	some difficulty (but not a lot)	a fair amount of difficulty (quite a lot)	great difficulty

b) This happens:

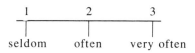

1	2	3
seldom	often	very often

Melvin J. Sorkowitz

11
Business Aspects of Hearing Aid Dispensing

With changing philosophies and codes of ethics, more and more audiologists are becoming directly involved in the dispensing of hearing aids. Unfortunately, there are few graduate programs in Audiology to provide us with the financial orientation necessary to run a successful business.

Melvin Sorkowitz was trained as an audiologist and has been a hearing aid dispenser for more than ten years. In his chapter he provides a basic business orientation and philosophical set for the audiologist who dispenses hearing aids. It is an excellent primer, but it is not an end-all. As Mel would say, the first thing for an audiologist to do is to employ a good lawyer and a good accountant.

MCP

The first requisite for the professional dispenser is commitment. Dispensing hearing aids is a difficult, arduous, anxiety-provoking task. You are "selling" a product to a population that is basically negative toward you and the prothestic device. The reasons for this negativism are multifaceted. You, as a dispenser, however, must be prepared to sell yourself and the device to the hearing aid user with all the gusto you can muster. By selling, I mean selling in the rehabilitative sense, not selling for selling's sake. After all, you are charging a substantial fee for your professional services and it is your responsibility to deliver. You are selling a product and service that is unwanted, for the most part, and the only way to be comfortable in dealing with the rejection and elation of helping the hearing-impaired is to know within yourself that you understand what you are doing and to know that you are earning your income because of someone else's misfortune—but in the most honest, efficient manner possible. It is only to your benefit, therefore, that you realize that the minute you accept his or her money, you accept the responsibility for your client. Also, you will be making all or most of your income from the sale of hearing aids. Therefore, you will have to charge significantly more than you pay for the product. *If you do not plan to make a profit, don't sell hearing aids.*

METHODS OF DISPENSING

The method by which you choose to dispense will be largely dependent on several factors. These factors, as I view them, are: 1. geographical location and need for services; 2. availability of capital; 3. the market; and 4. your own particular personality and desires. There are various settings in which hearing aids can be dispensed: on your own; with a large institution; or with private physicians. Certainly, the most fragile of these and probably the most financially rewarding is the free-standing office totally financed and operated under your sole aegis. It is to this particular dispensing environment that I will address myself, because of my ten years of dispensing experience in this area. All of the suggestions made can be extrapolated to suit the other environments, as you wish.

You must, if you are going to be successful in your business, be willing to admit what you don't know and to solicit help from those capable of helping you. You must enlist the aid of an attorney and an accountant to assist you in setting up your business. Don't be afraid to pay for advice, because you have no choice: one way, or the other, you will pay! The cost of undoing mistakes is more than paying initial fees to these professionals.

PHYSICAL SETTING FOR THE OFFICE

The decision regarding the physical aspects of your office depends entirely on your tastes. I suggest however, that you *keep the geriatric patient in mind when decorating.* For example, soft-cushioned sofas and chairs are contraindicated in a hearing aid dispensing office. In fact, straight back chairs are best. I found that old fashioned dental chairs are excellent in the consultation rooms because you can hydraulically control the height for mold work, etc. These chairs can be purchased very reasonably from most dental supply houses. Also, considering your clientele, you should display pictures and art work that engender nostalgic feelings. Flashy, noveau art tends not to instill the warmth needed to win patient confidence. I found, for example, that an old lithograph of the famous RCA picture "His Master's Voice" within eyeshot of the patient can be of tremendous value in establishing rapport.

I think the ideal physical arrangement for an office is a five room configuration. This consists of a reception/waiting room, small consult room, large consult room, repair labs and storage, and private office.

In your reception/waiting room you should have the necessary chairs, tables, lamps, and magazines for your clients. Your secretary/receptionist should have a large desk, copy machine, bookkeeping system, typewriter, scheduling book, and telephone.

The small consultation room should serve for post-fitting visits, spot repairs, mold adjustments, etc. It is not necessary to have a sound room, but a good portable desk-top audiometer is useful for quick threshold assessments. All necessary hand tools should be accessible in this room. Table 11-1 is a list of what I consider to be the necessary tools and accessories for a hearing aid office.

The large consultation room is where you make your initial contact with your prospective client. Attention to proper detail is of utmost importance. A sound room, to your specifications, is required with the proper audiometric equipment that suits your methods of assessing amplification needs. I will not influence you with my attitudes toward hearing aid evaluative techniques, except to say be comfortable with whatever method you choose. If it works for you, stick with it.

PROCEDURES FOR EVALUATION

My procedure in performing the hearing aid evaluation is the following.

1. *Thorough case history.* This is critical because many times the hearing aid candidate is accompanied by a relative, and taking this information establishes rapport with all parties. Many potential hearing aid users have negative attitudes. Since hearing loss is a family as well as a personal problem, you must deal with the family as well as the client.

2. *A complete audiological assessment.* This should be done, including air/bone and speech studies along with any special tests that may be indicated.

3. *A hearing aid evaluation.* This is needed to determine gain, output, and frequency response needs.

4. *A complete explanation of all findings and recommendations.* Include in this the uncomfortable subject of fees. The best approach is a direct one, and I have always found it more effective to bring up the subject myself. We each have our own particular methods of dealing with this subject, compatible with our own personalities.

5. *Closing the session.* Set up an appointment for the final fitting and consultation session. I strongly recommend a 10 to 14 day interval between evaluation and fitting. This allows enough time for you to get the mold (if one is required) and the appropriate instrument. I see no real need to stock instruments, unless it is part of your evaluative methodology. In addition, the user will have the

Table 11-1
New Office Supplies

Stock molds	Dummy cases
Earmold attachments	Presentation cases
Anvil for hinge screws	Instruction booklets
Scissors	Hand mirror
Blunt end tweezer	Glue
Hot air blower	Earmold box labels
Hand blower	Earmold mailing boxes
Earmold reamer	Earmold order forms
Test tips	Repair forms
Earmold box—plastic	Audiograms
Tubing—all sizes	History forms
Earmold material	Temple tips
Syringe	Filters
Packing instrument	Ear defenders
Mixing cup	Price lists
Spatula	Dri-Aid
Battery tester	Cetylcide
Files	Eyeglass cleaner
Screw drivers	Dental lathe and accessories for buffing
Pipe cleaners	Stapler
Otoscope	Paper clips
Mold material	Charts and holders
Cotton	Ultrasonic cleaner
Needle nose pliers	Battery envelopes
Taps	Wire cutters
Drill bits	Razor blades
Wire strippers	Vials for swim plugs
Acetone	New dealer kits from manufacturers
Tweezers	Tissues
Crochet hook	Dental drill
Screws	Batteries—all sizes

feeling that his aid is being built to "prescription." My personal bias is that if you have performed your job properly, the user's feeling is close to correct.

So, the first visit is over. You have won the confidence of the client; he or she has given you a good faith deposit and has an appointment to see you within two weeks.

At the initial visit, you should require a $50.00 deposit to cover your costs. You should explain that the balance is payable at the time of delivery. *Do not assume that the patient realizes that automatically.* If the patient cannot pay the balance of your fee, you can arrange for one-half payment and 60 days for the balance at no interest. Anything over 60 days should be financed at the bank. You should be able to work out some arrangements with your bank or you can also offer credit card arrangements.

COUNSELING THE HEARING AID USER

When the aid and mold arrive, your secretary should prepare a packet for the fitting orientation session. This packet should contain all information pertinent to the aid and your services.

It is extremely important that you standardize your presentation to the user. In fact, you may want to prepare a check list to give the patient. This accomplishes several things: first, it serves as a guideline for you in the session; second, the user can refer to it along with family members at home; and third, it is a defensive maneuver in that the user cannot blame you for "not telling me that."

Keep the instructions simple. Do not try to communicate every possible eventuality that can occur because invariably that which will never occur will be what is remembered—mostly out of context! Use your instructional check list to the letter. It may become excruciatingly boring, but it will save you hours of post-fitting frustration.

After you have talked about the product and explained about amplification in general, perhaps the hardest job is ahead—getting the user to physically put the aid and mold on the ear.

I always find it best to tell the patient that it is difficult to learn, but I follow it up with the statement that, "everybody eventually learns how." You can use a model ear, which is available from most earmold laboratories. This learning on the part of the user, however, is kinesthetic learning and extremely difficult to communicate, especially to the elderly. I say something such as, "did you ever hit a nail with a hammer?" The answer is usually, "yes." Therefore, I say, "the first few times were difficult, weren't they?" Again, the answer is "yes." "Why do you suppose it was difficult?" Answer, "I don't know." My response, "well, if you think about it, you really didn't know how high to hold the hammer, how hard to hit the nail, how firm to hold the nail, etc.—well, it's the same with your new aid; you must develop a touch." This analogy seems to work well.

You are then ready to test the patient with the aid. Again, I am not going to "prescribe" the procedure except that I always find that anything I can do to instill confidence in family members, and the user, is very important. Recorded word lists or information read from current periodicals requiring patient response are always helpful, if the patient is lucid enough to respond.

Do not allow the user to leave your office until he or she knows how to manipulate the instrument and earmold. You may want to "get rid of him," but don't! The reason is that he will be back and he probably will have reinforced some bad habits making it even more difficult to teach him correctly. If you are fortunate enough to have a competent secretary or assistant, have them bear some of the "brunt" of orientation, so that you can stay fresh for your next customer.

APPROACHING THE MARKET

The remainder of this chapter is designed to help you in the business of hearing aids and the business of practicing the "art" of dispensing. I will try not to be too simplistic; however, the "how to" approach seems the best method for explaining the various subjects. Let's start from the very beginning.

The Market

Your marketing plan is going to be directly related to the mode you choose in dispensing. There are three modes to choose from: private practice, an institution, or a physician's office. Of course, combinations of the three are also used in some situations.

If you choose the private practice avenue, your marketing thrust must be in two directions: toward the physician and toward the consumer. In a free-standing office, your physician contact should be the otolaryngologists. It is not advisable to solicit general practitioners and pediatricians because they are the source of many otological referrals and you start infringing on your own potential referral relationships.

I do not advise direct mailings to consumers; however, announcements to newspapers, physicians, nursing homes, senior citizens groups, etc., are perfectly legitimate and potentially profitable.

If you choose the private practice mode, make sure you have enough potential referral sources to "support" you. The best way to determine this is to, by direct contact, simply ask, "Doctor, how many aids do you refer a month?" and, "Would you refer to me?" It's a good idea to stack your referral sources by age. By this I mean that you should have young, middle-aged, and older otologists' referring to you because young doctors see young patients and so forth.

In the hospital or institutional setting, the market is slightly different because you aren't in jeopardy of offending the physician as easily. Therefore, you must contact all of your potential referral sources and offer a total rehabilitation package. Education is the key to this market. For example, a lecture to OB-gyn or pediatric residents relative to infant screening helps you get your foot in the door for hearing aid referrals. All the other positive aspects of good human relations are necessary, regardless of the mode you choose.

If you choose to dispense from a physician's office, he or the physician group is the market and is easily defined. All you have to do in this market is develop good working relationships with your coworkers and satisfy your customers.

Capitalizing the Business

After you have established the market and mode of dispensing, you must prepare financial pro forma statements, etc. to allow you to see exactly what you are doing and where you are going. The following should help in this task (Walsh 1979).

PRO FORMA PROFIT/LOSS STATEMENT

The amount of money needed to start a business of this nature can vary greatly; but if we assume that most dispensers would like to begin in a position of reasonable investment and realize a reasonable return, we can develop a sequential formula that will lead us to a "base capital need" figure. The fixed (regular and nonvarying) costs will be determined by the location to a great degree. If you are located in proximity to a medical environment, there is generally not much latitude in a rent figure. A good-sized office is about 500 to 800 square feet. Anything more than that would be a bit of a luxury when starting new. Add to the rent the other estimated operating expenses: heat, electricity, telephone, insurance, postage, etc., and a reasonable salary. This would be projected over the first year, by month. The same would be done with sales projections, by dollars, by month. From this is subtracted the cost of sales, hearing aids, batteries, etc., which will give us a projected gross profit or loss (Table 11-2). If the operating expenses are greater than the gross profit, the company is in a loss position, and capital (cash) will be needed to supplement the business until that time when it at least breaks even. A reduction in salary would, of course, be comparable to injecting that amount of capital. But, one additional step to determine the total capital (cash) needs must be taken, and that is a cash flow projection.

CASH FLOW PROJECTION

Expenses are paid with cash, not profit. A cash flow or cash budget is predicted on a month by month basis with incoming and outgoing cash being considered. (Table 11-3). In a new business of this nature, the "trap" that the unwary seem to fall into, other than the difficulty of predicting sales volume, is in not realizing the effect of a cash "gap" in accounts payable (cash due on the merchandise and hearing instruments to suppliers) and in accounts receivable (cash owed by customers for merchandise and services you have supplied). Figure 11-1 describes a potential 90-day segment in business, dealing with one patient. At day 15 the customer is evaluated and a hearing aid and mold ordered. The aid is shipped and *billed,* which begins the 30-day term that is most suppliers' policy. (Some have shorter payment terms.) The shaded area represents the 30 days, and payment is due on the 15th of the following month. If there

Table 11-2
Pro Forma Profit/Loss Statement,* 10 Months

	Months									
	1	2	3	4	5	6	7	8	9	10
Estimated sales										
Number of sales, instruments and fees	7	10	10	10	12	13	14	15	15	15
@ $300 each sales dollars	2100	3000	3000	3000	3600	3900	4200	4500	4500	4500
Cost of goods sold—instruments and molds	1050	1500	1500	1500	1800	1950	2100	2250	2250	2250
Gross profit	1050	1500	1500	1500	1800	1950	2100	2250	2250	2250
Estimated expenses										
Operating expenses	900†	800†	600	600	600	600	600	600	600	600
Salary	1000	1000	1000	1000	1000	1000	1000	1000	1000	1000
Estimated expense total	1900	1800	1600	1600	1600	1600	1600	1600	1600	1600
Estimated profit or (loss)	(850)	(300)	(100)	(100)	200	350	500	650	650	650

*Without consideration for capital equipment.
†Extraordinary starting expenses.

is no "down payment" received at the time of fitting, there is a 15-day "cash gap" created between the time the supplier is paid, and the time you receive payment from the patient (day 45 to day 60). If your cost of an instrument and a mold comes to $150, then, depending upon your sales success, there could be $1500 to $3000 floating at all times just on instrument sales. Any extended receivables beyond 60 days obviously compound the problems.

The accounts payable—accounts receivable cash flow determination will be mostly influenced by your philosophy of doing business. It's always best to begin with a firm payment policy and maintain it. Asking the customer for payment is the most difficult chore that most new dispensers contend with; they are much more uncomfortable than the customer. Table 11-3 represents a 10-month cash flow projection based on the sales projections shown in Table 11-2 (pro forma profit and loss). Estimated is collecting 100% of receivables each month (very optimistic), and projected is a cash shortfall in the first five months of $3,950.00. If collecting of receivables drops to 80% of total, per month, $1,294.00 must be added to that need for the five months.

Table 11-3
Cash Flow—10-Month Projection

	Months									
	1	*2*	*3*	*4*	*5*	*6*	*7*	*8*	*9*	*10*
Cash sales	1050	1500	1500	1500	1800	1950	2100	2250	2250	2250
Receivables from previous month	0	1050	1500	1500	1500	1800	1950	2100	2250	2250
Estimated receipts (incoming cash)	1050	2250	3000	3000	3300	3750	4050	4350	4500	4500
Operating expense	900	800	600	600	600	600	600	600	600	600
Accounts payable	1050	1500	1500	1500	1800	1950	2100	2250	2250	2250
Salary	1000	1000	1000	1000	1000	1000	1000	1000	1000	1000
Estimated payments (outgoing cash)	2650	3100	3100	3100	3400	3550	3700	3850	3850	3850
Cash Required	(1900)	(750)	(100)	(100)	(100)	200	350	500	650	650
Safety Level*	200	200	200	200	200	200				
Working capital surplus or (Shortage)	(2100)	(950)	(300)	(300)	(300)	(—)	350	500	650	650

*Minimum amount of cash on hand for unanticipated contingencies.

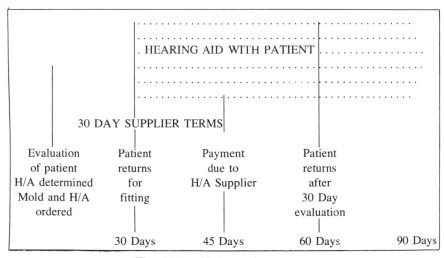

Fig. 11-1. 90-day patient sequence

CAPITAL EQUIPMENT NEEDS

We are now in a position to consider the capital equipment needs. You need $3,950.00 cash *during* the first five months of operation, plus you must acquire sound room, audiometer, office furniture, tools, etc. (Table 11-4). Listed is what would be considered basic equipment needs to open a dispensing business. There are, of course, other areas of testing and evaluating that could generate fees and enhance business, but they can factored in as the need (market) arises. This equipment would be satisfactory to begin operations.

Table 11-4
Capital Equipment—Estimate

Two-Channel Audiometer	$2500.00
6 ft × 6 ft sound booth with speakers and amplifier	7700.00
Hearing aid evaluator	2000.00
Impedance audiometer	2000.00
Office furniture	3500.00
Tools and miscellaneous	300.00
	Total $16,000.00

FINANCING ALTERNATIVES

There are three basic methods of obtaining funds for capital equipment. Listed in order of desirability, they are:

1. Outright purchase from your own funds.
2. Outright purchase with funds borrowed from a bank or lending institution; the equipment would be used for collateral.
3. Leased from a leasing company.

In method 1 you save monthly payments and you have a four-year depreciation tax write-off of $4,000.00 each year against the profits of the business. Your advantage would be the difference in interest between what you would receive on your money if left in a bank or savings institution, and what you might pay in interest in other plans. The difference would run 6–10 percent to your advantage. In method 2 (Table 11-5), tax write-offs are both the four-year depreciation and the interest on the loan. The cost of this method is less expensive than method 3 (Table 11-6), leasing, but sometimes more difficult to obtain if money is in short supply. Many times, the Federal Government's SBA (Small Business Administration) Program can be helpful when an individual is having difficulty obtaining funds. This is a program where the government guarantees payment of the loan to a bank if the borrower defaults. The negative aspect is the red tape that must be waded through, and there is the potential extended time element to obtain the loan, plus the extra paperwork each month that SBA demands. In

Table 11-5
Method Two—Bank Loan

Amount	$16,000
Term	4 years
Interest	12% annual
Monthly payment	$421.35
Total cost	$4,224.80

essence, you have taken on a partner, but in this era of tight money it may be your only alternative.

In method 3 (Table 11-6), the lease company retains ownership of the equipment during the term of the lease, (four years), and then there is some prearranged buyout by you. Usually it's a percentage amount; in this case, 7 percent of the original. This arrangement is the easiest to obtain, so is usually the most costly. The lease payments are business expenses (tax deductible). What you are paying for is the ability to terminate the agreement at any time, but you are giving up any equity potential.

By this procedure we have backed into the financial considerations of creating a pro forma profit and loss and cash flows without a consideration for capital equipment. At this point, you can take the capital (cash) you have available, deduct the cash you will need to operate the business, and then decide the best method of financing the capital equipment. This exercise would, of course, apply when you are considering a free-standing private practice or a medical clinical partnership.

What we have explored here is a system of sequential steps, an outline, which, when you "plug in" the facts and figures relevant to your prospective area, could give you some direction. The next move would be the preparation of a professional presentation or, perhaps, two—one to a bank or lending institution, and another to a medical group or private hospital. They will want to know the market, sales prospects, prospective investment and return on investment, profit potential, and cash needs. You now have a better understanding of the terminology and the interrelationship of some of those financial forms and methods.

Table 11-6
Method Three—Lease Plan

Amount	$16,000
Term	4 years
Monthly payment	$440.00
Buy out after 4 years, 7%	$1,100.00
Total cost	$6,220.00

One last bit of advice—the use of professional help, e.g., attorneys, accountants, etc.—is money well spent. *Financial arrangements, tax laws, and contractural agreements are critical to the operation and success of a business and should be handled by qualified experts.*

How to Maintain the Business

There is an old adage that "it is much easier to build a business than it is to maintain one." The reasons for this are myriad; however, what the statement probably directly relates to is that once a business is built, some people become "too comfortable" with their success and this comfort can gradually erode the business. The purpose of this section is to give you direct ideas on how to maintain your business.

INVENTORY

Your inventory needs are going to probably be in direct relationship to your philosophical ideas about the evaluation of hearing aids. For example, if you choose to do conventional hearing aid evaluations, such as the modified Carhart technique, you will need a substantial inventory representative of many manufacturers in order to complete a valid hearing aid evaluation. On the other hand, should you choose the master aid or any other suprathreshold testing technique that allows you to measure the physical perimeters of sound, you will need a very limited inventory. All you have to do after utilizing suprathreshold sound pressure measurement test techniques is call and order the appropriate hearing aid you desire, and reschedule your patient for several weeks for a hearing aid fitting. This, for me, works very well and I personally feel very comfortable utilizing the technique. Remember, the hearing aids you purchase are not producing revenue for you even though you will sell the hearing aids at some point in time. In addition, in this modern electronic age, there are many methods and pieces of equipment that are very valuable in assessing a person's hearing without a live hearing aid.

SERVICE

You have several alternatives. First, you can try to provide most of the service yourself. This necessitates your being technically qualified, or hiring someone who is technically qualified, to service and repair the hearing instruments. I used this method for about six years and found it to be very costly and very difficult to manage. The reason for this is that as you become busier dispensing, evaluating, and counselling your patients, you find you have less and less time for the tedium of repairing hearing instruments. Therefore, if you hire someone to do it, you are introducing another variable into your office, meaning a particular individual with all the concomittant problems of any individual working in your office. In other words, you are inviting personnel problems. The third reason I don't recommend doing your own repairs is that it is virtually impossible to repair all models and makes of hearing aids as well as the manufacturer. Therefore, suppose that you do a spot repair and change a microphone. You charge a reasonable fee for this service and give your user a six-month warranty. Suppose that four months later the user reports back to your office and you diagnose the hearing aid as having a defective amplifier. It is neither in your best interest nor the user's to do this service, therefore, you send it back to the manufacturer for repair. Naturally, the manufacturer is going to charge you for replacing this amplifier and, in addition, you are going to have to pass the charge along to the user. You are therefore inviting a difficult confrontation between you and user and the dialogue could go something like this: User, "I thought you told me this hearing aid had a six month warranty." Dispenser, "I did, but that was just for the repair of the microphone." User, "I thought that it meant that if it was repaired, it was under warranty for anything that happened in six months, etc. etc." It is quite apparent that you are inviting difficulty by trying to repair your own hearing instruments.

I find it much more efficient to invest in a "loaner" stock. By doing this, I am able to simplify the operation for everybody. Consider yourself—if you had a hearing aid and something was wrong with it, would you rather have it repaired and have to wait two or three days for it or would you rather have a loaner and have the instrument sent to the factory for a complete overhaul with a warranty on the repair? I think the answer is evident. Figure 11-2 illustrates the form I have the user sign for loaner instruments. I have rarely had a problem with a hearing aid user abusing the loaners—in fact, I believe I make quite a few friends by providing this particular service for them.

At the end of this chapter, a reference sheet is presented on hearing aid trouble-shooting that should prove useful in solving many user problems.

In the event of loss or damage as a result of my negligence, I _____ accept responsibility for this hearing aid model # _____ serial # _____.
This does not mean normal deterioration or mechanical failure.
This hearing aid has a value of $ _____.

        Signature (patient) _____

        Signature (ACI)   _____

        Date   _____

Fig. 11-2. Form for loaner instruments

BATTERIES

Your hearing aid users are going to require batteries at various intervals and it is certainly not to your advantage to tell them to obtain them from some other source. Figure 11-3 illustrates the battery program I utilized in my dispensing office. The program took a long time to develop and evolved after much trial and error. The advantages to this program are the following: 1. All money for

---

SERVICE AND BATTERIES
POLICIES AND PRICES

In order to maintain your hearing instrument at maximum efficiency and provide you with batteries at a reasonable cost, our policy is as follows:

1. A *Free* package of batteries is provided at the time of delivery of any new hearing instrument.

2. Batteries can be paid for in advance. This allows you (7) packages of batteries at the cost of (6). In addition, you need write only one check for your batteries. Your hearing instrument requires # _____ batteries at a prepaid cost of $ _____. All you have to do is call whenever you require batteries and after you have received your (6) packages your bonus pack will be sent. Individual packages cost $ _____ per package, however no bonus batteries are provided unless batteries are paid for in advance. These prices include postage and handling.

3. We request that you visit our office at six month intervals to assure maximum efficiency of your instrument. It is important that all aspects of your hearing aid be closely observed in that even slight changes in your hearing, mold, or instrument can produce negative results. We will send you periodic reminders to come in for this service. There is no charge for routine office visits.

We believe, if you follow our suggestions, you will experience the best of amplification at a reasonable cost and a minimum of inconvenience to you. Please feel free to call our office if you have any questions.

Sincerely yours,
Audiological Consultants, Inc.

Fig. 11-3.   Battery program/policies and prices

batteries is paid at one time and only one accounting transaction is required; 2. The user only has to pick up the telephone and request batteries; 3. The user is protected against the inflationary spiral of prices because he has purchased his batteries at a predetermined price; and 4. The user need write only one check for roughly one year's supply of batteries. The program itself consists of the user paying for six packages of batteries in advance and obtaining seven.

There is another old adage in the hearing aid industry; *"You know you have arrived when you are paying your rent on your gross battery sales."* This program, if utilized properly, will get you there fast because you are getting money without expending money for the product. In other words, the patient paid you for six packages of batteries and you have not given him anything yet. Figure 11-4 illustrates the card used to keep track of the batteries as they are shipped upon request. It is imperative that you keep accurate records because the only problem with this particular method of dispensing batteries is the potential argument over whether or not a person received his or her batteries. Figure 11-5 illustrates the form sent to the user along with his sixth package of batteries and his free bonus package. It is very nice to open the mail in the morning and receive these "small checks." It substantially increases your cash flow position. In addition, it makes for continued patient or user contact over the years. It is important that you do not price your batteries out of the market, however you should realize a substantial profit from the sale of batteries. Table 11-7 illustrates the battery program rationale.

```
┌─────────────────────────────────────────────────────────────────────┐
│                         BATTERY CLUB CARD                             │
│  NAME _____ PHONE   _____         │
│  ADDRESS  _____ ACCT#   _____         │
│           _____ 3rd PARTY _____       │
│  DATE FIT  _____ AID _____         │
│  BATT _____ POT ADJ _____         │
│  DATE PAID    #PAK/DATE MAILED                                        │
│  _____  1. ____ 2. ____ 3. ____ 4. ____ 5. ____ 6. ____ 7. ____  │
│  _____                                                           │
│  _____                                                           │
│  _____                                                           │
│  ____                                                                 │
└─────────────────────────────────────────────────────────────────────┘
```

Fig. 11-4. Battery club card

RECALLING PATIENTS

Figure 11-6 illustrates the initial recall I use prior to the expiration of the factory warranty on the user's hearing instrument. This particular recall serves several important functions. First of all, it is considerate—how many items have you purchased in your life where you have been reminded that the warranty was about to expire? Secondly, it is a defensive maneuver in that should something happen to the hearing instrument within the first several years, you can remind the user that you did indeed take the time to send him a warranty recall before his factory warranty expired. Thirdly, you cannot imagine how many users express their pleasure that you have informed them about the warranty on their particular hearing instrument. Lastly, it is an excellent vehicle for reselling or reevaluating. For example, suppose you thought initially that your user would be a good binaural candidate, but because of many other reluctances on his part you did not want to pursue the issue. If the user is, at present, happy with his hearing instrument, it may be efficacious to evaluate the possibility of his wearing a second aid. In addition, many patients who have worn their hearing aid for almost a year find that they would like to obtain a second one, perhaps in a pair of sun glasses or an all-in-the-ear for various listening situations. Therefore, it is very important that you maintain constant contact with your hearing aid users, and the recall systems work excellently. Figure 11-7 illustrates the recall used at least once a year following the initial fitting. Figure 11-8 illustrates the card used when

```
┌─────────────────────────────────────────────────────────────────────┐
│  Our records indicate that this is your 6th package of batteries.     │
│  Enclosed is your bonus package.                                      │
│  If you wish to continue with the battery program, please send a      │
│  check for $ _____.                                              │
│  Please call our office if you have any questions.                    │
│                                                                       │
│                               Sincerely yours,                        │
│                               Audiological Consultants, Inc.          │
└─────────────────────────────────────────────────────────────────────┘
```

Fig. 11-5. Form sent to user with the sixth battery package/bonus package

Table 11-7
Battery Plan (Jan. 3, 1979)

Prepaid Plan (Seven Packages)	User Saves	Individual Packs
13—$25.00	$4.40	$4.20
41—$26.00	$4.45	$4.35
74—$29.00	$4.95	$4.85
312—$22.00	$3.90	$3.70
675—$24.00	$4.00	$4.00
401—$14.00	$2.45	$2.35
AA—$18.00	$3.00	$3.00

Dear

Just a note to advise you, that the warranty for your hearing instrument expires _____
If you are having *any* problems at all, or would like your instrument checked, please make an appointment *before* expiration date of warranty, so there will be no charge to you for repair.

Sincerely yours,

M.J. Sorkowitz

Fig. 11-6.   Initial recall card

Dear

Our records indicate that your hearing instrument is now almost _____ years old.
We have purchased sophisticated test equipment to measure and record the response of your instrument and to eliminate all guesswork from providing you with the best amplification available. Therefore, we ask that you call our office at 885-6680 and make an appointment to have your instrument thoroughly evaluated. This is important in that even slight changes in your hearing, mold or instrument can produce negative results.

You are under no obligation to do anything except assure yourself the best hearing possible. There is no charge for this service or for any other routine office visit. We hope to see you soon.
Kindest personal regards.

Sincerely yours,

Audiological Consultants, Inc.

Fig. 11-7.   Recall used following initial fitting

	Delivered 11/2/78

Doe, Julia (Mrs.)
603 Main Street Philadelphia, PA 19144

Date	Recall	Date	Recall	Date	Recall

Fig. 11-8.   Card used when recalls are sent

recalls are sent, as well as how to keep track of whether or not your recall system is efficient.

A visit to your local dentist or dental specialist could prove worthwhile in your establishing your own particular recall, or patient contact, system. The dental profession is very "systems oriented" and you can implement many of their ideas. However you do it, it is imperative that you maintain at least yearly contact with your hearing aid users.

PROMOTION AND ADVERTISING

This area must be compatible with your particular personality. I find that yearly cocktail party/dinner meetings with all my potential referal sources, with some topical item being discussed, are productive in promoting my business. I do not do any advertising in the conventional sense. If, for example, you would like to demonstrate to the potential referral sources some new product or test equipment, most manufacturers would be more than happy to cooperate with you in any promotional seminar-type session and, in fact, may even help you to defray the expenses.

By utilizing this method of promotion, not only are you promoting an idea, but you are making a direct eye-to-eye contact with your referral sources at least on a yearly basis. You cannot become too friendly with referral sources.

The other method of promoting your business is to constantly write letters as you see your patients. For example, I purchased a small hand-held dictating machine and dictate a letter on every single patient I see, whether for the first or the fifteenth time. This method has several advantages. First of all, it is a means of keeping your name in front of the community and your market. Secondly, it allows your referral sources to know that you are interested in your work, and that you are aware of the fact that they sent the patient to you originally. Thirdly,

I find that to dictate right in front of the patient is an extremely effective method of letting the patient know you are in contact with his doctor and are interested in him as a hearing-impaired person.

Any other promotional ideas you may have can and do work. Don't be afraid to advertise yourself and your business in any reasonable way. The worst thing you can do is "keep your business a secret." Many people make the mistake of trying to insulate themselves and make themselves more professional than they should. Display and line ads in the Yellow Pages can be an effective advertising tool. On the other hand, when considered against actual returns, newspaper ads will usually not prove efficient. Direct mailings often prove useful as a way of keeping your name in the minds of the people you are aiming toward. Also consider contacts with other speech and hearing professionals in your area. They can and should be cultivated as potential referral sources. Figures 11-9, 11-10, and 11-11 are examples of additional promotion materials that are effective.

RESELLING AIDS

The next subject is an important one and relates to the reselling of hearing aid users. About the third or fourth year of operation, you will find an inordinate amount of reselling to be done. The reason for this is that many people have now realized that amplification is an integral part of their lives. Consequently, they want to obtain a second, or backup, hearing instrument. Secondly, many people are hard on their hearing aids and are in need of a new product. Thirdly, as you become more adept at fitting, you will find many more occasions for binaural use as the years go on. It is also a fact that many people just want a new product every three or four years. In this sense, a hearing instrument is no different than a car, a watch, or any other consumer item. In addition, the hearing aid industry is always evolving new products and most people like to have the latest, whether it be a coat, suit, or hearing instrument.

I find that a very effective method of reselling is to incorporate the repair or renovation of the "old hearing aid" into the fee for the new instrument. Suppose, for example, your fee is $425.00. If you send the old hearing aid back to the manufacturer for repair, it's going to cost you approximately $35.00 or $40.00 for a complete overhaul with a six-month warranty. By including this renovation with the purchase of the new hearing instrument, the user feels that he is getting a bargain, and he is. Most people like to feel they are getting a bargain, and, from a cost point of view, you can easily afford to do this. It's just as easy to take care of one person with two hearing instruments as it is to take care of one person with one hearing instrument.

Dear Dr.

As a relatively new member of the audiologic community in Philadelphia, we would like to extend our heartiest welcome to you. In addition, we would like to acquaint you with our facility and philosophy regarding aural rehabilitation.

The main purpose of Audiological Consultants, Inc. is to provide you with a convenient, logical solution to your hearing care problems.

As you may know, we assume the responsibility of dispensing hearing instruments. We have simply concluded that hearing impaired persons who cannot benefit from medical or surgical treatment, should have the opportunity to receive professional counsel when acquiring an aid. Furthermore, we are convinced that these persons have the right to expect competent, responsible follow-up care, fair treatment, and informed decisions from the person who recommends and dispenses the aid. The clinical audiologist, by virtue of his training and experience, is uniquely qualified to perform these integrated functions. By adhering to the following policies, we have every reason to feel that this long neglected aspect of hearing care can be attended to without compromising any accepted standards of clinical or professional judgment.

1.   Patients will be seen on a referral basis only, and should have otological clearance by their physician.

2.   No solicitations of hearing aid prospects through the mass media, no mailing campaigns, no door to door canvassing, or similar activities.

3.   Only those instruments that have proven to be of high quality will be used.

4.   Patients incapable of benefiting from amplification, despite our best efforts, will be expected to return the instrument to us. A reasonable, specified service charge will be the only fee.

5.   Your patients will be urged to contact you sometime after obtaining the instrument to report on their experience with it, and to give you an opportunity to re-evaluate them.

Audiological Consultants, Inc. is located in the Northern Medical Offices, directly across the street from Albert Einstein Medical Center, Northern Division. All patients referred here will be seen by me, personally. I was graduated from the University of Wisconsin in 1966 with an M.A. degree in Speech and Hearing. Prior to opening Audiological Consultants of Philadelphia, I was clinical audiologist at the Albert Einstein Medical Center and practiced itinerent audiology in the Philadelphia area.

We are looking forward to providing our services for you and your patients. Please feel free to visit our office at any time, and to contact us if you wish any further information about our policies or services.

Kindest personal regards.

Very truly yours,

Melvin J. Sorkowitz
Audiological Consultants, Inc.

Fig. 11-9.   Additional promotional material

Dear

Enclosed is a brochure explaining our general concepts and philosophies regarding the fitting of hearing aids.

For many years this particular area of aural rehabilitation has needed better trained, more competent people. We feel that academic training in audiology is essential and uniquely qualifies the audiologist to fill the need so necessary to perform this important job with professional skill.

As members of the paramedical field, we are eager to cooperate with you and your patients requiring amplification.

Please scrutinize this brochure and feel free to call us regarding any of our services and policies.

Sincerely yours,

Melvin J. Sorkowitz
Audiologist

Fig. 11-10.   Additional promotion material

PROBLEM SOLVING

The next "how to" section relates to particular problems that I have encountered in my dispensing career and how to solve them. It is my intention to utilize narrative dialogue in hypothetical situations to effectively delineate problems. Make no mistake about it, you will have problems on a daily basis! I can assure you that if you utilize some of the dialogue that follows in your rehabilitation approach, your life will be made much easier. These problems are in direct relation to the previous section of this chapter on how to maintain your business effectively.

Dear

We have been, for the past few years, fabricating custom made swimming plugs for those patients who previously could not enjoy swimming because of post surgical or allergic conditions.

These plugs are molded and delivered to the patient in one visit to our office. Our results have been quite successful in both adults and children.

If you desire any further information, please call.

Sincerely yours,

Melvin J. Sorkowitz
Audiologist

Fig. 11-11.   Additional promotional material

Presenting Fees

The first problem that comes to mind is the presentation of your fee for dispensing the hearing instruments. You must be confident and positive in presenting your fee because people do have a right to know how much they are going to have to pay. Do not assume that they will automatically write you a check. I strongly suggest, following whatever evaluative techniques you utilize, that you bring up the subject of fees. This allows you to effectively neutralize this delicate subject and approach it head on. I accomplish this by saying something such as: "Mr. Jones, my fee, including all the tests done today, all of your future service calls, and any service I may render to you or your hearing aid is $xx.xx. This includes all future office visits here and all services rendered during the warranty period. Of course, after the warranty period, you will be charged for repairs because I will be charged from the factory." It is important to maintain direct eye contact with your user while presenting this fee and to not just give a number and remain silent. You must be confident and positive in presenting this to the user and also do it in as nonchallant a manner as possible. Certainly, you are going to get some people who will balk at your fee even if you were charging $50.00. However, if you use this approach, you'll minimize your difficulty. Another related approach to presenting fees is presented in Figure 11-12.

It is not advisable to fit a hearing aid at a lower price and charge for service calls. If you choose to do it in this manner, you will undoubtedly lose your patient because somebody else will perform the same services you will, for nothing. Again, we can take a lesson from the dental profession, which has historically presented one particular fee for service regardless of how many visits were required.

Collecting Fees

The potential problem is directly related to the presentation of fees:—getting your money. Remember, you are not a banking or lending institution. You are a single proprietorship and cannot afford to be a money lender. I strongly advise that you fit a hearing aid in two visits. The first visit should consist of the evaluation and explanation of the problem and what you intend to do about it, and how much it will cost. At the initial visit, you should require a $50.00 nonrefundable deposit to cover the costs of time and materials expended. You should then give a patient a 10-day to 2-week interval before he is fit with his hearing instrument. It should be explained at the initial visit that the balance is due upon delivery of the hearing aid. This is not an unreasonable request. If you think about it, how many items can you obtain from any particular institution and not pay for it at the time of delivery? I can't think of any!

If the patient relates that he is going to have a problem paying, you can, if it is written up properly in a contract, extend him 60 days to pay the balance, if, at

---

HEARING AID INFORMATION SHEET

You may have suspected a hearing loss because you had difficulty hearing people speaking softly, hearing them in groups or in noisy situations, or hearing television when other people have it adjusted to their own comfortable loudness. Today's Audiological evaluation has confirmed that you have a significant hearing loss. Having a hearing loss does not mean that you are deaf, but, rather, that speech is not loud enough and you may have difficulty understanding it.

The U.S. Food and Drug Administration (FDA) regulations pertaining to the sale of hearing aids recommends that you be examined by a physician, preferably one specializing in diseases of the ear, prior to purchasing a hearing aid. The physician's examination must be performed within six months prior to the hearing aid purchase. If the doctor finds that your hearing loss cannot be improved with medication or surgery (or if you do not want medical treatment) he can sign a statement that you can be considered a candidate for a hearing aid.

The FDA regulations allow you to purchase a hearing aid if you do not want a medical opinion concerning your hearing loss, and you are over 18 years of age, if you sign a medical waiver. We believe that it is in your best interests to have a medical examination and do not recommend the waiver.

Our hearing aid program has been designed so that we may offer to each of our patients who need amplification a program of consistent high quality including: selection and fitting of the hearing aid; continued patient follow-up services; the most possible convenience; and a competitive pricing structure.

THE PROGRAM

1. A HEARING AID EVALUATION will compare your abilities to hear and understand speech with and without a hearing aid. If improvement in your ability to hear and understand speech is demonstrated, we will recommend that you use a hearing aid for several weeks to determine its benefits to you in your daily life situation.

2. In addition to the services offered by PACIFIC HEARING SERVICES, as described below, you will also incur charges for the EARMOLD(S) and HEARING AID EVALUATION. As part of our hearing aid program, these services are offered through Valley Ear, Nose and Throat Medical Group, Inc., and/or some agency other than PACIFIC HEARING SERVICES. Fees for the earmold(s) and/or hearing aid evaluation are not included in the price of the hearing aid or other charges of PACIFIC HEARING SERVICES.

   Generally, the HEARING AID EVALUATION will be performed at the Audiology Department at Casa Colina Hospital in Pomona or at Valley Ear, Nose and Throat Medical Group in Upland.

Fig. 11-12.   Hearing aid information sheet

the time of delivery, he pays you half of the balance. Relating back to Figure 11-1, you can see that if you do not get your money at the time of delivery, you are going to put yourself into a considerable cashflow deficit and find it very hard to meet your current bills.

You can check into some of the credit card programs; however, in my experience most of the elderly patients dealt with in a hearing aid dispensing office do not have credit cards. Again, this is one of those problems that manifests itself mostly because of the insecurity of the dispenser in talking about the "nasty subject" of money. I implore you to be direct and confident in a rehabilitative sense in dealing with this problem. There is no avoiding discussing

VALLEY EAR, NOSE & THROAT MEDICAL GROUP, INC. has no financial interest in PACIFIC HEARING SERVICES, and derives no financial benefit from the sale of hearing aids by PACIFIC HEARING SERVICES.

3. The 30 day initial use period allows you to take the aid home and use it in your daily life routine. This time is for you to adjust to the hearing aid and determine if it is going to benefit you significantly.

    a. At the beginning of this period, you will be asked to pay for the hearing aid.

    b. During the 30 day period of time we will see you periodically to make any further necessary adjustments on the aid and to help you to adjust to it.

    c. ANY TIME during the 30 day time you may cancel the hearing aid purchase contract for any reason and receive a refund of all but $40.00 (per aid) of what you paid for the aid(s). The $40.00 constitutes a rental fee for the hearing aid.

4. The price of the hearing aid includes:
——the hearing aid.
——any visits related to your use of the aid for 6 months following the fitting.
——complete service during the warranty period.
——an initial supply of batteries.

5. At the time of the hearing aid evaluation, then, you will have to make two payments—one to PACIFIC HEARING SERVICES for the hearing aid and the other to Valley ENT Medical Group/Casa Colina Hospital for the evaluation fee.

6. Below is a breakdown of the approximate costs involved in our program, excluding fees for the hearing test and medical examination.

    a. EAR MOLD (per ear) $_____ (payable at the time of the impression)
    b. HEARING AID EVALUATION $_____ (payable at the time of the evaluation)
    c. HEARING AID $_____

I am acknowledging receipt of this information sheet by signing below. This is NOT a contract and in no way obligates me to buy or rent a hearing aid.

_____   _____

    DATE   SIGNATURE

Fig. 11-12.   Hearing aid information sheet (continued)

money and there is no way anybody else can do it for you. You have to step up to the task and be confident that you are going to earn the fee, charge for it, and most importantly, get paid for it at the time it is rendered. *If you are in business to make a living, you have to ask for and receive monies owed you.*

User Acceptance

The next problem that may appear at the time of delivery of the hearing instrument is this question from the user: "What if this hearing aid doesn't work or if I don't like it?" You should never bring this question up yourself! If the user asks this question, the best response is, "If you can not adjust to this hearing instrument within 30 days, for whatever reason, all you have to do is come back to this office and I will refund the entire fee less my dispensing costs." Be sure you specify exactly what your dispensing costs are. In addition, on the contract you give the user, write down the terms of return privileges.

The user must understand that there is a tacit trust involved with you and his hearing aid fitting. He must further understand that this trust must be predicated on his trusting you, not you trusting him. After all, you have an office, a staff, and are a substantial member of the business community. He, on the other hand, is off the street, and you don't have time to do a financial check on him, so you must have your money. In addition, if there is going to be a trust, have the user trust you.

I would go as far as to say that if a user is not satisfied with this particular arrangement, it is highly likely you do not want to deal with him. Of course, certain situations will arise where you have to deviate from this particular policy. However, as a general rule I stick hard and fast to full payment at time of delivery and refund in 30 days, if necessary.

After you have fully oriented the patient to all aspects of hearing aid use and care, it is time to write your letter to the referral source. You can utilize any form you desire; however, the physician is busy, so keep it short and to the point. As I mentioned earlier, it is important to correspond with referral sources at all times either by writing or by telephone calls.

I always end the final consultation and fitting session with a statement such as this: "Okay, now we have fit you with your hearing instrument and it is my impression that it is the proper instrument and everything should go fine. I don't anticipate any problems; however, if you have a problem I will have no way of knowing about it unless you tell me. If you come back here in 30 days and demand your money back, I will give you your money back with no questions asked; however, I will be angry with you. The reason I will be angry is that after you walk out of here today, I'm not going to think about you until you tell me you have a problem. If you tell me you have a problem, I will do everything in my power to solve it. Occasionally, there are some patients who just do not adjust to amplification and have to have their money refunded. I don't think you are one of them; however, I want you to come in and see me next week and let me know how you are doing. At that time we will make any adjustments that may be necessary. You see, I am going to charge you, even if the hearing aid fitting be unsuccessful. You have already paid, so you may as well take advantage of it. What you are paying for is my ability to make you hear and I can only do that if you tell me there is a problem."

After the patient leaves, if you have done your job properly, chances are there will be no problem with refunds; however, should the patient come back in 30 days and state that he cannot hear with the aid and demands his money back, you can try to counsel him into continuing with the instrument. But, he may be so vehement against hearing aid use that it is propitious to just refund the money.

Make the refund in a very professional manner and, preferably in front of the patient, dictate a letter to the referral source stating that the hearing aid fitting has not been successful, letting the patient hear exactly what you have to say to the doctor. This particular approach accomplishes several results. First of all, the patient knows that you have contacted his doctor or audiologist and that you are not afraid to admit failure. Secondly, he cannot go back to the referral source and say that you did not try or that you did not care about him. It is most important to protect yourself in dealing with the public at large and especially the hard-of-hearing population. The one thing you don't want said about you is that you took advantage of anybody. You can, by employing the preceeding approaches, rest assured that you have done your best to make this person hear.

The patient is then on his way to aural rehabilitation through the use of a hearing aid; you have written the doctor a letter; and now you must take care of his hearing aid demands for the life of the hearing instrument.

Repairs

There are many problems that will occur with each individual, and every day will be a new learning experience for you. I will not get involved with any of the technical things that can occur with hearing aids, molds, etc., except to say, make sure you give each patient enough time to fully evaluate the problem. During the warranty period or the first year, I do not, as a rule, charge patients for anything except batteries. If, however, after the warranty period, the need arises for service, I find the easiest way to charge for servicing a hearing aid is to charge the manufacturer's repair invoice cost plus a certain fee for handling the hearing instrument. Remember you have overhead in running your office, and you cannot afford to repair a hearing aid for nothing. The patient does not expect it, and again I defy anybody to explain to me how they can provide goods or services at no profit. There is no such thing as no profit. If you repair a hearing aid for a user at the manufacturer's cost, you are operating at a loss.

I think it only fair to state that you are a businessman and being a businessman implies that you make a profit. You cannot afford anything unless there is a profit involved. *If this offends you, you should not be dispensing hearing aids.*

Cosmetic Acceptance

Another problem you are undoubtedly going to combat is that of consumer reluctance to wear a hearing instrument. The problems in dealing with this issue are deepseated psychological problems and all I intend to offer at this point is superficial solutions to the problem without becoming psychoanalytic. I have found that especially during the initial interaction with the user, it is important to relate hearing loss as a family communicative problem. I also found it extremely effective to use the ''sense of guilt'' to force the user who is reluctant because of the cosmetic aspects into wearing a hearing instrument. The dialogue goes something like this: "Mr. Jones, do you realize you are being selfish?" Mr. Jones, "What do you mean?" "Well, why should you or I or anybody else expect people to walk around yelling at us when all we have to do is wear this device and people will be able to talk to you in a normal tone of voice." Mr. Jones, "I don't know, it seems to me that if people speak up, I can hear them." "Mr. Jones, don't you realize that people are speaking up, in fact they are even shouting. I don't know about other people but I find it easier not to talk to hard-of-hearing people than to have to yell at them, especially if they can be helped with a hearing instrument. Therefore, you owe it to yourself and your family to wear a hearing device. In fact, I may even hang a sign up in this office that says, 'Wearing a hearing aid is a sign of consideration for others.' " In this way you are encouraging the person to take responsibility for his communication.

Monday Morning Club

Another problem that may be more of a myth than a problem is "Monday Morning Club." It is my strong belief that if you do your job properly in fitting and counseling, your "Monday Morning Club" will be minimized; however, there are certain hearing aid users, who, because of their age, loneliness, or inability to adapt, will be persistent visitors to your office. By "Monday Morning Clubbers," I mean the people you know are going to call on Monday morning to complain about their hearing aid because they have been shut in all weekend or alone and just need someone to talk to, or those who chronically put the battery in backwards, or kink the tubing.

In the beginning of your dispensing practice, you have plenty of time to talk to these people; however, as time goes on and you become busier, it becomes impossible for you to give the time to these people that they demand. Consequently, it is very important that you pinpoint the problems and spot your potential "Monday Morning Clubbers" early and relate directly to them. I do not mean by this that you have to be nasty, but simply direct. You can say something such as, "Mr. Jones, I understand that you feel you have a problem; however, I have examined your hearing instrument and your hearing, have looked in your ears, and checked your earmolds, and there really doesn't seem to be anything wrong. However, should you have this problem by the end of the week, I would appreciate hearing from you." This lets the user know you are still interested in them and that you have given them permission to call you later in the week. Many times, by doing this you are utilizing the idea of latency to minimize a potentially difficult situation. Possibly, by the end of the week they will be feeling better physically and mentally and in all probability will not call you. This is not a foolproof approach. There will always be certain people who demand more of you than you are willing to give. This "goes with the territory," and again, you must be thick-skinned enough to withstand it. I must reiterate that if you have done your job to the best of your ability, your Monday Morning Club will not be nearly the headache you think it will be. In addition, the more proficient you become and the more experience you gain in dealing with the hard-of-hearing public and fitting hearing aids, the less "Monday Morning Clubbers" you will have.

CONCLUSION

You have embarked, or are about to embark, on a very exciting adventure. The exhilaration of making a satisfactory hearing aid fitting and the positive reinforcement you receive is well worth the battle. I hope that the ideas I have presented in this chapter will help you avoid many of the problems. I encourage you to be innovative and perceptive enough to evolve your own particular methods of doing whatever is possible to encourage the hearing-impaired to wear amplification, so that they can become a communicating member of society again.

Make no mistakes, the job is a difficult one, requiring enormous patience, salesmanship, and tenacity to withstand all magnitudes of blows to your ego. If you are prepared to withstand the difficulties in fitting the hearing-impaired and taking care of their rehabilitative needs, you will enjoy a highly successful, profitable, spiritually rewarding life. Keep in mind that you are running a business; there is nothing wrong with that, so long as you are providing the best services to your clients possible. Profit is certainly not a dirty word. Our country was founded on the profit motive and it is probably the prime motivating factor in all of our lives. Just remember, the minute you start thinking you are doing something for nothing, you are doing it for less than nothing. Profit and peace of mind in knowing that you have done a good job are all important.

TROUBLE-SHOOTING GUIDE FOR IN-HOUSE
EVALUATION OF HEARING AIDS

This section is presented as an outline for trouble-shooting minor repair problems in the office, to avoid having to send the instrument in for repair.

1. Battery contacts
   a. Weak (always use new batteries when making evaluations)
   b. Intermittent (there can be a difference in size of battery-check evaluation of aid using both a 76 and 675 type battery. You may have to adjust the battery contacts between a 76 and 675 battery.)
   c. Oxidized batteries or contacts may cause distortion or weakness in an aid.
   d. Dirty battery contacts may be cleaned by using an eraser.

2. Volume control
    a. Dead spots in volume controls may sometimes be cured by manipulating the volume control from the low and to the high end very rapidly several times. Most volume controls are self-cleaning.
3. Switch (mike-tel, on/off)
    a. Switch problems may sometimes be cured by manipulating the switch several times.
4. Feedback (see Chapter 2)
    a. To see if feedback is in the aid, listen to the aid using *personal* earmold. A perfectly fitting earmold is needed to determine if feedback stops. When properly coupled, check tubing to assure a tight fit over the receiver coupler, pinch the tube off about one inch up from the receiver coupler, and hold the aid to ear with volume full-on. If feedback is audible, it should be sent to the factory for service.
    b. Minute cracks in the elbow (conduction unit) or tubing may cause feedback.
    c. Loose fitting earmolds can cause feedback.
    d. Tubing that couples the hearing aid to the earmold must fit tight.
    e. Be certain that tubing or elbow (conduction unit) has no splits.
    f. Directional microphones
        1. Make sure both the front port and top port are working properly.
        2. Plugged screen over top port microphone can cause the aid to be weak. To clean, use a soft brush and be certain aid is held upside down so that dirt will fall away from screen.
    g. Potentiometer adjustments (external)
        1. On some aids, you have adjustments that set gain, pressure (MPO), and curve characteristics.
        2. With the volume control full-on or near full-on, use a small screwdriver, with your personal earmold, with tube attached to the receiver coupler, and adjust the potentiometer from the high to low end to make sure the response changes.
        3. While adjusting these potentiometers, you may hear a grinding sound. This is normal, and should not be a cause for sending the aid back to the factory.
    h. In-the-ear aids
        1. Wax accumulation may cause aid to be weak, distorted, or dead.
        2. If there is a wax guard, remove and clean with a Q-tip or vacuum.
        3. Look into receiver canal and inspect for additional wax. If wax is found, use very small needle to bring wax to the surface.

TEN-STEP LISTENING CHECK

1. Battery (weak, dead, intermittent)
2. Volume control (self cleaning)

3. Switch (mike–tel, self cleaning)
4. Feedback (aid, earmold, tubing)
5. Directional mike (top port, front port)
6. Pot (curve)
7. Pot (MPO)
8. Pot (gain)
9. Microphone (gain pressure)
10. Receiver (gain pressure)

BIBLIOGRAPHY

Walsh S: A guide for the person considering hearing aid dispensing. Hear Instrum 30:12–35, 1979

Kenneth E. Smith

12
Professional Relationships

Over the years there have been various groups of professionals and para-professionals who have been directly involved in the diagnosis and rehabilitation of the hearing-impaired: audiologists, otologists, teachers of the deaf and hard-of-hearing, and hearing aid dispensers. It is rather ironic that there has been such a great lack of communication between these individuals, all of whom work with communication disorders. Starting with the premise that the audiologist should be the case manager, Ken Smith presents rationales and suggestions for improving the relationships between the audiologist and the other team members. While some of his proposals will meet with disagreement from various quarters, Ken's suggestions will undoubtedly lead to much discussion and, hopefully, facilitate improvements in these professional relationships.

MCP

When I wrote this chapter for the first edition of this book, I was a university professor with a limited clinical load. My teaching, administrative, and supervisory responsibilities limited my direct contacts with hearing-impaired patients. As each semester progressed, students were given more and more direct responsibility for the evaluation of the patient and followup services. Professional relationships were relatively easy to establish, and my involvement with hearing aid evaluation and follow-up was limited to five or six cases per month.

For the past three years, I have been in private practice, having daily contact with 7−12 patients, and direct responsibilities for 10−15 hearing aids *per week*. My professional relationships now have a direct impact on my business and on the quality of care provided to hearing-impaired patients and their families. Understandably, my experience has had a profound effect on my understanding of, and approach to professional relationships, and accounts for a rather dramatic shift in the content of this chapter.

The "Hearing Health Team" is a concept widely referred to in the commercial and professional literature on hearing aids, and is routinely described to students as a reality and as being beneficial to the patient. However, public feuding between the American Academy of Ophthalmology and Otorhinolaryngology, the American Speech, Language and Hearing Association, The National Hearing Aid Society, and various branches of government make this concept less and less credible. Instead of working together for the benefit of the hearing-impaired patient, there appears to be a struggle in progress for the rights "to" the patient as opposed to the rights "of" the patient.

In my experience, this struggle almost always relates to an economic or territorial motive. Basic problems relate to the quality of services provided to the patient (i.e., hearing aid dealers discount the value of audiological evaluation), the cost of such services (i.e., the otologist may ask, "Is audiological evaluation and management justified, based on the cost?" . . . etc.); competition for patients (i.e., the resultant income generated by patient visits, surgery, evaluation, hearing aids, etc.); and a struggle for control of the patient's loyalties (i.e., the physician and audiologist may disagree about whether a hearing aid will be helpful to the patient).

At this point it is important to understand that an economic motive behind hearing health care is not objectionable. Without patients, income, markup, and profit, there would be no hearing health services. The objectionable fact is that, at times, the economic motive seems to be the primary motive underlying the management of the patient. The best interests of the patient may be lost, and the result is less-than-effective rehabilitation. One must wonder if the patient's best interests are assuming more importance as the FDA and FTC regulations go into effect,[1] as manufacturers and dispensers of hearing aids improve their self-regulation, as more otologists and audiologists enter directly into hearing aid dispensing, and as hearing aids and hearing aid accessories continue to improve.

ASSUMPTIONS UNDERLYING PROFESSIONAL RELATIONSHIPS

Professional relationships are based on transactions between groups of people, between professional organizations representing those people, and between individual professionals. While interorganizational relationships receive

[1]The FDA regulations affect prior medical clearance for amplification, required or recommended examinations, and establishes guidelines for information to the consumer and were in effect as of August, 1977. The FTC Recommended Rule for the Hearing Aid Industry of November 19, 1978 has been circulated for comment. This document may be obtained by writing the Public Reference Branch, Room 130, Federal Trade Commission, 6th and Pennsylvania Ave., N.W., Washington, D.C. 10580. The FTC Rule would establish a buyer's right to cancel within 30 days of purchase and would restrict various sales and advertising techniques.

the most publicity, relationships between individual professionals probably have the greatest effect on the hearing-impaired patient and the quality of habilitative/ rehabilitative services.

There are several assumptions underlying professional relationships that affect the evaluation and delivery of the hearing aid.

1. That a hearing health team exists
2. That all professional activity relates to the patient's best interests
3. That there is a "best" source of management for the hearing-impaired patient and his rehabilitation program
4. That professionals are capable of relationships and communication that can have a positive effect on the patient and his rehabilitation program

A review of current professional and trade publications, and more specifically of the positions assumed by professional organizations, makes the concept of the hearing health team questionable. The medical community argues that the point of entry as well as supervision of the rehabilitation program rests with the physician. Audiologists and hearing aid dispensers argue that "nonmedical" hearing problems are best handled by members of their own disciplines, and that the physicians have inadequate training in, or understanding of, communication needs of the hearing-impaired patient. Traditional hearing aid dispensers complain about physician or audiologist statements that a hearing aid will not be helpful to the patient.

The hearing aid industry argues that they alone have the expertise to dispense and fit the aid, while the audiologists complain that the hearing aid dispensers are undertrained and motivated purely by economic factors.

Even the government seems to contribute to the weakness of the team concept. Current FDA requirements specify examination by a physician before a hearing aid purchase, but do not mandate clearance for amplification by the otologist—the medical specialist best qualified to examine the ears and hearing problems (FDA, August 1977).

While one can argue effectively that the hearing health team does not exist, successful professional relationships between the audiologist, hearing aid dispenser, and the otologist suggest that the hearing health teams *do* exist. When these specialties cooperate, when the relationship promotes quality patient care, and when the economic interests of all three professions are satisfied, the patient's interests and rights can be managed successfully. The patient's interests relate to restoration or improvement of auditory communication skills through the use of a hearing aid and his or her right to a quality product, efficient service, a fair price for the hearing instrument, and an understanding of his or her hearing loss and hearing aid. In short, the patient must receive professional quality services at each stage of the process; professionals must communicate, understand, and respect each other; and the territorial limits of each group must be carefully observed. It *is* possible and it *does* exist.

My own experiences with a team demonstrate that cooperation can be a reality. I have worked directly with two otology groups by providing the otologist's patients with audiological services. I had direct responsibility for interpretation and recommendations to those patients. Patients were then referred to a hearing aid dispenser who followed directions, made good decisions, and kept the medical-audiology team well informed. The result was a professional quality service to each patient.

Discussion of the patient's best interests almost always relates to the discipline of the professional leading the discussion. I can hardly ignore my own experience and the experience of colleagues regarding the fitting of inappropriate hearing aids, deceptive sales practices, failure to identify significant medical conditions requiring the physician's attention, and the failure to give the patient realistic expectations for use of the hearing aid as well as appropriate follow-up services. To make matters worse, our knowledge of hearing aids, their affect on human hearing, and the manner in which the human ear processes the amplified signal is limited. One can only be amazed how little we know about hearing aids, the fitting process, auditory training, training of students in the fitting of hearing aids, and the number of research questions that remain unanswered. Despite this reality, the impression is given that the "best" procedures and the "best" professionals to be responsible for the fitting of the hearing aid lies within a single discipline. My own bias is that the physician and audiologist probably have the most complete knowledge (by training, not experience) to evaluate, prescribe, and fit the hearing aid. Dispensing in a medical-audiological setting would appear to be the trend in hearing aid fittings (Bailey and Winston 1978).

While this is certainly the trend, it is not a current reality, nor is it always in the patient's best interest. A lack of knowledge of the day-to-day problems of the hearing-impaired patient and his hearing aid and a lack of time available to counsel, train, and rehabilitate limits the effectiveness of the audiologist and/or physician as the dispenser(s) of the aid (Pratt 1978). An experienced, trained hearing aid dispenser who can and will follow recommendations can be one of the most important factors in successful adjustment to a hearing aid when conditions necessitate the involvement of the traditional hearing aid dispenser.

In summary, although hearing health teams appear to exist, the patient's best interests may be undermined because of a lack of training, experience or time and there is no "best" source of management for every patient. Still positive, productive professional relationships are possible despite what you read.

PRIMARY RELATIONSHIPS AFFECTING THE AUDIOLOGIST

The Otologist

FDA Regulations, effective August 25, 1977, require prior medical clearance before the patient can be fitted for a hearing aid. While the patient may sign a waiver of medical clearance, and while the regulation requires only a "physician'' (a specialist in diseases of the ears, nose, and throat is suggested but not mandatory), I believe that most audiologists have referred and will continue to refer patients to the otologist. Several factors affect the relationships between the otologist and the audiologist.

The audiologist may be seen as a technician or 'dial twister' relegated only to obtaining test data with a minimal role in interpretation. This attitude is apparent when one considers the number of physicians who use nurses or nonprofessional persons to test hearing. In my opinion, at least part of this attitude relates to the inadequate training of the clinician to perform as a professional, and the fact that audiology (at this point in time) is expensive. To complete a thorough job of assessment, the otologist must purchase expensive equipment and pay a salary and other overhead expenses to the audiologist, unless the audiologist functions as an independent contractor.

Rarely does the audiologist generate patients for the physician. Couple these factors with the fact that audiological fees charged to the patient (not all patients seen by ear, nose, and throat specialists require audiology) are enough for the service to "break even" and one can understand the physician's attitude toward the audiologist. Again, the "non-cost effectiveness" of audiological services is not always the case, but it is the rule rather than the exception.

The independent audiologist (i.e., not an employee of the physician) involved in both evaluation and hearing aid dispensing may be perceived as "competition for ears" by the otologist. This situation applies also to the general community most often when the audiologist sees a patient and makes a direct referral to an otologist, bypassing the referring physician or the patient's previous physician. This apparent ignorance of courtesy and medical ethics often justifies the physician's attitude toward the audiologist.

Otologists often see themselves as responsible for the total management plan for the patient. This attitude is sometimes generalized and encourages the physician to make recommendations that might better be handled by the audiologist or hearing aid dispenser. This attitude is not uncommon or unjustified (considering the life and death problems the physician-surgeon must deal wth on an every day basis), but it is to the audiologist's advantage to gradually shift some of this responsibility from the physician, particularly in the areas of hearing aids and rehabilitation. This can only be accomplished through a direct contribution to patient management by the audiologist.

In private practice, the medical community is the most consistent and productive source of patients for the audiologist. Without positive medical relationships, the survival of the audiologist in private practice is questionable. Aside from the economic impact on the audiologist and of physician referrals, the patient can benefit directly from coordinated medical and supportive care, remembering that the "ultimate" authority to many patients is the physician. Thus, active positive support from the physician can have a direct effect on successful use of the hearing aid.

Developing productive relationships with the otologist involves a knowledgeable, professional approach to evaluation and management of hearing and the hearing aid. In the diagnostic phase of the process, audiological data are used to make the diagnosis and to affect treatment. Interpretation of the data, and the quality of information given to the patient can affect the course of treatment; the audiologist can assume a direct role in time-consuming interpretation and follow-up services, which benefits the patient and reflects directly on the physician.

Once the economic, territorial, and time factors of the relationship are accounted for, the beginnings of a hearing health team can be seen. When the audiologist establishes himself as a professional and as a contributor, his fees are justified, he generates patients for the practice, and the relationship between the physician and audiologist becomes cooperative rather than supervisory. It can and *does* happen, but both the audiologist and physician may need to alter preconceived attitudes.

The Traditional Hearing Aid Dispenser

The traditional hearing aid dispenser ("nonaudiologist" or "nonphysician") presents a peculiar challenge and dilemma for the audiologist. In many cases, a good relationship with one or more dealers may be beneficial to the patient, and economically practical. The audiologist may not have the time, interest, capital, or business know-how to dispense and service the hearing aid. However, most audiologists feel that they know more about hearing and the hearing aid than the dispenser.

This superiority complex is seen most often in the educational audiologist who may have no experience or knowledge of the business world. While this attitude is sometimes justified, the resulting transactions in this type of relationship rarely result in effective communication or benefit to the patient. A "superior–subordinate" relationship between the audiologist and the dispenser can be explosive. Conflicting information and recommendations to the patient can result in confusion and a lack of confidence in *all* of the professionals included in the hearing aid fitting.

In establishing a positive relationship with a hearing aid dispenser, the audiologist should remember the following:

As the current controversy over responsibility for the hearing-impaired patient and his hearing aid continues, the audiologist poses a direct threat to the "professionalism" and the income of the hearing aid dispenser. Many dealers view the audiologist as unnecessary in the dispensing process (except for some children and certain medically related cases). They may court the audiologist only as a source of referrals, but the courting procedures (appropriate in the business world) may appear unethical to the audiologist. Such procedures may include free meals, gifts, and other incentives to refer patients for hearing aids. Acceptance of such incentives poses an ethical dilemma for the audiologist, and should be carefully evaluated on an individual basis. A business luncheon is appropriate for discussing business, hearing aids, or specific patients, but alternating responsibility for the check can alleviate any ethical problems.

In April 1978, the Supreme Court of the United States ruled that a professional society's canon of ethics having the effect of limiting competition among the society's members is illegal (United States versus National Society of Professional Engineers, 1978). As a direct result of this decision in July of 1978, ASHA's Executive Board recommended that all restrictions on the making of profit by ASHA members through the sale of hearing aids be suspended.

Resolution 53, approved by the Legislative Council of ASHA at the 1978 Convention meeting in San Francisco, supported the Executive Board's recommendation. Specifically, that approved resolution states that:

1. The hearing aid must be dispensed as part of a rehabilitation plan.
2. The cost of the product and the dispensing fee must be itemized for the consumer.
3. The consumer must be given freedom of choice for the source of services and products.
4. Consumers must be informed about fees prior to service delivery.
5. Services and products provided by the audiologist must be evaluated.

In summary, the audiologist can now fit and dispense hearing aids in a competitive market at a profit. Following the announcement in this change in the Code of Ethics, the National Hearing Aid Society welcomed ''rank and file ASHA members'' (Fortner, 1978), suggesting a new spirit of cooperation and growth.

For the first time since the debate over dispensing began, the audiologist and traditional hearing aid dispenser are direct competitors. The long-term effects of this change in ethics on training and professional relationships cannot be predicted at the present time. However, a major source of friction (i.e., ''no profit'' dispensing) appears to have been eliminated.

While the dispensing audiologist may now compete directly with the traditional hearing aid dispenser, a cooperative relationship may be beneficial. The audiologist may be unable (or unwilling) to provide follow-up services in the home or to the nonambulatory patient. He may also find it helpful to learn the ''art'' of hearing aid dispensing from an experienced dispenser. Training institutions simply are not prepared to teach these day-to-day skills that are so critical to successful hearing aid practice.

It would also appear that the audiologist is now free to enter into business or contractural relationships with traditional hearing aid dispensers. The frequency of advertisements in the trade journals seeking to employ audiologists in hearing aid outlets has increased dramatically during the past year. Considering this shift in product delivery, training programs are in need of immediate program and practicum changes to meet new roles and relationships of the audiologist in private practice.

Hearing aid dispensers and, particularly, manufacturer's representatives, often approach the audiologist with a condescending attitude. I frequently hear complaints about the lack of knowledge about hearing aids and fitting demonstrated by audiologists, and such complaints are often justified. Training in the fitting and evaluation of the hearing aid has not been a major emphasis of the audiology training programs, and the new graduate is, too often, unprepared for anything but a technical or philosophical discussion of hearing aids. Bluffing one's way through a discussion of hearing aid fitting is not conducive to developing a mutual respect between the audiologist and dispenser.

Perhaps one of the most positive results of the interorganizational struggle, the FDA–FTC regulations, and the audiologist's emerging role as a hearing aid dispenser, will be an increasing emphasis on the hearing aid in our training programs.

One of the major goals of the Academy of Dispensing Audiologists is to have a direct impact on training programs by developing curriculum guides for "professional audiology" training programs. Such an impact must involve training in business, business ethics, hearing aid fitting, hearing aid technology, rehabilitative measures and professional relationships. These changes in training can only benefit the patient, whether the audiologist elects to dispense the aid directly or work through the traditional hearing aid dealer.

The audiologist who elects to work through the traditional hearing aid dispenser must:

1.   Be knowledgeable enough to make specific recommendations for both the hearing aid and fitting.
2.   Select hearing aid dispenser(s) who will keep him informed of changes in or problems with the fitting recommendation.
3.   Select hearing aid dispenser(s) who are capable of making changes in the fitting when they will be beneficial to the patient.
4.   Define, carefully, the process of and responsibility for follow-up of the patient once the aid has been fitted. For example, in my own practice, when a patient is referred to a hearing aid dispenser, I see the patient on at least three separate occasions: at the time of the initial evaluation, on the day the hearing aid is first fitted, and at the end of the trial/rental period. The dispenser may be asked to adjust the fitting at any stage of the process.
5.   Provide the dispenser with information (other than the hearing aid recommendation) that may be helpful to the dealer in the fitting. For example, special problems with work environment, manual dexterity, ear preference, family influences, etc., can be critical to the success of the hearing aid fitting, and this type of information exchange can only be effective at a "professional" level of communication.
6.   Have a specific method for evaluating the manner in which the dispenser has affected the rehabilitation of the patient. This evaluation process is critical

since the actions of the dealer reflect directly on the audiologist or physician who referred the patient for the aid fitting.

Finally, in my opinion, the practice of arbitrarily rotating hearing aid referrals between several dealers is irresponsible. If the interests of the patient are of primary importance, selection of the dealer becomes a matter of convenience for the patient. The personality of the dealer and the patient, competence of the dealer, products dispensed by the dealer as well as cost factors to the patient associated with the hearing aid are important.

Despite the best of intentions, professional relationships between the audiologist and hearing aid dispenser will remain strained until positions and territories are better defined by the hearing aid industry, the audiologist, the medical specialists, and the third parties who underwrite the cost of medical examination and treatment, audiological services, and the hearing aid.

Teachers and Educational Specialists

Professional relationships with educators present the audiologist with special problems in the management of children with hearing aids. Successful use of the hearing aid depends heavily on both the parent and the person directly responsible for the training of the child—the teacher. Yet, the audiologist's contacts with the teachers are often sporadic (at best). Teachers complain about the lack of detailed information from the audiologist about the use and care of the hearing aid, while the audiologists complain that the teacher's main desire is an ''ideal'' setting for the hearing aid.

Teachers may also feel the need for guidance in the use of group auditory trainers in the classroom, and may ask for the audiologist's assistance in the design and implementation of auditory training programs. Unfortunately, the audiologist may not be well-trained in either area. Admittedly, there has been a trend toward more rehabilitation activity from the audiologist, and new emphasis is being placed on speechreading, auditory training, language development, and educational planning. However, most audiologists are employed in a clinical or teaching role, and not directly involved on a daily basis with the education of the child. Because of this lack of support, the teacher may feel isolated from the audiologist, and may resent or resist his suggestions. Again, the patient's best interests are not served.

Remembering the economic factors and the best interests of the patient, proper management of the hearing aid in the classroom can prolong the life of the aid, minimize service needs, and accelerate the auditory learning of the child through constant and consistent amplification.

One of the most opportune times for the audiologist to establish a working relationship with the teacher is during the hearing aid trial fitting period. Since the young child lacks the language to give the audiologist a definitive basis for the selection and fitting of an appropriate aid, the feedback from the teacher about the child's classroom performance can be critical. The audiologist should remember that the teacher or educational specialist is a professional with multiple responsibilities and generally less-than-optimum remuneration. His or her time is valuable, and requests for data on hearing aid performance should be organized for maximum efficiency and a minimum of paper work.

If the teacher uses behavior modification techniques in the classroom, rate data can be collected comparing hearing aid with no hearing aid conditions. Collection of these data usually requires an existing data recording program or the use of an aide or teaching assistant. If rate data recording is not feasible, I ask the teacher to collect and return data presented below on a weekly basis throughout the trial period.

APPENDIX: TRIAL AMPLIFICATION FEEDBACK FORM

Name ——————   Date ——————

1. *Response to voice.* Does the child respond more readily, more accurately, etc., when he is fitted with the hearing aid than when he is in the unaided condition?
2. *Response to environmental noises.* Is the child more aware of clickers, doors, etc., with the hearing aid on than without the hearing aid?
3. *Visual contact.* Is there an increased sensory awareness (visually) when the child is wearing the hearing aid?
4. *Behavioral changes.* Are there any overt changes in the child's interactions with the teacher or his parents when he is wearing the hearing aid?
5. *Does the child show any tolerance reactions* to the hearing aid with which he is fitted? Does a clicker, loud voice, slamming of the door, etc., cause the child to pull the earmold out, turn the hearing aid off, bring tears to his eyes, screaming, etc.?
6. *Vestibular effects.* Is there any apparent decrease in the child's motor coordination or his balance abilities when he is fitted with the hearing aid?
7. *Aggression toward amplification.* Does the child show any overt rejection of the hearing aid which could be costly to the parents over an extended period of time?
8. Are there any *special problems* demonstrated by the child which might indicate modification of the hearing aid arrangement. For example, if the child has cerebral palsy, is his frequent falling a hazard to the hearing aid function?

The teacher is then included in the decision about whether or not the aid is really making any difference in the child's performance. In this way, the relationship between the teacher and audiologist is productive and beneficial to the patient.

In-service workshops, telephone consultation, and classroom visits can mean the difference between a sporadic contact and a meaningful relationship between the teacher and the audiologist. The goal is creation of a line of communication that is both easy and productive. As this relationship is achieved, everyone benefits.

In summary, professional relationships that are productive and in the best interests of the patient require time, effort, and an understanding of the prejudices affecting each profession. A willingness to be flexible when inevitable conflicts occur in meeting the patient's communication needs is critical. While this chapter reflects current conditions affecting the physician, audiologist, hearing aid dispenser, and the teacher, these conditions are susceptable to immediate change. Such changes will occur as a result of research, economic, legal, and consumer issues and, hopefully, as a result of our perception of the "patient's best interests."

BIBLIOGRAPHY

Audiologists voice opinions on proposed dispensing rule change. ASHA 20:542−549, 1978

Bailey H, Winstom M: The role of the physician in clinic dispensing. Ear Nose Throat J 57:51−59, 1978

Fortner M: ASHA bows to anti-trust laws on dispensing policies. Audecibel 27:107−108, 1978

United States vs National Society of Professional Engineers, No. 76−1767. ASHA 20:542−549, 1978

Resolution #53 of the Legislative Council of the American Speech and Hearing Association, San Francisco, California, 1978

Pratt L: Why physicians may regret a decision to dispense hearing aids. Ear Nose Throat J May, 1978

Hearing Aid Devices. Professional and Patient Labeling and Conditions for Sale, Department of Health, Education and Welfare, Food and Drug Administration, Federal Register, Vol. 41, No. 78, April 1976

Recommended Rule for the Hearing Aid Industry. November 19, 1978. Available from the Public Reference Branch, Federal Trade Commission, Room 130, 6th and Pennsylvania Avenue, N.W., Washington, D.C. 20580.

Appendix

Acoustical Society of America Standard Specification of Hearing Aid Characteristics S 3.22−1976*

1. INTRODUCTION

1.1   This standard describes hearing aid measurements that are particularly suitable for specification purposes. Whenever possible, the conditions and procedures of existing American National Standards, in particular S3.3−1960 (R-1971), "Methods for Measurement of Electroacoustical Characteristics of Hearing Aids," and S3.8−1967 (R-1971), "Method of Expressing Hearing Aid Performance," or modifications of these, are employed. Consideration was given to various IEC Recommendations or proposals where applicable, as well as to proposals supplied by the Hearing Aid Industry Conference, Inc., and the Food and Drug Administration of the U.S. Department of Health, Education, and Welfare.

1.2   The procedures of this standard differ significantly from existing standards in the establishment of a *reference test gain-control position* (see 6.6) to which the hearing aid is adjusted for certain measurements, such as frequency response, harmonic distortion, and equivalent input noise level.

1.3   The reference test gain-control position considers that the gain control setting for certain tests should be related to the saturation output capability of the hearing aid. Among the advantages of the gain-control setting specified herein are (1) the gain control is set closer to a typical "use" setting than with the S3.3 method particularly for high-gain aids, (2) harmonic distortion measurements are made with a setting appropriately related to the maximum output capability of the hearing aid, and (3) a reference test gain is specified that is more representative of the "use" setting than is the "full-on" gain setting of S3.3 and S3.8. A modification of the "full-on" gain measurement is retained for tolerance setting purposes.

NOTE: A somewhat different reference test gain-control setting method was originated by the National Bureau of Standards (NBS) for the Veterans Administration (VA). With the NBS method, a random noise signal with a long time average spectrum distribution resembling speech is used to produce a 60-dB sound pressure level in the free field where the hearing aid is placed. The hearing aid gain control is set to produce an output of 12 dB below saturation sound pressure level with this signal. Because of the difficulties that have been found in accurately reproducing the specified random noise spectrum in a variety of hearing aid testing systems, including "sound boxes," a pure-tone averaging method that is capable of providing accurate measurements and reproducibility in existing measurement systems has been substituted for the random noise method. It has been found to give results very close to those obtained with an accurately shaped random noise signal.

2. SCOPE

2.1   This standard is intended to meet the need for specifications of hearing aid performance parameters and their tolerances. The quantities suggested for specification and tolerance are considered to be useful for specifying, selecting, or fitting a hearing aid.

2.2   Tolerances are given relative to specified characteristics for a particular model supplied by a manufacturer. The procedures are more appropriate to "standard" than to "made-to-order" models. The latter usually require individual test data to be supplied with each hearing aid. In some cases of made-to-order hearing aids, the proposals will be useful; in others, special procedures or the manufacturer's established procedures for such aids may be appropriate.

2.3   This standard describes certain hearing aid measurements and parameters that are deemed useful in determining the electroacoustical performance of a hearing aid. Some of these lend themselves to setting of tolerances for the purpose of maintaining product uniformity and for compliance with the performance specified for a model.

2.4   It is not the intent of this document to restrict the variety of hearing aid performance available nor to inhibit in any way advances in the state of the art.

2.5   This standard is limited to the specification of electroacoustical characteristics. It is felt that further study is required before standard test procedures relating to mechanical and environmental performance can be established.

3. DEFINITIONS

3.1 Supply voltage

The supply voltage is defined as the voltage measured at the battery terminals of the hearing aid with the hearing aid turned on, with the gain control at the reference test position, and with no input signal.

3.2 Saturation sound pressure level for 90-dB input sound pressure level

The saturation sound pressure level for a 90-dB input sound pressure level is defined as the sound pressure level developed in a 2-cm³ earphone coupler when the input sound pressure level at the microphone sound entrance on the hearing aid is 90 dB *re* 20μPa, with the gain control of the hearing aid full-on. The abbreviation for this term is SSPL90.

NOTE: It is recognized that the true saturation level may occur with more, or occasionally with less, input sound pressure level than 90 dB. However, the differences are usually small over the frequency range of interest and the single input sound pressure level of 90 dB makes automatic recording of the SSPL90 curve very simple.

3.3 High-frequency-average saturation sound pressure level

The high-frequency-average saturation sound pressure level is defined as the average of the 1000-, 1600-, and 2500-Hz values of SSPL90. The abbreviation for the term is HF-average SSPL90.

NOTE: The prefix "HF" is used to differentiate this quantity from the "output" as defined in S3.8-1967 (R-1971), which uses 500, 1000, and 2000 Hz for averaging.

3.4 Full-on gain (pressure)

The amount, in decibels, by which the sound pressure level developed by the hearing aid earphone in a specified coupler exceeds the sound pressure level at the microphone opening of the hearing aid is defined as the full-on gain (pressure).

3.5 High-frequency-average full-on gain

The high-frequency-average full-on gain is defined as the average of the 1000-, 1600-, and 2500-Hz values of full-on gain. The abbreviation for the term is HF-average full-on gain. (See Sec. 6.4 for measurement conditions.)

3.6 Reference test gain control position

The reference test gain-control position is defined as the setting of the hearing aid gain control so that the average of the earphone coupler sound pressure levels at 1000, 1600, and 2500 Hz with a pure-tone input sound pressure level of 60 dB *re* 20 μPa is 17 dB less than the HF-average SSPL90, or, if the gain available will not permit this, the full-on gain-control position of the hearing aid.

3.7   Reference test gain

The reference test gain is defined as the gain of a hearing aid when its gain control is set to amplify a 60-dB sound-pressure-level input signal to a level in the coupler that is 17 dB below the saturation sound pressure level of the hearing aid. Gain and saturation values are determined on the basis of the average of the 1000-, 1600-, and 2500-Hz values. If the gain available will not permit this, it is the full-on gain of the hearing aid. (Refer to Sec. 6.6.)

3.8   AGC hearing aid

A hearing aid incorporating means (other than peak clipping) by which the gain is automatically controlled as a function of the magnitude of the input signal is defined as an AGC hearing aid.

3.9   Sound pressure level

Throughout this standard all sound pressure levels are referred to 20μPa.

4.   TEST EQUIPMENT

4.1   General

The test equipment described in this section conforms in many respects to the requirements for measurements described in American National Standard S3.3 − 1960 (R-1971). Details are added where necessary for the additional tests or test conditions required in this standard. In particular, the standard considers the input sound pressure level as that at the microphone opening of the hearing aid instead of that in free field as in S3.3 − 1960 (R-1971).

4.2   Test space

Unwanted stimuli in the test space, such as ambient noise or stray electrical or magnetic fields, shall be sufficiently low so as not to affect the test results by more than 0.5 dB. Equipment meeting the conditions of Secs. 4.3 and 4.4 shall be available.

NOTE: A test space having high sound absorption is preferred and generally used.

4.3   Sound source

The sound source, in combination with a calibrated control microphone or other means, shall be capable of maintaining the requisite sound pressure level at the hearing aid sound entrance opening with ± 1.5 dB over the range 200 − 2000 Hz and within ± 2.5 dB over the range 2000 − 5000 Hz. The sound source shall be able to deliver sound pressure levels between 50 and 90 dB at the position of the sound entrance opening. For response measurements, the total harmonic distortion of the source acoustic signal shall not exceed 2%. For harmonic distortion measurements, the total harmonic distortion of the source acoustic signal shall not exceed 0.5%.

4.4   Control microphone system

The frequency response of the system used to determine the sound pressure level at the position of the sound entrance opening of the hearing aid, applicable to its mode of use, shall be flat within ± 1 dB over the frequency range 200–5000 Hz. The calibration of the microphone system at any stated, selected frequency between 250 and 1000 Hz shall be accurate to within ± 1 dB.

4.5   Frequency accuracy

The indicated frequency of the sound source shall be accurate to within ± 2%. The indicated frequencies on a recorder chart shall be accurate within ± 5%. The paper speed and the pen speed on a recorder shall be such that the indication does not differ by more than 1 dB from the steady state value over the required frequency range.

4.6   Earphone coupler

4.6.1   A 2-cm³ earphone coupler in a closed configuration and suitable for the particular hearing aid being tested is to be chosen from among those described in American National Standard S3.7–1973, "Method for Coupler Calibration of Earphones." Reference is made to Secs. 4.5.2, 4.5.2.1 (HA-1), 4.5.2.2 (HA-2), and 4.5.2.3 (HA-2 with entrance through a rigid tube), except that a flexible tube may be used. The coupler and tubing employed are to be stated.

4.6.2   Microphone used in earphone coupler. The pressure frequency response of the microphone used in the earphone coupler, along with its amplifier and readout device, shall be uniform within ± 1 dB over the frequency range 2000–5000 Hz. The calibration of the microphone system shall be accurate at any stated, selected frequency between 250 and 1000 Hz to within ± 1 dB.

4.7   rms response

Test equipment used for measuring sound pressure levels shall give readings, for nonsinusoidal signals required to be measured, equivalent within ± 1 dB to the readings that would be obtained with true rms responding equipment.

5.   STANDARD OPERATING CONDITIONS

5.1   Standard ambient conditions

temperature: 23 ± 5° C (73 ± 9° F);
relative humidity: 0% to 80%;
atmospheric pressure: 760 (+35, −150) mm of Hg.

Actual conditions at the time of test shall be measured and recorded.

5.2   The following operating conditions for the hearing aid under test shall be stated by the manufacturer and shall be used for all required measurements unless otherwise specified in this standard.

5.2.1   Supply voltage. The type of power source used, the supply voltage, and, in the case of a power supply, the internal impedance, shall be stated. Either an actual battery of the type normally used in the hearing aid, partially discharged to avoid typical high initial voltage, or a suitable power supply that simulates the voltage and internal impedance of real batteries of the type normally used may be employed.

5.2.2   Type of insert earphone (if applicable).

5.2.3   Acoustic connection to the earphone coupler. For insert earphones, the HA-2 earphone coupler shall be used, in which case the acoustic connection is automatically defined. (Refer to 4.5.2, 4.5.2.2 of S3.7−1973.)

For aids with internal earphones, the HA-1 earphone coupler of the HA-2 earphone coupler with entrance through a tube may be selected, as appropriate. (Refer to Secs. 4.5.2, 4.5.2.1, and 4.5.2.3 of S3.7−1973.) If the HA-2 earphone coupler with entrance through a tube is employed, the tube may be rigid or flexible. However, the tube dimensions must be maintained at 2.5 cm (0.984 in.) long ± 4% and 0.193 cm (0.076 in.) diam ± 2%.

5.2.4   Accessories, such as earhook type, insert filter type, etc. The particular accessories to be used shall be described fully. An earhook is to be employed if required in actual use.

5.2.5   Basic settings of controls. Tone control settings should be chosen to give the widest frequency range. All other control settings should be chosen to give the greatest HF-average SSPL90 and the highest HF-average full-on gain. If this is not possible, the setting giving the greatest HF-average SSPL90 should be selected. If varying degrees of AGC are available in an aid, tests are to be made with the greatest amount of compression, even if a reduced HF-average SSPL90 results.

6.   RECOMMENDED MEASUREMENTS, SPECIFICATIONS, AND TOLERANCES

The results obtained by the methods specified below express the performance under the conditions of the test, but will not generally agree with the performance of the hearing aid under actual conditions of use. The difference between actual and test conditions must be kept in mind in interpreting the test results. In the area of gain, particularly, the use of higher frequencies for averaging will usually give a higher number than the S3.8−1967 (R-1971) or HAIC gain.

6.1 Curves

It is recommended that all published curves of gain, response, or output versus frequency be plotted on a grid having a linear decibel ordinate scale and a logarithmic frequency abcissa scale with the length of one decade on the abcissa equal to the length of 50 ± 2 dB on the ordinate.

6.2 SSPL90 curve

With the gain control full-on and with basic settings of controls, record or otherwise develop a curve of coupler sound pressure level versus frequency over the range 200–5000 Hz, using a constant input sound pressure level of 90 dB (Fig. 1). From the above curve, determine the maximum sound pressure level. This maximum sound pressure level shall not exceed that specified by the manufacturer.

6.3 HF-average SSPL90

Average the 1000-, 1600-, and 2500-Hz SSPL90 values. Tolerance: the HF-average SSPL90 shall be within ± 4 dB of the manufacturer's specified value for the model.

6.4 Full-on gain

Full-on gain shall be measured with the gain control of the hearing aid set to its full-on position and with a sinusoidal input sound pressure level of 60 dB, or, if necessary to maintain linear input-output conditions, with an input sound pressure level of 50 dB. For AGC aids, the input sound pressure level shall be 50 dB. The input sound pressure level shall be stated. The full-on gain is the difference between the coupler sound pressure level and the input sound pressure level.

6.5 HF-average full-on gain

Average the 1000-, 1600-, and 2500-Hz full-on gain values. Tolerance: the HF-average full-on gain shall be within ± 5 dB of the manufacturer's specified value for the model.

6.6 Adjustment of the gain control to the reference test position

With an input sound pressure level of 60 dB, adjust the gain control so that the average of the 1000-, 1600-, and 2500-Hz values of the coupler sound pressure level equals the HF-average SSPL90 minus 17 dB, within ± 1 dB. If the aid does not have enough gain to permit this adjustment, set the gain control full-on. For AGC aids, set the gain control full-on.

NOTE: The long-term average sound pressure level for speech at 1 m approximates 65 dB re 20μPa. Speech peaks are typically 12 dB above the average level. By adjusting the gain control to give a cuupler sound pressure level 12 dB below the saturation level for a 65-dB input sound pressure level, a very rough estimate can be made that speech peaks should not exceed the saturation sound

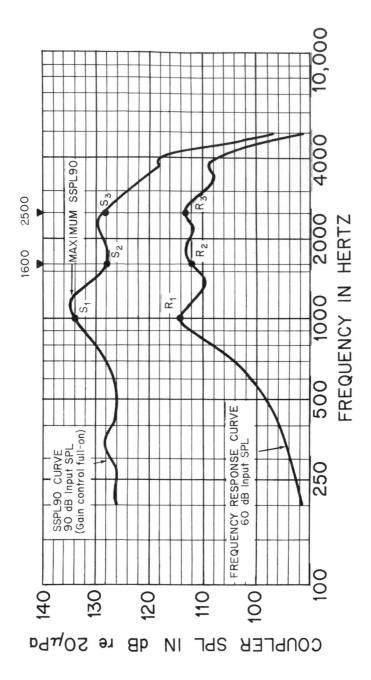

Fig. 1. Example of SSPL90 and frequency response curves: HF-average SSPL90 = $(S_1 + S_2 + S_3)/3$. Reference test gain control position is determined by $(S_1 + S_2 + S_3)/3 - (R_1 + R_2 + R_3)/3 = 17$ dB.

pressure level available in an aid. The use of 60-dB input sound pressure level and a 17-dB gain control setback from the SSPL90 value gives essentially the identical setting, but simplifies measurement with generally used test equipment.

6.7 Reference test gain

This is normally determined by subtracting 77 dB from the HF-average SSPL90. For information purposes, the reference test gain shall be stated on specification sheets. For hearing aids with gain less than the value so determined, the reference test gain is taken with the gain control full-on as the HF-average full-on gain per Sec. 6.5

6.8 Frequency response curve

With the gain control in the reference test position as defined in 6.6, and with an input sound pressure level of 60 dB, record or otherwise develop the frequency response curve over the range 200−5000 Hz or a lesser range determined by limits 20 dB below the average of the 1000-, 1600-, and 2500-Hz response levels (Fig. 1). For AGC aids an input sound pressure level of 50 dB is to be employed.

6.9 Tolerance method for frequency response curve

6.9.1 Tolerance range. The following procedures shall be used:

(a) From the manufacturer's specified frequency response curve determine the average of the 1000-, 1600-, and 2500-Hz response levels.

(b) Subtract 20 dB.

(c) Draw a line parallel to the abcissa at the reduced level.

(d) Note the lowest frequency, f_1, at which the response curve intersects the straight line.

(e) Note the highest frequency, f_2, at which the response curve intersects the straight line, if this is less than 5000 Hz.

6.9.2 Frequency range. For information purposes, but not for tolerance purposes, the frequency range of the hearing aid shall be considered as being between f_1 and f_2 as indicated in Fig. 2 (even if f_2 exceeds 5000 Hz).

6.9.3 Tolerance. The tolerances in two bands shall be as follows

	Frequency Limits	Tolerance
Low band	$1.25f_1$ to 2000 Hz	± 4 dB
High band	2000−4000 Hz or $0.8f_2$, (whichever is lower)	± 6 dB

6.9.4 Compliance template. Compliance with the tolerances may be determined using a suitable template with upper and lower limits that are derived from the manufacturer's specified response curve for the model. Vertical adjustment of the template on the response curve of the measured hearing aid is permitted. Horizontal adjustment up to 10% in frequency is permitted. Following these adjustments, the entire portion of the curve between $1.25f_1$ and 4000 Hz or $0.8f_2$, if lower than 4000 Hz, must lie between the upper and lower limit curves (Fig. 2.)

6.10   Harmonic distortion

With the gain control in the reference test position and with an input sound pressure level of 70 dB, measure and record the total harmonic distortion in the coupler output for input frequencies of 500, 800, and 1600 Hz.

In the event the response curve rises 12 dB or more between any distortion test frequency and its second harmonic, distortion tests at that test frequency may be omitted. Tolerance: The total harmonic distortion under the above test conditions shall not exceed that specified for the model.

6.11   Equivalent input noise level (L_n)

With the gain control in the test reference position, determine the average of the coupler sound pressure levels at 1000, 1600, and 2500 Hz for an input sound pressure level of 60 dB. Remove the acoustic input signal and record the sound pressure level in the coupler caused by inherent noise.

If L_{av} is the average sound pressure level in the coupler due to the 1000-, 1600-, and 2500-Hz signals and L_2 is the sound pressure level in the coupler due to noise, then the equivalent input noise level is

$$L_n = L_2 - (L_{av} - 60) \text{ dB}$$

NOTE: this method is not appropriate for AGC aids.

Tolerance: The equivalent input noise level shall not exceed the maximum value specified for the model.

6.12   Battery current

With the gain control in the reference test position, measure the battery current with a pure-tone 1000-Hz input signal at a sound pressure level of 65 dB. Tolerance: The battery current for the above test conditions shall not exceed the maximum value specified for the model.

6.13   Coupler sound pressure level with induction coil

With the gain control full-on and the hearing aid set to the T (telephone input) mode, the hearing aid is placed in an alternating magnetic field having a frequency of 1000 Hz and a magnetic field strength of 10 mA/m and is oriented to produce the greatest coupler sound pressure level. This sound pressure level is recorded. Tolerance: The measured value of the coupler sound pressure level shall be within ± 6 dB of the manufacturer's specified value for these test conditions.

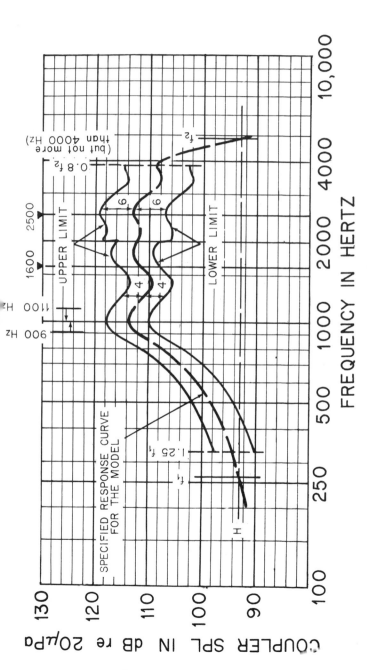

Figure 2. Example of construction of tolerance template for frequency response curve: horizontal line H is 20 dB below the average of the 1000-, 1600-, and 2500-Hz levels on the specified response curve. In use, the template must be kept square with the graph of the measured curve but may be adjusted vertically any amount and horizontally up to ± 10% in frequency. Lines on the template at 900 and 1100 Hz show the maximum allowable horizontal movement referred to the 1000 Hz ordinate on the measured curve. After adjustment of the template, the measured curve must lie between the upper and lower limits on the template.

6.14   Automatic gain-control hearing aids

The following tests apply to AGC aids:

6.14.1   Input-output characteristics. Using a pure-tone test frequency of 2000 Hz, measure the coupler sound pressure level for input sound pressure levels from 50 to 90 dB in 10-dB steps. Plot the coupler sound pressure level along the ordinate against the corresponding input sound pressure level along the abcissa on a grid having linear decibel scales with equal-sized divisions for both ordinate and abcissa. With the measured and specified curves matched at the point corresponding to 70-dB input sound pressure level, the measured curve at 50- and 90-dB input sound pressure levels shall not differ in output sound pressure level from the specified curve by more than ± 4 dB.

6.14.2   Dynamic AGC characteristics. With the gain control full-on and using a square-wave-modulated pure-tone input signal of 2000 Hz, which alternates abruptly between sound pressure levels of 55 and 80 dB, determine the attack and release times from an oscilloscope pattern. The attack time is defined as the time between the abrupt increase from 55 to 80 dB and the point where the level has stabilized to within 2 dB of the steady state value for the 80-dB input sound pressure level. The release time is defined as the interval between the abrupt drop from 80 to 55 dB and the point where the signal has stabilized to within 2 dB of the steady state value for the 55-dB input sound pressure level. Tolerance: The attack and release times shall each be within ± 5 ms or ± 50%, whichever is larger, of the values specified by the manufacturer for the model.

6.15   Interpretation of tolerances

The tolerances of Sec. 6 apply to the performance of the hearing aid as determined with perfectly accurate measurement equipment. To ensure that performance is within a specified tolerance when using imperfect measurement equipment, the tolerance on the measured value must be less than the specified tolerance by the maximum error of measurement. To be sure that performance is outside of the specified tolerance when using imperfect measurement equipment, the tolerance on the measured value must be greater than the specified tolerance by the maximum error of measurement. As an example, suppose that the microphone system in the coupler, along with acoustic errors in the coupler, has a tolerance of ± 1.5 dB. The HF-average-SSPL90 would have to be within ± 2.5 dB of the specified value to be sure that ± 4 dB was being achieved. Also, in checking an aid for compliance of this parameter, using test equipment with accuracy no better than ± 1.5 dB, the allowable tolerance would have to be ± 5.5 dB.

Index

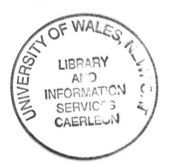